Pharmacology – Research, Safety Testing and Regulation Series

POISONS: PHYSIOLOGICALLY ACTIVE SUBSTANCES

Pharmacology – Research, Safety Testing and Regulation Series

Antibiotic Resistance: Causes and Risk Factors, Mechanisms and Alternatives
Adriel R. Bonilla and Kaden P. Muniz (Editors)
2009. ISBN: 978-1-60741-623-4

Poisons: Physiologically Active Substances
S. B. Zotov and O. I. Tuzhikov
2009. ISBN: 978-1-60741-973-0

Pharmacology – Research, Safety Testing and Regulation Series

POISONS: PHYSIOLOGICALLY ACTIVE SUBSTANCES

S.B. ZOTOV

AND

O.I. TUZHIKOV

Nova Biomedical Books

New York

For permission to use material from this book please contact us:
Telephone 631-231-7269; Fax 631-231-8175
Web Site: http://www.novapublishers.com

Library of Congress Cataloging-in-Publication Data

Zotov, S. B. (Stanislav Borisovich)
Poisons : physiologically active substances / S.B. Zotov and O.I. Tuzhikov. -- 2nd ed.
p. ; cm.
Includes bibliographical references and index.
ISBN 978-1-60741-973-0 (hardcover)
1. Poisons. I. Tuzhikov, O. I. II. Title.
[DNLM: 1. Poisons--pharmacology. 2. Poisons--history. 3. Poisons--toxicity. QV 600 2009a]
RA1211.Z6813 2009
615.9--dc22

2009024598

Published by Nova Science Publishers, Inc. ✦ New York

Contents

Preface to the Second Edition

It has been four years since the publication of the first edition of this book (Zotov, S.B., & Tuzhikov, O.I. [2005]. *Poisons: Physiologically active substances* [First Edition]. Volgograd: VolgGTU, RPK Polytechnic [Russ.]). During this time, the authors received a series of reeqeusts from readers about expanding the circle of problems to discuss, including an examination of ecologically dangerous products of human activity and questions about the destruction of chemical weapons. Therefore, the present edition includes two new chapters concerning aspects of problems of destruction of chemical warfare agents and persistent organic pollutants (POPs) in the environment. The history of these issues and perspectives on the problems they present in today's environment were addressed by a Russian convention, culminating in a signed exectutive order prohibiting development, production, accumulation and application of chemical weapons and their destruction; and the Stockholm Convention on Persistent Organic Pollutants in 2001 addressing ecologically clean removal of POPs. Illumination of these important questions stipulated not only the international governmental obligations of the Russian Federation, but treatment of the actual consequences of the worsening conditions of life activities connected with soil pollution.

Each of the book's chapters has been revised and updated with new structures of physiologically active substances (PhAS). Essential alterations and additions conclude that, along with the known conjectures in the mechanisms of PhAS effects ("key-lock" theory, theory of competitive inhibition and others), in recent years the attention of chemists and medical professionals has been drawn to a new theory connected with the existence of exfoliating effects in the area of contact between PhAS aqueous solution and biomembrane-containing receptors. It is necessary to emphasize that this has not examined volumetric effects, but effects in a subtle layer of solution applied to the substrate. Life and its manifestations form fermentative chain reactions in water solutions. Exfoliation of a solution or separation from it of some component inevitably leads to a cessation of reactions that had been running with participation of substances separate from the solution. A hypothesis about toxic bond action with exfoliation of water solution, i.e., displacement of equilibrium solutions membrane complexes under action, for example, of more hydrophobic compounds, was discussed for the first time in 1982. S.P. Gabuda, doctor of physical-matematical sciences, a well-known specialist in the area of NMR spectroscopy, had been studying the properties of condensable phases and molecular movement near phase transition. A definitive contribution to the development of this theory came in 2005, when K.K. Kalninsh made discoveries regarding the catalytical activity of water and L.P. Pavlova researched the effect of the bioactivity of water on different organisms.

This has allowed explanation of a number of facts and given new explanations for the essential action of poisons, including such a delicate peculiarity as a connection between activity and conformation of the inert part of a molecule and with the presence of salts in biological solution.

Each chapter has essentially completed references published until the middle of 2008 (334 instead of 195); moreover, each reference is cited only once per chapter at its first appearance, and not repeated later.

The authors express gratitude to postgraduate student of Volgograd State Technical University, A.S. Berezin, for technical help in preparing the manuscript, and professor of chemistry, M.O. Tuzhikov, for help with the translation.

A book such as this may not ever reach completion, since developments and the appearance of new facts in science take place perpetually, which require reevaluation of preceding knowledge. This book could be useful as an additional textbook for postgraduates and students of chemical, pharmaceutical and medical universities and colleges, and as a reference book for ecologists and specialists in the area of research and modification of modern medicines.

The authors hope that this book will awake the interest of young investigators to the very difficult but extraordinarily interesting area of synthesis of new, highly effective medicines, an area in which there is still much to be done. The outlook seems impressive.

— S.B. Zotov and O.I. Tuzhikov

"Dedicate Bright memory of Teachers
Nemec Vulf Grigor'evich,
Sochilin Evgeniy Georgievich,
Smirnov Vadim Viktorovich"

"All things are poison and nothing
is without poison, only the dose permits
something not to be poisonous."
Theophrastus Paracelsus

Introduction

This book does not provide full discussions about every presently-known physiologically active substance (PhAS); it is collection of essays describing the history of finding the structure, synthesis or revelation of the interconnection between the structure and physiological impact of the most interesting and peculiar poisons and their groups. These essays differ from each other both in the volume of information and in the aspects of examined questions and, unlike the other descriptions of poisons and medicines, they answer some questions from the point of view of the chemists-synthesists and technologists and, of course, reveal the scientific interests of the authors. The finding and synthesis of any structure of PhAS is connected with intense systematic and trial-and-error work and, sometimes, with long-term failures and unexpected breakthroughs. The authors sincerely believe that the reader feels amazement and excitement in the atmosphere of findings and discoveries.

Since humans began to realize that they differ from animals with the opportunity to think and draw conclusions and inferences from various facts surrounding him, they used gathered data to improve their life. From this time, poisons—or, in the modern definition, physiologically active compounds—became known. When foraging for food, mainly vegetables, both the ancient human being and his domesticated wild animals sampled a great variety of fruits, stalks and plant roots. As a result, all edible food was selected, and poisonous and unhealthy items were rejected. Together with plants, many animals are also poisonous. Based on incomplete data from world-wide health protection organizations, about half a million people suffer from snakebites; this is an estimated one-twentieth of all injuries from poisonous animals. Bites and pricks by aculeate poisonous insects incur much greater mortality than snakebites. In antiquity, the number of poisonous animals and plants was obviously greater than nowadays. Their populations were not under the influence of industry, urbanization or agriculture. Experience led human beings to use poisonous plants and animals appropriately by taking the opportunity to use poisons for hunting, for affecting the organism with the purpose of changing its normal functions, and for medicines. Since then, poisons and medicines are concepts inseparably connected with each other, embodying the struggle and unity of two opposing forces, like good and evil, and life and death. Therefore, viewing predominantly poisons, the history of their perception and evolution, we are obliged to touch on their opposites—medicines and remedies. In this connection, we could rather call the subject of this examination "physiologically active substances (or compounds)" (PhAS), but we have kept the historically-developed name of that vast group of substances— "poisons."

Chapter 1

Poisons in Mythology

The knowledge of poisonous plants and the ability to predict the consequences of poisoning and its effects were vital information for primitive human beings. Control over his surroundings exalted him. It is reasonable to assume that knowledge about the effects of poisons, medicines or remedies, their sources, methods of isolation and application was veiled in obscurity and mystery. Along with the knowledge regarding physiologically active compounds came assumptions about both poisons and medicines that identified correspondingly with evil and good spirits and black and white magic. The most ancient knowledge was passed from one generation to the next at first in oral form and then with the beginnings of written language in shorthand form in myth and ritual, performed during national celebrations. Evidence of this has been found during archeological excavations on vases, seals, cups, shields, temple walls, tapestries and similar objects. Among the myths known in the present day (Egyptian, Cretan, Palestinian, Babylonian, Indian, Chinese, Japanese, Hittite and others), Egyptian myths are the most studied, the most extensive of which concern problems and phenomena, and most are variations of original versions of some myths. The time period of the appearance of myths could be estimated from about 5000 to 1000 years B.C., before the origin of patriarchy. Further, mythology is a history of the ancient world known to be more complete and better as far as it was recorded and noted by authors (historians, chroniclers and others) living at that time, but they were not always fully objective in their stating of events.

Consideration of a wide variety of ancient Greece myths, specifically containing mentions of physiologically active substances, methods of their application and effects was provided to us on the basis of one the most fully complete myths in the presentation of Robert Graves. He was a talented and erudite mythologist with the imagination of a poet. He aspired to provide an entire picture of the world that could satisfy both scientists working in this or other closely-related spheres along with a wide range of readers. It should be emphasized at this time that, in contrast to the level of our usual educational endeavors, readers should make a personal effort beyond the basic knowledge of chemistry to reach deeply into this world and value its original beauty and variety.

From the mythological description of poisons' properties, it follows that their action was connected first of all with the magic of one or another god and not with the presence of any poisonous substance. It is not possible to directly identify the exact first mention of physiologically active substances (PhAS) because there is no accurate correlation of event with time. Therefore, in order to identify the first mentions, in our opinion, it is necessary to consider the use of PhAS as antidotes during ecstatic episodes for priests, bacchants, maenads, witches and other "assistants" in the world of the gods—their retinue, the persons carrying out this or that cult or religious practice.

Originally used as a remedy for excitation, for example, maenads used not only wine (which was extended only after the statement of a cult of Dionis), but they also chewed narcotic leaves of laurels, an ivy, or burnt in the flame of oil lamp placed in a closed space barley grain, hemp and laurels leaves. However, it is more probable that they simply placed hemp, laurel and barley in the hot ashes that remained from burnt-down charcoal, which is easier and more effective for ingestion of narcotic smoke. Available data on the presence of calcium cyanide in laurel leaves contradicts modern representations that the latter can be the substance responsible for the stupefying effect. In Greece, up to the Roman epoch, there was a taboo on the chewing of bay leaves by everyone except a priestess-prophet. In fact, Dionis was brought up with honey, and his attendant-maenads had thyrsus (the pine branches twined with ivy), which can indicate that before another intoxicant drink was used: fir-tree beer seasoned with ivy and sweetened with honey. The honey drink, possibly, was the "nectar" that was cooked from fermented honey and which the gods continued to drink on the Homeric Olympus. By the way, the ivy had special importance also because it, as well as other four sacred trees—a prickly oak of Silt on which is found cochineal, an alder of Foroneja, a rod and a pomegranate of Dionis—was used in manufacture of the red dye applied in painting, and also for painting the faces of cult participants in fertility rituals. In Rome this custom has remained in the form coloration of the face of the victorious, and even in recent times the tradition remained whereby rouge was applied to the face of English kinds during official ceremonies.

The poppy appears among the most ancient knowledge of plants containing PhAS. Under the certificate of Ovidiy, flowers that were collected by the Cora were poppies. On many images found at excavations, Demetra holds poppies in her hands, and heads of poppies are twisted in her hair or passed to her daughter, Cora. In those times, poppy seeds were probably added to bread, but the Cora collected them and accepted them as a soporific, and it was considered a symbol of revival after death because of the scarlet color of the petals. Mint was used during funerals together with rosemary and myrtle to stifle the smell of decay. Barley drink, which was imbibed by Demetra, was also seasoned with mint. To Tiffon, the biggest monster ever born, three goddesses of destiny offered "gentle" fruits, declaring that with their help he could restore his power, although the fruits were actually lethal. Possibly, it was the usual "death apples" that often appeared in myths (compared to the poisoned apple in the Russian fairy tale "About a Dead Szarevna and Seven Heroes" or their opposite, "rejuvenate apples," in the fairy tale "About Ivan-Czarevitch and a Grey Wolf"). The white Narcussus flower with the red aureole, which, according to Pliny's *Natural History*, grew on the spot where a drop of blood fell from Narcissus after his suicide, is used in the preparation of an ointment for the treatment of ear illnesses (though its application is often followed by a headache), and as remedy for treatment chilblains. This flower is now known more as a drug. The image of Pan's flagellation by sea onions on the occasion of unsuccessful hunting is interesting. The sea onion contains, along with cordial PhAS, the poison-irritant used for extermination of mice and rats, and also as a cleaning and a diuretic remedy that was taken before certification rituals. Therefore, Pliny considers it a symbol of clarification and liberation from the influence of wicked powers. One of the main goddesses—Artemis, Apollo's twin sister—as well as her brother, could inflict a plague and rapid death on people, and also treat them. At the same time she considered it a main inconvenience of her position that women in childbirth would exasperate her with entreaties and requests for childbirth without pain, as her mother, Leto, had painless pregnancies and childbirth.

A salutary universal remedy of Athena was mistletoe (*ixias*), a word closely connected with the name *Iskhiy* (force) and *Iksion*. East European mistletoe, or *loranf*, is the plant parasite that grows on oak, as opposed to its Western counterpart that grows on poplars or apple trees. Mistletoe was considered the genitals of the oak tree, and when druids ritually cut it off, they engaged in symbolic emasculation. The dense juice of its berries was perceived as oak sperm, a liquid attributed with enormous regenerative possibilities. Aeneas visited the world of dead with mistletoe in his hand and, thanks to it, he returned to the world of the living. The grass that allowed Glavk to lift from a tomb and to bring back to life the corpse of Ippolit, based on the description, was most likely mistletoe. The last act belongs to demigod Asklepiy, killed by Zeus during an instigation of intriguer-gods. Iskhiy, Asklepiy, Iksion and Poliid are actually the same mythical character personifying salutary properties which the chopped-off genitals ostensibly possessed. The art of medicine was inherited by both of Asklepiy's sons, whose authority was very high. The Asclepiads, the descendants of Asklepiy, became famous for the art of doctoring. This is confirmed by events during the Trojan War, when one of his sons, doctor Makhaon, was wounded in a skirmish after which the Greeks took flight. In another example, Filoklet suffered from a wound that would not heal for long time. One of his brothers washed it with fresh water, and after Filoklet had fallen asleep, he cleaned the wound with a knife and numbing substances, filled it with wine, applied curative grasses coiled around a stone and then the patient quickly recovered.

Willow was also considered a tree with great strength. Bitter medicine prepared from willow bark historically has been used in the treatment of rheumatism, and ancient Greeks who settled moist plains had access to it. However, branches of one of willow variety with which the Spartan Asklepiy was identified—specifically *Agnus castus*—was put into a box that was placed on women during a fertility holiday, ostensibly to frighten off a dragon, as confirmed by Arian in *Stories of Animals*, though actually most such spirits were thought to present themselves in the form of snakes. Therefore, it is not accepted that priests of Asklepiy's specialized in the treatment of barrenness, and that's why his cult was widely known.

With the help of wild olive, evil spirits were banished in Greece, and in Italy and north Europe birch was used for the same purposes (remember birch broom and Russian bath). Worship of trees was widely practiced in mythology, which is reflected in objects of different works of antiquity found during archaeological excavations. After the events of the Greco-Persian Wars, winners of the Nimey games were no longer crowned with olive, but instead rewarded with a diadem consisting of parsley, which was a symbol of mourning. Persistent dark associations with parsley are evident in the fact that the plant everywhere is known as a treatment to induce miscarriage. There is even an English saying: "Parsley magnificently grows in the garden of the cuckold." Women of many countries to this day use parsley as a non-surgical method of interruption of undesirable pregnancy.

Chiron was famous as a doctor, scientist and prophet. He was called a descendant of Iksion, which brought him the second name "Filira's son" ("lindens"). Linden flowers, then as well as now, were widely used as a tonic. In a myth about the Argonauts, Medea, the well-known sorceress, skillful doctor and compiler of every possible drug, calmed a hissing dragon, the guardian of the golden fleece, and with help of magical charms and freshly-cut juniper branches splashed sleep-inducing drops onto his eyelids. Then Jason was able to take the fleece from an oak and go to "Argot." Medea quickly cured the wounded men with her medicines. Medea's crocus of Colchids is a poisonous *Colchicum*, or a meadow saffron, which ancient people used, as well as now, as a true antigout agent. Magical views about it are attributed to Medea and her reputation. Mythologists of the classical epoch could not decide for themselves whether Medea was an illusionist, cheater or magician. The "copper of rejuvenation," ostensibly used by her, is found everywhere in Celtic myths and Slavic fairy tales. Perhaps, therefore, Medea calls herself a hyperborean goddess—in other words, the goddess from the north known at that time. Notably, the art of poisoning was inherited (according to Homer) by just one grandson of Medea—Mermer. Another hero of mythology, Achill, treated Teleph for a wound by scraping rust from the spear that wounded him and sprinkling it over the wound, which healed, but not without a help of a grass called *achilleos,* a curative plant that he found. Achille's treatment of the wound with a spear is based on an ancient homoeopathic principle—"similar treats similar." Mynos, an inhabitant of Melamp, is considered to be the first mortal (unlike immortal gods) endowed with the gift of prophecy, the first doctor, the first builder of temples of Dionis in Greece, and the first to dilute wine with water. Greek doctors considered that althaea (*althaia,* from *althainein,* "to treat") had medicinal properties, about which they were not mistaken, and it was the first spring flower from which bees collected honey. It, as well as the ivy flower, has special mythical importance. The leaves and bark of and elm, according to the illustration of Pliniy, were used as a medicinal product. It was considered that medicines produced from them would be more effective if, for their manufacture, the raw materials were taken from trees growing on tombs of tsars or the leaders who had died from wounds.

Adonis, the spirit of the annual awakening of nature, was given birth by a myrrh tree which was known as a stimulant. It is highly difficult to give definition to "a magic grass of moly," found in Homer. Sorcerers name it "wild rue," though the description given in the *Odyssey* allows identifying it as a wild cyclamen, which is difficult to find. It typically has white petals, a black bulb and very sweet smell. Late classical authors designate the plant with the word "moly," a plant similar to garlic and having a yellow flower. According to legend, it grows (as onions, sea onions and usual garlic) under the waning Moon; therefore, it was used against the lunar magic of Gekata. The Babylonian hero, Marduk, smelled a magic grass in order to cover the disgusting smell of the sea goddess Tiamat; however, in the epic there is no description of this grass. Marduk simply periodically put the grass to his nostrils and smelled it—in other words, the respirator, a prototype of a gas mask, was actually invented. A similar description of the use of such magic grass is given in a known myth about Hercules during the suppression of a revolt of the giants against the gods. Thus, Hercules in such a way neutralized the breath of Alkyoney, the leader of the giants. Prokrida, beloved of

Mynos (the governor of Crete at the beginning of the second to the end of the third millennium B.C.), presented to him, in a sign of gratitude for gifts, a special potion—a broth from the magic grasses made by the magician, Kirka. Prokrida forced Mynos to drink it in order to make him safe from reptiles and insects, and the potion was effective. In myths, there are a number of allusions to the magic grass that is capable of restoring life to the dead. Glavk observed its vivifying effect on fish, and some sources spoke about placing the grass on a dead hare or dragon, which slowly, restored them to life. Having tried this grass, Glavk became immortal. In the Babylonian legend of Gilgamesh, we can find a similar revival of a snake. The flower of eternal life was stolen from him by a dragon that shed its skin and became young again. Not having managed to keep a flower, Gilgamesh saw his own fate as death. In its description, the grass resembles buckthorn, which the Greeks applied as a depletive before participation in mysteries. By the way, the magic grass planted by Kron, one of the first Supreme gods of the Golden Age, greatly resembles the magic *herbe d'or* of the druids. One of the patronesses of the Olympic games was Moliona (the tsarina of Moly), from whom the word *moly* was given to the plant used against lunar magic. She is also known by the name Argameda (multiclever), and is called the sorceress-daughter of Avgiy, who knew "as many curative grasses, as many the earth rises" (Homer, the *Iliad*).

According to mythology, a considerable contribution to the knowledge of poisons was made by the hero Hercules. In the last and the most difficult feat, he captivated Cerberus, a dog protecting Hades, the kingdom of the dead. During his capture by Hercules, the saliva of Cerberus dripped onto green fields, and from those spots a poisonous plant, aconite, grew. The plant is also called hecatine, as it was first used by Hecate. In a myth about Tesey, Plutarh specifies that this plant is called "aconite" because it grows on naked rocks. Egey, according to a myth, was to offer Tesey a bowl of wine prepared in advance by Medea. The bowl contained aconite, the poison from a plant that she had brought from Aherusia. Aconite is a poison with a paralyzing action, used by Thessalian sorceresses in the preparation of an ointment "for flights": it numbed the feet and hands, giving a feeling of isolation from the earth. But as it was also an antipyretic, Hercules, carrying a fever during his labor of driving away the Stymphalian birds, could quite be attributed to the revelation of this flower. There are data in Tibetan and Chinese sources about use of poisonous aconite both for hunting animals and for medical purposes. With the exception of aconite, Hercules found the grasses "heraclion or wild origan for treating all illnesses"; Siderians heraclion, having a thin stalk, a red flower and leaves similar to those of coriander, grows on lakesides and banks and effectively heals all wounds placed by iron; henbane causes dizziness and insanity. Nymph's heraclion, having a root similar to the age-old weapon—a nightstick with a reinforced end—is so-named after the nymph who was abandoned by Hercules and died of jealousy. It is said to deprive men of strength for twelve days (Pliny, *Natural History*).

In myths, the overwhelming number of mentioned physiologically active compounds has a phytogenesis and that is not casual; the reasons for this, in our opinion, are the environment and living conditions of human beings at that time. The "cradle" of mankind is connected, first of all, with the vegetation characterized by a rather large variety of poisonous plants (nowadays more than 10,000 toxic plants have been identified). There are fewer mentions in myths about poisons of animal origin, among which the leading place is held by snakes. The casual death from a snakebite is most often found in mythology. The first victims were the wife of Orpheus, Eurydice; a number of characters of Trojan War; the Argonauts and other characters of Greek mythology; the Egyptian, Ra, who is a hypostasis of Osiris, who was also bitten by a snake; and Libyan. Every instance was a bite to the heel. The following is a typical description of the poisoning of the Argonaut, Mopsus, who stepped on the Libyan snake: "His eyes became clouded with a fog, his hair began to fall out, and he died in agony." The water snake bit the foot of the well-known archer, Filoklet, during a sacrifice. Neither ointments nor poultices helped—the wound became more awful, the cries of the victim became louder and his associates could not help. Odysseus landed unluckily on the deserted coast of Lemnos. There, he eventually was recovered and lived for several years, shooting birds for livelihood. Along with the accidental poisoning from a snakebite in the lower extremities, there is a description of a purposeful poisoning of a stream by means of a snake. Used for drinking, this water led to a mass poisoning of the thirsty. Along with water, wine was used as solvent of poisons. At the same time, the method of checking wine for the presence of poison is described (for example, the Ion made a sacrificial libation to gods, and by the arrival pigeon, having enjoyed the spilled wine, fell dead after that).

The first mention of suidice by means of poison in Greek mythology is the story of Alkestida who, out of love for her husband, poisoned herself and fell into Hades in place of her husband. Along with snakes in myths, insects are also noted—in particular, a scorpion from whose sting Orion (in one of the myth's versions) perishes. The story by Plutarch of the god Set sending a scorpion to kill the child Gor, the son of Isida and Osiris, during the hottest period of summer, explains the death of Orion from the sting of a scorpion and proves the appeal of his patroness, Artemis, to Asklepiy (Plutarch, *About Isida and Osiris*). Orion resembles the Babylonian Hercules, Gilgamesh, whom the tenth table of the calendar epos said was attacked by a human-scorpion. This myth tells how the tsar-priest was mortally wounded on the day when the sun starts to rise in the constellation of the Scorpion (August). The well-known Odysseus, as well as the prophet Teresiy, predicted that he would be killed by his own son, Telegon, who attacked Itaka by mistake. Odysseus, protecting Itaka, was wounded on the shore by a spear which, instead of a tip, had a skate's thorn. Almost the same destiny was met by Rodose's Katrey, whose son unintentionally wounded him with a spear on the sea coast. Spears with a skate's thorn, used also in Polynesia, inflict long suppurating wounds, which the Greeks and Romans considered incurable (Elian, *About Animals*); by the way, the skate is found throughout the Mediterranean Sea.

The story of Filoklet's death due to poison—in other words, Hercules's arrows moistened in the blood of the Hydra—is possibly the most ancient. Euripides notices that the Hydra was so poisonous that her breath alone and even a trace of her smell could destroy all life. According to myth, Hercules split a trunk into pieces and put his arrows into the venomous bile of the Hydra. Even a small wound caused by such an arrow became deadly. Though the Hydra on the surface resembles the sea dragon killed by Perseus, its prototype was, possibly, a fresh-water monster, as well as the majority of those mentioned in Irish and Welsh mythologies, called *piastres* or *avanks*. Another such monster is based on a Homeric epithet of Lacedaemon, specifically *cetoessa*—in other words, a "water monster," undoubtedly living in any deep reservoir. For example, it was common practice to sacrifice the bodies of dead Spartan tsars, tied with branches and thrown into the river Evrot, to a monster living there. The poisonous arrows of Hercules, stuck into a knee or a foot, were a cause of death of many heroes and characters of myths. For example, in the description of the fourth labor of Hercules, it is said that the arrow that was shot by Hercules passed through the hand of Ellat and landed in the knee of the centaur Chiron. Out of grief for the arrow hitting his old friend, Hercules pulled from his knee the arrow tip, and though Chiron, a doctor, prepared medicines for the treatment of his wounds, in this case they appeared to be useless and he, groaning, left for a cave but did not die because he was immortal. To resolve this conflict, it is noted that later Prometheus agreed to become immortal instead of him and Zeus confirmed this exchange. At the funerals, which were arranged by the centaur Phol, the latter took one of the arrows of Hercules and began to examine it. "Such a large creature has died from such a scratch," he said in surprise. But here the arrow dropped out of his hands, pierced a foot, and he fell dead. In general, many centaurs and heroes suffered from the arrows of Hercules, and the principal operation of a poison in an organism by a prick of a poisoned tip of an arrow was extensive enough. Many myths describe variations of such a method. To kill Achilles, the adopted son of Chiron, Paris gives Thessaly Apollo's killing arrows (Thessaly, as well as her ally Ethir, was well-known for her poisons). And, at last, when Philoklet avenges Achilles and kills Paris, he uses one more arrow from the quiver of Hercules. It is rather probable that in Thessaly the tsar-priest was killed by an arrow impregnated with snake poison which the special assistant stuck into a foot between the heel and ankle. Some sources say that cause of Thalosis' (a metal copper giant) death is his wound in an ankle bone with the poisoned arrow of the Argonaut Peant (Platon, *Minos*). By the way, there are instructions, that both "sacred" and "profane" in primitive religions mean the same or two sides of the same. Thus, tabooed animals in the book *Levit* were considered profane because they were sacred; the tomb of the human crushed with lightning or poison was fenced as a place of burial for cattle who died of Siberian ulcer.

Along with arrows, poison can be inserted into an organism without visible damage by penetration through a coverlet (in modern terms, with cutaneous injection). Following is a quotation from a myth about Hercules: "...He sent the ambassador to Dayanira (wife of Hercules) in order to deliver to her an elegant tunic for carrying out a sacrificial ceremony. Dayanira was not so young and, to charm her husband, decided to give him a tunic moistened, according to centaur Ness, with a love talisman which actually was the strongest poison (a solution of poison from the blood of a hydra, Ness). Hercules put on the sent tunic and began a ceremony; he had already sacrificed to the gods a hundred foals of cattle, but suddenly he let out a heart-rending cry as if he were bitten by a snake. Heat dissolved the poison of the hydra in the blood of Ness, and the tunic stuck to the body of the hero, causing terrible spasms. Inexplicably, from intolerable pain, Hercules overturned the altars. He tore the clothes from himself, but it had grown so strong in him that together with it the flesh was pulled, baring white bones. His blood hissed and bubbled, as if spring water in which red-hot metal was being tempered. Hercules rushed to the nearest stream, but poison began to burn down even more strongly...." Since then, stream waters are scalding hot and places from which they flow are called *Thermopylae*, meaning "hot gate" (Sophocles, *Scholy*). Discounting the magical character and fantastic exaggerations of the above-stated description, it has to be said from modern point of view that such a poison had high toxicity not only via intramuscular or intravenous injections (arrow), but also via cutaneous administration. A similar example of a poisoning through a coverlet appears in a myth about the Argonauts, wherein Medea presents Kreus with a beautiful dress impregnated with poison, and its fitting led to the death of the competitor.

The third possible source of physiologically active compounds is natural mineral substances. In myths they are presented very sparingly, although plant and animal poisons also act as hypostases of poisons and medicines. In many sources, it is emphasized that the waters of the River Styx (the river of the kingdom Hades) are poisonous. Pavsany gave one variation of the death of Alexander the Great in which he was poisoned with water from the River Styx. Teuphrant, one of de Missy's tsars, recovered from leprosy by means of the curative properties of a stone antipathos (Greek *anti*—against; *pathos*—suffering, a pain). Dolphins are depicted as children of the sea (dog-headed and flipper-bearing beings) who interfered with weather by means of sorcery, creating fogs and spoiling crops, and using sulphur and water from the River Styx. The Stymphalian birds destroyed by Hercules spoiled crops with their poisonous dung. Clearly seen here is the opportunity to influence by physiologically active compounds not only real living organisms but all of nature and, first of all, vegetation, which interferes with the ecological equilibrium of the environment and leads to negative consequences for all beings living in it, including humans. It is possible to state that there were instructions in myths regarding the possible use of various agricultural insecticides, pesticides and fertilizers. Subsequent examination of PhAS has shown that they consist of two indissolubly united parts; in other words, they could be used both for destruction of vegetation and crops and for maintenance and increase in crop yields, and for stimulation of growth and development of plants and destruction of its enemies—plant pests.

Finishing this discussion of myths, it is necessary to point out that all of them were connected to the real world of the Greeks at that time. And in one myth about Midas, Moskhy's Macedonian tsar who was famous for planting pink gardens and transforming into gold anything that he touched, there is a question regarding an Atlantic continent and physiologically active compounds based on the phytogenesis of this continent. The old satyr, Sylen, tells Midas wonderful fairy tales about a huge continent behind the ocean stream that is completely separated from Europe, Asia and Africa. According to the tale, the satyr gives Midas the following description: "There is a place where two rivers flow nearby: the trees growing on the coast of one river bear fruit that force the human to groan and cry, although he won't waste away by eating them. But the fruits growing on coast of another river return youth even to very old people." In modern representation, these are clear indications of the possibility of the existence of the American continent and the taking by its inhabitants of phytogenic drugs with typical "breakdown" and euphoria. Eratosthenes, Mela, Cicerone and Strabon argued this point, and Seneca predicted the discovery of this continent in the second act of his *Medea*. It is said that this part of the play had a great impact on the young Christopher Columbus. Considering the physiologically active compounds mentioned in ancient myths—the first records of which concern the first millennium B.C. and, for example, the *Iliad* and *Odyssey*—as scientists regard the first documentation as dating from the time of Pisistrat (second half of the sixth century B.C.), it is necessary to emphasize that work on their texts has never been interrupted and has proceeded further, especially with the efforts of the scientists from Alexandria during the Hellenistic era (after Alexander the Great). There is a great variety of hypotheses about the origin and reliability of myths, including Homeric poems, and it is possible to become fully acquainted with this topic in A.F. Losev's work

Homere. Taking into account the fantastic form of myths caused by the aspiration to create interest and thus aesthetic admiration—in spite of the nearly universal themes surrounding blood and death—we notice that they have incorporated some actual historical experiences of the surrounding world and, in particular, poisons or, generally, physiologically active compounds: their finding in nature, methods of application and effects. It would be not reasonable to ignore this experience, especially because it contains sources based on a broad range of modern sciences: chemistry, pharmacology, toxicology, biology, ecology and many more fields of medicine and other branches of knowledge. Consideration of myths, legends, fairy tales and other sources of oral creativity has shown that PhAS can exist and be used in various aggregate conditions: in the form of liquids, gases and solid substances. Their main and unique source is nature—flora, fauna and natural materials. Methods of delivery of poisons to an organism depend on their aggregate condition: gases and steams arrive mainly through respiratory tracts and coverlets; liquids through a gastroenteric path, mucous membranes (cavities of the nose, eye, etc.) and coverlets; solid substances through a gastroenteric path or, in the form of dust, through mucous and respiratory pathways. In order to become a poison from a natural chemical compound—in other words, to show its toxic or other physiological effect—such a substance must enter the human body either naturally or violently (for example, by an arrow prick). Although the basic methods of penetration of poisons into an organism had already been known even in mythology, they were not limited to the methods listed above and, as we will see further, they were constantly improved and became more and more various. In mythology, naturally, there are no quantitative laws regarding poison (i.e., the concept of "dose", or the specific quantity of the poison entering an organism), but qualitative laws are noted: i.e., the general interrelation between the specific poison entering an organism and the effect (for example, aconite both for paralysis of an organism and as an ointment for "flights"). Revealing the conditions of the interaction of a poison with an organism and the interrelation with effect will be, in a later chapter, a basis for the major section on the science of poisons, i.e., the general toxicology.

Chapter 2

Poisons in the Ancient World

According to the data we have examined, there are mentions of poisons in the manuscripts of Egypt, in ancient books of India, and in sources from the ancient Greeks and Romans. The transition to a settled way of life, urbanization and formation of the first states, and the fierce and ruthless struggle for existence and power led to a wide demand for poisons that gave a push to an intensification of their study. The great demand for poisons could no longer be satisfied by searching for and gathering the corresponding plants and animals; it was easier to organize their constant reproduction in special carefully-protected territories. The first "gardens" of poisonous and curative plants mentioned in ancient myths appeared in Colchis (the gardens of Medea), Iberia and, especially, Thessaly. *Pharmacids* were engaged in the preparation of poisons and medicines in these gardens. They were magicians with knowledge of the secret actions of poisons and medicines (from here came the scientific name for the action of medicines—pharmacology). The insidious art of preparation of various poisons arose in the ancient East, and with the conquests of Alexander the Great were spread worldwide. And though empire of Alexander the Great was short-lived and was divided up after his death, an important accomplishment had been achieved. The exchange of knowledge as a result of a mixture of cultures against a background of constant requirement for poisons led to the widespread practice of producing poisons, secretly or obviously—as a rule, at imperial courts—as a tool of political struggle for the whole millennium (from 1.5 thousand years B.C. to 1–1.5 thousand years A.D.). However, poisons also continued to be widely used later in the political culture of the Middle Ages and up to the present day. After the campaigns of Alexander the Great, the Asian knowledge of plant poisons was quickly and widely extended throughout all of the Hellenistic world. The East has shown the broadest possibilities of application of natural physiologically active substances as medical products. Tea, rhubarb, *Ricinus communis* L., man's fern, tannins, wormseed, opium, henbane and other plants were known and were taken for medical purposes as early as extreme antiquity. But there is much greater historical documentation of the conclusion that poison causes death, and tsars and the nobility began to use it to solve their problems. Especially known in history were the governors of Pergamsky and Pontius kingdoms. The last tsar of Pergamum, Attala III (second century B.C.), left a mark in history of botanical "achievements." In his big garden, henbane, ramson, hemlock, foxglove, delphinium and aconite were carefully grown. Poisonous medicines personally made by him were usually checked by doctors, although a sad fate was not avoided by his friends. In this sense, an unlucky commander, the governor of the Pontius kingdom on the Black Sea coast who was at war with Rome for a quarter of the century, was even more well known. The father of Mitridat died because of poison, and the heir, from an early age, decided to do everything possible to avoid a similar fate. The gardens of Mitridat exceeded the botanical oddities of Attala: the Pontius monarch devoted all of his free time off from military campaigns to the cultivation of poison and the search for antidotes. Just in case, he trained his body to withstand the actions of poisons and he succeeded in it. Subsequently, the phenomenon of tolerance of poisons was given the name *mitridatism*. It, however, did not help the eternal loser. When Pompey finally destroyed his armies, Mitridat poisoned his entire family and tried to poison himself, but the he sustained even a "horse's" dose of poison and it was necessary to him to accept death by the hand of the slave.

During the time of the dictator Antonia—based on the example of the courts of the eastern rulers—the post of a slave checking the food served to the lord of Rome was documented. But poisonings during the imperial epoch were applied on such a wide scale that food-checking personnel united, like other craftsmen, in a special board similar to modern trade unions. At that time, a beautiful custom appeared in which a ring of glasses filled with wine are clinked. This custom is still practiced today. But ancient Romans clinked glasses much more strongly, watching that wine from one cup splashed into another. In such way the absence of poison in wine was assured. The most widespread poisons of antiquity were aconite (varieties of this perennial grass of the buttercup family with a flower in the form of a helmet number about three hundred, and all of them are poisonous), along with hemlock and cicuta. Athenians traditionally took a great interest in water hemlock—infusion of its root killed in minutes. In 399 B.C., the 70-year-old philosopher Socrates (300 judges pro, 250 con) was killed democratically most possibly with this poison for the seduction of impressionale youth with his ideas. Almost one hundred years later, the great orator, Demosfen, plotting against Tsar Phillip, father of Alexander the Great, died. At the same times, Athenians in prison poisoned the strategist Fokiona with hemlock for his sympathies with Alexander the Great. In Rome there was a tradition to solve important problems with the help of poisons. In 331 B.C., a sequence of sudden deaths fell upon the patricians, stately citizens. Some respectable Roman matrons created a unique club: they gathered and created potions and poisonous substances with which they killed the bothered husbands, both their own and others. According to historian Tit Libya, a big investigation was held which led to the conviction of 170 women. This was the first case of legal prosecution of murder by poisoning in Roman history. Before the approach of a new era, during an epoch of civil wars when even the lives of aristocrats-patricians were being depreciated, the authorities more often encouraged suicides of politically-prosecuted citizens. It was absolutely legally possible to receive from the authorities a broth of hemlock or aconite to avoid the shame of public execution. During the epoch of the emperors of Ancient Rome, there were a great many episodes in which experts in the making of deadly mixes showed their worth in a struggle for power even among close relatives. Following are some typical examples. The Emperor Tiberius poisoned his adopted son, the well-known commander Germanius, on whose body before death dark blue stains broke out and foam flowed from his mouth. Subsequently, Tiberius inflicted a mass punishment, having learned that his son Drusus was poisoned by his own wife in collusion with the head of the guardsmen. Only the death of Tiberius stopped the sequence of tortures and executions of the crowned "inspector." Apparently, it was not done without the participation of his grandson, Caligula, whose relatives Tiberius had killed. In avenging his relatives, Caligula furtively poisoned his grandfather. Caligula had a reputation for being an expert on poisons and personally invented new structures and methods for their application. When a gladiator named Pigeon was wounded in a duel, the emperor under pretext of treatment inserted a poisonous mix into his wound, after which he gave the poison the name "pigeon" and added it to his list of poisons. After the murder of Caligula, a huge chest filled with different poisons and detailed recipes was found, and though Claudius (who replaced Caligula) destroyed this warehouse, it did not stop the solemn procession of poisons. He also was poisoned. Poison was poured for him by his wife, Agrippina. In her opinion, the emperor was mistaken in the appointment of the successor, and after his death she appointed as emperor her own son, Nero. Taking the throne at the age of 17, Nero quickly quarreled with his mother, who pretended to actively participate in the management of the empire. Going too far, Agrippina flagrantly poisoned the head of a province of Asia (the proconsul Silane) at a feast, and she threatened to poison young Britannicus, the heir-apparent of Claudius. Nero did not argue with his mother and simply poisoned Britannicus. In general, Nero killed many prominent Romans, sending to them poisoned delicacies for the purpose of occupation of their property and replenishment of treasure, which he was rampantly squandering. He exhausted the wealth of his rich aunt. He ordered that a huge dose of a laxative be given the ailing elderly woman. His teacher, the philosopher Seneca, was rescued from poisoning by drinking only water and eating the most simple food and fruits in which it was difficult to mix anything. In the ancient Roman literature, there is evidence that Nero and his mother resorted to services of Lucusta, a well-known producer of deadly poisons. For her merits, the felon-emperor rewarded the accomplice with rich estates and allowed her to have apprentices, but her life eventually was terminated on an executioner's block.

Numerous similar examples, even on a large scale, are known in the history of eastern countries—for example, in Persia. Artaxerxes III (fourth century B.C.), in order to occupy the throne, poisoned not only his brothers and son but also 80 more people who, in his opinion, posed a risk. Attempts to prohibit the cultivation of aconite in gardens even on penalty of strict punishments (Emperor Trajan) did not lead to a reduction in the scale of application of poisons for mercenary and political purposes. In addition, in ancient Rome, the phytogenesis of poisonous substances had already become known and was widespread. Also, the poisons of animals (snakes, toads, scorpions and salamanders) were known. There was even primitive knowledge of poisons of mineral origin—arsenic, lead, mercury, and green copper. The Egyptian, Zosima, in approximately 300 A.D. wrote an encyclopedia of 28 books containing all current knowledge of chemistry that had been collected during the previous five to six centuries. Although the value in terms of current knowledge is limited, there are interesting data on mineral poisons, in particular arsenic, and about methods of extracting lead acetate. Zosima showed that some poisonous compounds have sweetish taste (the name "lead sugar" has survived to the present). By the way, production of metal salts, in particular of acetic acid, was one of the first acids that ancient Greeks and Arabs learned to extract from substances of plant or animal origin. Mineral acids (sulfuric and strong nitric) and methods for their extraction were not discovered in Europe until approximately in the fourteenth century. Discovery of strong mineral acids became the most important chemical achievement after the successful extraction of iron from ore approximately 3,000 years earlier. But the victorious procession of natural PhAS was based on the preceding phytogenesis. Emetics and depletives (milk, quince, lemon, centaury, and begonia) were involved as antidotes. The well-known *teriyakis* (in translation from the Greek "remedy from snake poison") came from the East. It consists of a mix of opium with tens of other components and was used widely right up to the eighteenth century. The previously-mentioned Agrippina took teriyakis for prophylaxis after each meal daily. Medicines and poisons contained in plants are mentioned in the compositions of Theophrastus (ca. 300 B.C.); and descriptions of poisonings take a considerable place in the works of well-known physician Galen and doctor Dioskorida (second century B.C. to the first century A.D.), but the majority of other authors of antiquity—Homer, Demosthenes, Aristotle, Veratius, Plato, Apulia, Pliny, Ibn Sina (Avicenna) and others—fully and vividly write about motives of crimes and conditions in which they were made but do not pay enough attention to the medical picture of poisoning, methods of introducing and quantities of poison, or the characteristics of the poison. Let us point out that Avicenna (980–1037) was the last great scientist of the Arabian world of that time and the one alchemist who did not believe in the transformation of other metals into gold. In the course of six hundred years, up to the eighteenth century, his outstanding work, *Canon of Medicine*, was considered the basic manual for doctors of Europe. It is the encyclopedia of medical science that places the name of its author at the level of Hippocrates and Galen. The *Canon* was published for the first time in Latin in 1483. In the sixth part of the Canon, entitled "The General Reasoning on Poisons," there are data about poisonous animals, their poisons and methods for the treatment of poisonings.

A time of decline was coming. The devastating attacks of the Tatar-Mongolian hordes moved the centre of scientific thought to Europe. However, the development of numerous recipes for poisonous mixes (many thousands) in the ancient world had already been prepared not only for achievement of the fastest, desirably instant death, but also from the smallest amount of poison possible, taking into account methods of application along with the features of the human body. In order to complicate or make impossible the identification of a poison based on taste or smell when used with food, wine or water, poisoners varied the composition of poison, adding substances to hide any unpleasant taste or smell. The same poisoners, as a rule, made antidotes, and at that time the greater the number of poisons it "resisted" the more complicated the antidote was. Thus, for Nero, his doctor made an antidote of 70 components. Emperor Karkalla (third century A.D.) received poisons from distant Asian provinces, paying hefty sums for especially intricate mixes and structures. One hundred years later, Constantine the Great transferred the capital of the Empire to Constantinople, where a powerful caste of highly professional poisoners were employed. An increase in the efficiency in the manufacture of poison was reached by two basic methods: 1) making (including multicomponent structures) poisons by mixture, both in the liquid and solid form; and 2) "boiling" a poison, a determinative of which was an increase in the concentration of the active ingredient by evaporation of the initial product (as a rule, it was a water solution). Following is a typical example of the use of the second method: Nero, having received poison from Lucusta issued an ordered to serve it to Britannicus during lunch, but the dose was not strong enough and Britannicus was merely weakened. Then the emperor ordered

Lucusta to boil a stronger poison. She, in the presence of Nero, tested the poison on a goat; it died in five hours, which did not satisfy the master of Rome. After the next boiling, the poison was given to a pig, and it died immediately. Then Nero ordered a poison to be served "... at the table and to give it to Britannicus during dinner with Nero. From the first drink, he fell dead. ..." By the way, the description contains one of the first examples in ancient history of the use of experimental animals for an estimation of the efficiency of a poison. Subsequently, this method of estimation of toxicity would be developed both qualitatively and quantitatively, and led to basic toxicology. In sixth century, according to the laws of Justinian, manufacturers of poisons and love potions, as well as black magicians, were to be burned, crucified or put at the mercy of wild animals. Nevertheless, the Byzantium art of preparation of various poisons survived to medieval Western Europe and Russia.

Before beginning a discussion of the development of the science of poisons in the Middle Ages, it is necessary to note that the first, imperfect attempts at using poisons as a weapon of mass destruction during military operations had already been undertaken in the ancient world. All of the previously-presented information concerns poisons for "individual application" and, although in myths the idea of poisoning water for mass destruction of the opponent is suggested, such an attempt was not actually realized until 600 B.C. Armies of the Amphictionic League, headed by the tyrant Cleisthenes of Sicyon, besieged Kirrha, a city on the bank of the Pleistos river. At first, Cleisthenes gave an order to partition off the river to leave the enemy without water, and when it did not help, he ordered the armies to gather roots of hellebore—a plant containing (as will be established later) helleborein, the extremely poisonous glycoside. These roots, in great numbers, were thrown into a formed dam, and after a while the poisoned stream was directed into a former channel. The besieged, exhausted with thirst, drank the water. An epidemic poisoning began and they were easily overcome by the Amphictionics. The Roman historian Justin described a similar example in which live venomous snakes were used as a chemical weapon. Commander Hannibal, in a naval battle against the governor of Pergamum known for his poisons (see above), issued an order to collect a great number of poisonous snakes in clay pots. At the height of battle, these vessels were thrown onto the enemy ships and spread horror among the ranks of the defenders. Bitten and simply frightened seamen rushed about in a panic along the ships, plunged into the sea and soon surrendered. In this case, the reason for the victory was not the mass poisoning of the seamen, because not many were actually bitten. More likely, they surrendered because of the horror of so unusual a weapon and the panic that ensued.

Time was passing, and alchemy was being practiced; after a promising beginning, the discipline began to fall out of favor for the third time (for the first time by the Greeks, and the second time by the Arabs). Experiemnts in the transmutation of accessible metals into gold were permeated by mysticism and swindle. In 1317, Pope John XXII anathematized alchemy, and honest alchemists, being compelled to hide what they were doing, began to cloak their endeavors in even more mystery, cheating in the hope that alchemy would prosper as before. But the winds of change had already come to Europe. The Byzantine Empire had seen its last days, and in 1453 Constantinople fell and became Turkish forever. Greek scientists escaped to Europe. The traditions and knowledge that they brought with them became a powerful stimulus of rigorous research and important discoveries in Europe. It is important to emphasize that European scientists did not come empty-handed. They had a lot of new, unknown or even contradictary knowledge to that of the great Greeks. Finally, this marked the beginning of the scientific revolution, which overtook the world of alchemy rather slowly in the form of basic mineralogy and medicine. Thus, even under consideration of its ancient history, it is obvious that the science of poisons was absolutely empirical during this time. It was in a state of germination, being limited mainly by the "art" of preparation and application of poisons, and its essence was reduced to the search for more effective mixtures and composition, both in toxicity and in counteraction to known poisons (poison-antidote). The search for such preparations was carried out with a method known as "casual happening" by mixing friable substances or solutions and their boiling evaporation of, as a rule, initial preferred components from any plant, animal or mineral raw materials. Taking into account that initial components had a different quality, both in the content of active substances and in the content of impurities; the lack of a standard system; the casual character of preparing the ingredients; and the extreme limitations of chemical and physical techniques and methods of purification and isolation of target substances; the overwhelming majority of these numerous "experiments" led to negative results. Although individual "successes," in practicality, could not be reproduced and were intended for one-time personal use, the first attempts in antiquity of the use of poisons as weapons of mass destruction and, simultaneously, as medical products have already been documented.

Chapter 3

Poisons in the Middle Ages

The entire period of the Middle Ages, as well as antiquity, abounds with gloomy patterns of poisonings that received extremely wide circulation in political conflicts and as instruments used in the resolution of personal disputes. Knowledge about the biological essence of the effects of poisons and antidotes was still at a basic level; it carried a fortuitous, empirical character and was not used in practice. Amulets and charms of all kinds, along with spells and various mystical plots, were widely practiced at that time. Against this background, the appearance of the work of two contemporaries living at the beginning of the sixteenth century—George Bauer (under the pseudonym Georgius Agricola) from Germany and Theophrastus Phillippus Aureolus Bombastus von Hohenheim (under the pseudonym Paracelsus) from Switzerland—was absolutely revolutionary. Agricola was engaged in mineralogy and its connection with medicine. His work, *De Re Metallica*, published in 1556, is a classic and, as a result, mineralogy was declared a science. It was the most important work in chemical technology for the next two centuries.

Von Hohenheim (more well known under the name of Paracelsus), along with Avicenna, considered that the basic objective of alchemy that dominated at that time was not searching for methods of producing gold; rather, it was the manufacturing of remedies. Before Paracelsus, plant preparations were used mainly as remedies, but Paracelsus piously believed in the efficiency of remedies made from minerals. Paracelsus began the important field of chemistry called iatrochemistry (sometimes called *yatrochemistry*, from the Greek word for doctor, ιατροδ). Iatrochemistry played an important role in the fight against the dogmas of scholastic ancient and medieval medicine. Iatrochemists promoted empirical progress, tried to find chemical basis for the existing theory of humoral pathologies, formulated the concept of acidity and alkalinity, began the first reproducible experiments (although they were not always methodically correct), and discovered many new compounds. Paracelsus and his followers—Jan van Helmont, Sir Francis Bacon, Angelo Sala and Andrei Libavy—virtually formed the basis of experimental chemistry based on the measurement of physical quantities, and ensured the development of the first universal scientific theory—the phlogiston theory. Nowadays, a well-known expression (an epigraph of this book) is attributed to Paracelsus, the pioneer of toxicology. The depth of his expression is impressive, and today it is the motto of many toxicological laboratories all over the world. Paracelsus understood and was the first to put in written form that it is important to determine the concrete quantity of a substance, including a medication, for demonstration of its poisonous character. After that, it is not so difficult to determine the lethal dose of any substance (not only medicine). Iatrochemistry made the development of applied chemistry during that period a little bit easier, because it used language not understandable by people unfamiliar with chemistry, and broke with the traditions of mystical theorizing. And as a result, the era of gathering and description of empirical material began. Paracelsus suggested the idea of the addition of chemistry to the "great mother," medicine, the universal science, and understood the relationship between a toxin and its dose and effect. His idea was supported by his apprentices and followers and ensured, first of all, the possibility for the development of a medico-physiological direction of toxicology. This science studies the results of the effect of toxins on an organism and particularly on people, and investigates agents to heal intoxicated organisms. At the same time, the chemical toxicological study of toxins—their extraction; testing compounds and structures; identifying the physical and chemical properties; and, most importantly, the relationship of the chemical structure of a substance with its biological activity—could not progress significantly because of the lack of a theoretical basis for modern chemistry concepts, i.e., elements, chemical bonds, etc. The period of iatrochemistry ended in the second half of the eighteenth century when phlogiston theory rose and then fell thanks to the work of Lomonosov, Lavoisier, Priestley, etc.

Robert Boyle (1627–1691) played an important role in support of this progress. He helped chemistry separate further from medicine by giving it a new direction for development: "I consider chemistry from completely new positions, not as doctor or alchemist, but as a philosopher." Boyle injected the term "analysis" into the work of chemists and urged them to draw conclusions based only on experiment. He introduced many new reagents and started to use chemical reactions for authentication of various substances. However, there was still a long way to go before the discipline of chemical toxicology would become an important branch of chemistry, so let us return to the cheerless and gloomy situation of the Middle Ages. The militant religious fanaticism, together with the ambitious machinations of the aristocracy in the fight for power and souls, generated a great number of intrigues, conspiracies and palace revolutions. The list of tsars, kings, princes, bishops, dukes and their retainers and relatives who were poisoned by or used toxins is extremely long. Killing for political reasons, for personal revenge and even for hire became the norm. The Renaissance in Italy, in the opinion of D.P. Kosorotov (a famous Russian toxicologist), was a period of poisonings and poisoners who in many respects had exceeded the achievements of the ancient world. We mention incessant murders under the order of Pope Alexander VI and his son, Caesar Borgia, only because all of them were inflicted mainly by toxins with a mineral origin, arsenium in particular. Arsenium has been called "toxin of Borgia" for some time. Henry VIII of England was so bothered by the constant poisonings of close aristocrats that he passed a law of 1531 whereby poisoners were thrown into boiling water. Poisonings in France and Spain were not less frequent. A significant contribution to the descriptions of poisonings and poisoners, along with historical chronicles of those events, were presented in the classical literature of different countries and time periods based on fictional accounts of the Middle Ages. Images of Milady in *The Three Musketeers* or Madame de Villefort in Alexander Dumas' *The Count of Monte Cristo* are widely known. Notable poisoners, according to the custom of their era, widely used toxins for resolution of arising problems.

Although the plots are amusing, modern experts of chemical toxicology only smile and take exception, because the wife of the royal prosecutor, for example, selects brucine as a poison and as a result another character in the novel develops immunity to it by swallowing it in small doses over a long period of time. Brucine, as well as the identical poison, strychnine, and the phenomenon of mithridatism are incompatible because of the ability of these toxins to have an effect, i.e., to cause intoxication even in small doses. In addition, brucine and strychnine can accumulate in an organism. Therefore, the events as written by the author of *The Count of Monte Cristo* cannot be associated with brucine in principle.

Shakespeare, describing the murder of Hamlet's father, refers to henbane, which has atropine in its compound as an active ingredient. The ghost of his father speaks of it as follows:

"...Sleeping within my orchard,
My custom always of the afternoon,
Upon my secure hour thy uncle stole,
With juice of cursed hebenon in a vial,
And in the porches of my ears did pour
The leperous distilment; ... "

In consideration, poisoning by (more accurately, overeating) henbane is characterized by the occurrence of psychic excitation; scopolamine would have been more accurately used by Shakespeare for this purpose, as scopolamine is related to atropine in chemical construction, has a calming action and is characterized by a nearly identical lethal dose. Datura and mandragora, containing scopolamine, were widely used earlier as a narcotic and hypnotic agent. Let us note an unusual route of injection of a toxin into an organism—through the ear. Significant contributions in the area of methods of injection of toxins into organisms along with the expansion of an assortment of toxins were made during the Middle Ages. In addition to traditional methods, poisoners began to use widely subjects of everyday practice which often and for a long time came into contact with the object of their attention: for example, linen fabric, dresses and suits, table serving objects, bed clothes, pillows, pins and, especially, books. Poisoners acted within the environment of the educated and prominent for whom it was customary to read before going to sleep. Thus, books, before the appearance of printing on paper, in the majority were handwritten and made of various materials—papyrus, birch bark, parchment, etc. Poisoners learned that these materials could be easily soaked with liquid toxins, which would retain their toxic features for a long time. The victim took and held the book in his hands whereby he or she was subjected to cutaneous administration and, in addition, while turning the poisoned pages during which he might wet a finger with saliva, ingested the toxin through the mouth (per os). Solutions of arsenic acids with the addition of other various agents were especially effective. This insidious toxin killed hundreds and thousands of people in many nations. Toffana, a professional poisoner of the seventeenth century, confessed to the killing of more than 600 persons, including two popes! She owned a store of toxins and one of her hellish mixes was called "Toffana's water" or "Neapolitan water." Judging by description, the toxin, which the druggist offered young Romeo, was also arsenic (Shakespeare's *Romeo and Juliette*). Arsenium and the history of Middle Ages are inseparable—numerous, at times contradictory, but always mysterious and dramatic descriptions of poisonings are always connected with the fight for power, with politicians and rulers, profit seekers and grabbers coming and departing in anonymity. The famous Soviet toxicologist, S.N. Golikov, in answering the question regarding why poison was so widely used in early history, cites the expressive phrase of Quentin: "A toxin is more difficult to identify than the enemy"; i.e., Quentin believed that a toxin has serious advantages in contrast to a weapon: there is no noise or blood. Therefore, the study of toxins as a means for use in criminal activities was considered for a long time as a part of judicial medicine. With cultural growth, the strengthening of state control over production and the use of toxins, they started to lose their ominous significance. But, on the other hand, they received a powerful stimulation for development in the nineteenth and twentieth centuries, which led to the creation of two new branches of the chemistry of physiologically active compounds: the chemistry of diversionary toxins and the chemistry and technology of toxic agents. A brief discussion about them will be given further.

The second industrial revolution after the production of iron took place from the tenth to the sixteenth century. Many technical processes, devices and constructions that stimulated the development of all branches of knowledge were generated. As one of the effects, a period of great geographical discovery arrived. Europe, in the person of Christopher Columbus, studied the coast of Africa and made a voyage around the continent to open the New World—South and North America. It is necessary to emphasize that all plants and animals (at least the overwhelming majority) typical for central Europe had been checked for the availability of biological activity by this time. In this sense, the flora and fauna of Africa and especially the American continent presented a new vast field for discovery and analysis. The first description of the primitive use of a paralyzing toxin, curare, for wetting arrows was made by the English traveler, Sir Walter Raleigh, when he encountered the Indians of the Orinoco River region in 1595. However, it was not until 1897 that Rudolph Boehm identified that this toxin consisted of quaternary ammonium organic compounds, which are responsible for the specific action of this toxin, and tertiary bases (amines), which don't have such activity. We will speak later about the interrelation between the activity and chemical structure of compounds similar to curare. Here it is necessary to accent the importance of these preparations in the practice of surgical anesthesia. Interestingly, the Indians of the Amazon Basin use the toxin curare as goods for exchange with other populations and continue to use it widely for silent and effective hunting with the help of an air gun, although they already have easy access to modern firearms.

With the exception of curare, the large and varied vegetation of the tropical zones of Africa and America provided many other physiologically active compounds to mankind that have found varied and wide use today, mostly as medicines.

Pharmacies were the main place for chemical research during that period. Outstanding chemists of Europe worked there. In 1581, the English Queen Elizabeth sent a court doctor, Robert Jacob, together with druggist Jetties Frenham, to Russia at the request of the Russian tsar. We can consider this year as the beginning of the origin of chemistry in Russia. The second drugstore was not opened until the seventeenth century in Moscow, and by the time of Peter I there were only eight of them, but they were not yet laboratories in which discoveries were made. A change in attitude toward the sciences and to chemistry in particular occurred in the time of Peter I, when the Academy of Sciences was opened in 1724 and the first pharmaceutical "garden" was planted. It was not until 1745 that the first professor of chemistry appeared in Russia in the person of Lomonosov. He became the first ethnic Russian academician. Quackery, which had dominated in the past, employed various poisonous grasses and powders. A doctor from abroad by the name of Bomely, who attended to Ivan Groznyy, was the most typical quack-poisoner. Seven of Groznyy's wives were poisoned, in the same way many seditious boyars were killed. Medieval Russia did not differ from Europe in this aspect and used toxins for the same purpose.

Misunderstanding of the basic chemical foundation of the action of toxins, the mystery surrounding them, and legends and superstitions sometimes held back development and rejected the progressive ideas of antiquity. A number of scientists, blind to other explanations and not understanding the concept of cause and effect held intuitively materialistic but also primitive opinions (for example, the existence of a "sharp sting" of a toxin by analogy to snakes, insects, etc.). Others attributed the effect of toxins to their spiritual nature. As a result, "universal antidotes" appeared, e.g., talismans, charms and amulets. As amulets, people used the horn of a unicorn, small horns of a horned viper and, with the development of mineralogy, agate, many jewels and even a bezoar stone (gallstone), which was also used in the form of a powder and even for intake. Bezoar gallstones generated a whole group of antidotes in sixteenth and seventeenth centuries called *bezoardics*. Nevertheless, doctors-practitioners successfully used simple and sure methods such as antidotes, which have been used in medicine up to the present. The method consists of inducing rapid and effective excretion of toxins from an organism with the help of emetic, sudorific, purgative and diuretic agents.

In summary, I would like to emphasize that the history of the development of sciences of toxins and antidotes in the Middle Ages was characterized by the following:

- the discovery of a great number of physiologically active substances with an extraordinarily wide spectrum of action, and
- the introduction into the exploratory practice of new techniques and devices, which led to a conversion from qualitative to quantitative characteristics, measurable and comparable data, and searches for a new fundamental foundation of chemistry.

All of this progress in knowledge was based on a new historical foundation, connected with the formation of large and intensively developing industry and with the occurrence and strengthening of the bourgeoisie. Industrial progress that had begun in the eighteenth century in Europe promoted significant qualitative and quantitative changes in knowledge, including chemistry. There came an era of atomic theory in classical and biological chemistry, the era of Butlerov's theory.

Chapter 4

Development of the Chemistry of Physiologically Active Substances (PhAS) in the Nineteenth and Twentieth Centuries

By the end of eighteenth century, experimental work which demanded systematization within a single theory had been gaining momentum. French chemist Antoine-Loran Lavoisier became a pioneer of such a theory. In 1789, he stated and, most importantly, experimentally proved the mass conservation law (a building block of nineteenth-century chemistry). In 1756, Lomonosov was the first to express a conjecture about the existence of this law, but his works were published in Russian and Western European chemists, including Lavoisier, could not read them. New approaches to the processes of oxidation and burning establishing that air is a multicomponent system (using not only data from his own experiments, but also the data of contemporary scientists) struck a blow not only to phlogiston theory and the theory of elements that dominated during that time, but also prompted a full revision of the theory of chemistry. In 1789, Lavoisier released his *Elementary Treatise on Chemistry*. He classified knowledge in chemistry accumulated by that time in his book, relying on new concepts and using nomenclature developed by him and other French chemists (de Morveau, Berthollet and Fourcroy). Actually, this was the first book about chemistry in its modern conception. Lavoisier's success showed chemists that using quantitative measurements could help to explain chemical reactions. French physiologist Claude Bernard (1813–1878) introduced an experimental method in medicine that allowed recognition not only of the external signs of poisoning but also the physiological mechanisms that underlie the process. In 1844, Claude Bernard, studying the action of the poison curare, was the first to show how it was possible to determine the action of a poison on an organism in experiments on animals. He also was the first to ascertain that curare does not affect the entire nervous system, but only the area of nerve endings connected with muscles. This experimental study of poisonings allowed toxicologists and chemists to obtain results quickly, which in scientific value eclipses all previous progress. The development of the scientific discipline of experimental toxicology (the science of the effects and treatment of poisons in an animal organism) is attributed to Claude Bernard.

Nowadays, toxicology, together with physiological analysis, widely uses biochemical, anatomic and other methods of research, including research at the cellular and molecular levels. This allows exploration and knowledge of the effect of poison in all its many-faceted occurrences, which will promote understanding of the mechanisms of action of PhAS and their interrelation with chemical structures. This, in turn, can allow specific regulation of the biological activity of a substance by synthesizing an active compound for a particular purpose before designing its construction of antagonist-antidote.

The history of evolution and formation of modern inorganic and organic chemistry is completely stated in numerous works of science historians. Domestic historiographers and chemists (see the bibliography) also made a large contribution to this subject. Therefore, we will focus on the key moments in the evolution of chemistry that significantly influenced modern chemical toxicology or, more exactly, toxicological chemistry. In 1861, Friedrich August Kekulé characterized organic chemistry as chemistry of compounds of carbon. Developing this idea, it is possible to characterize inorganic chemistry as the chemistry of compounds containing all other elements. This definition gained wide acceptance and is still in use today. Justus von Liebig, Friedrich Wöhler, Joseph Gay-Lussac and Jöns Berzelius specified possibility of isomerism, i.e., compounds sharing the same atoms but with different molecular structure and, accordingly, different properties.

The main points of theory of a structure of chemical compounds were stated by A.M. Butlerov in his 1861 report, "On the Chemical Structure of Matter," at a congress of German scientists-naturalists. He formulated rules for the identification of the structure of organic compounds, and explained the phenomenon of isomerism. Kekulé applied points of structure theory to aromatic compounds, and Archibald Scott Couper suggested a suitable graphic representation of structural formulas (chemical bonds in the form of short line). Experimental confirmation of the theory of chemical structure by Butlerov and his followers had huge significance for its verification. The most important contribution of A.M. Butlerov distinguishing his work from that of Kekulé and Cooper was statement about the inseparable interrelation between chemical structure and the properties of molecules. The same idea became the foundation of the periodic table of elements suggested by Dmitri Ivanovich Mendeleyev. This fundamental conception of Russian chemists was corroborated over the next 150 years of the development of chemistry and is still relevant. Jacobus Henricus van't Hoff and Joseph Achille Le Bel had suggested a tetrahedral model of the carbon atom that explained not only stereoisomerism but also optical isomerism (activity). Moreover, compounds with several asymmetrical atoms of carbon (bonded with four different groupings) always had a number of experimentally-found optically active isomers, according to the van't Hoff-Le Bel theory. At the end of the nineteenth century, an opinion was asserted that the stereo arrangement of bonds is typical not only for the carbon atom. Viktor Meyer, William Jackson Pope and, next, Alfred Werner proposed a coordination theory that could interpret and forecast numerous events of isomerism of coordination compounds, including optical isomerism. German chemist Johann Friedrich Wilhelm Adolf von Baeyer suggested a "strain theory" using an idea of a three-dimensional construction of molecules. This theory promoted an explanation of the instability of carbon rings with fewer than five carbon atoms and the dominance of five- and six-member carbon rings among natural cyclic compounds. Subsequently, an ability to build a ring of any number of carbon atoms (with five or more atoms) free of angular stress at the expense of the location of a tetrahedral ring of carbon in specified cyclic systems in *different* (not in one) planes was stated. The van't Hoff-Le Bel theory was finally verified in Emil Fischer's work on examples of optical isomerism of simple sugars, and by 1900 a three-dimensional model of a molecule was approbated by almost all scientists. Along with qualitatively new theoretical backgrounds, the nineteenth century was characterized by serious progress in a new field of chemistry—synthetic organic chemistry. German scientists Justus von Liebig, Felix Hoffmann, Otto Bayer, Carl Gräbe, along with English scientist William Perkin and others developed the foundations of synthesis, technique and equipment, and for the first time purposefully synthesized many natural compounds. This progress paved the way for the theory and technology of applied chemistry. As these occurred mainly in Germany, the country held a monopoly in synthetic organic chemistry before World War I. This fact, along with other premises, allowed Germany to become a world leader in chemical industry by the beginning of the twentieth century.

First Germany and then other countries participated in the development of the chemistry and technology of toxic agents (TA) with high toxicity for humans, for which compliance with many specifications was required. The main requirement was comparative simplicity and low cost of production with high efficiency of application. The chemistry and technology of TA and various problems related to them will be discussed later in a separate chapter. Vitamins, hormones and alkaloids were widely researched in the twentieth century, and in many situations the structures of their molecules were ascertained with the use of classical chemical methods of analysis, including microanalysis, and recently-discovered methods (infrared, ultraviolet and mass spectroscopy, chromatography, diffraction of X-rays, etc.). Richard Wilsstatter identified the structure of chlorophyll. Heinrich Wieland and Adolf Windaus investigated the structure of steroids and compounds related to them; Otto Wallach, the structure of terpenes; Hans Fischer, the structure of heme (the coloring agent of blood); and Paul Karrer, the structure of carotenoids (important plant pigments). Chemists started to synthesize specified structures of natural compounds of increasing complexity. Sir Robert Robertson began his research with the study of physiologically active alkaloids. He earned distinction with his discovery of the structures of morphine (1925) and strychnine (1946). This work of Robertson was corroborated in 1954 by the distinguished American chemist Robert Burns Woodward. Together with William von Eggers Doering, he synthesized quinine in 1944. William Perkin, in his own hunt for this compound, earned prosperity by accidentally discovering aniline purple, the first synthetic coloring agent, and leading its subsequent industrial production. Woodward, using research into the mechanisms of organic reactions as a basis, synthesized compounds with more and more complex structures: cholesterol, the most well known among steroids, and cortisone (a steroid hormone) in 1951; reserpine, the first tranquilizer, in 1956; chlorophyll in 1960; and derivative of the antibiotic tetracycline in 1962. Tetracycline itself had been synthesized for the first time by M.M. Shemyakin with collaborators around that time, and information about it was published in 1967. In his work, the American biochemist (native of Russia) Phoebus Levene established the structure of nucleotides, components of nucleic acids responsible for control of chemical processes in the human organism. In the 1940s and 1950s, Dr. Alexander Todd synthesized a line of nucleotides and related compounds and confirmed Levene's conclusions.

At the start of the twentieth century, the ability to use synthetic compounds was theoretically substantiated, and their use as medications began (arsphenamine [Salvarsan] for treatment of syphilis, sulfonamides for treatment of many infectious diseases, etc.). By the end of the Second World War, the technology of the production of penicillin (one of the most effective preparations for infectious diseases, extracted from a culture of a green mold by Alexander Fleming in 1929) was engineered. In 1958, chemists learned to modify natural penicillin by changing single radicals in it to other organic fragments. Such semisynthetic products had no analogues in nature and possessed higher antimicrobial activity in some situations. This method of a search for more effective biologically active compounds is also suitable for poisons. Some alkaloids can be "modernized" by changing one fragment to another, so that the general structure of the original "maternal" substance as a whole is preserved. Along with the progress achieved up to the present in the undoubtedly important synthesis of natural structures, chemical synthesis can yield compounds that are missing in nature but which possess some biologically active properties. Synthesis can also compete with biosynthesis. It was precisely this method that all highly physiologically active compounds were synthesized. Because of their complex properties, including physicochemical, they began to be considered not only as probable poisons but also as toxic agents for warfare. Hundreds of thousands, even millions, of new structures unknown in nature were synthesized. Their properties had already been tested by the beginning of the twentieth century. In addition to toxic agents with common poisonous effects (hydrocyanic acid, chlorocyanogen, arsenous and phosphorous hydrogen, carbon monoxide, etc.), others with suffocating effects (phosgene and its analogues), lachrimatory effects (the lachrimators—chloroacetophenone, brombenzyl cyanide, etc.), irritant effects (the sternites—diphenylchlorarsine, adamsite, etc.) and blistering effects (yperite, nitrogenous yperite, and lewisite) were revealed among them. The progress of the chemical industry by the beginning of the First World War, especially in Germany, allowed Germany to become a pioneer in the use of chemical products as warfare agents (CWA). This spurred other countries to keep up with research. As a result of this progress both in synthesis and in industrial chemistry, the assortment of known toxic agents increased. Also, CWA with a new type of effect: nerve-paralytic agents (tabun, DFP, sarin, soman, V-gases)—were discovered and produced. CWA were not applied during the Second World War; nevertheless, intensive research and searches for new structures, as well as the the development and perfection of a subset of the chemical industry—toxic agents—moved forward. Fascist Germany continued to work on research into chemical weapons and development of new products even on the threshold of its defeat. Similar research was carried out in England, the United States, and in France in the post-war years. The Soviet Union did not lag substantially behind other industrially-developed countries in increasing its defensive potential in chemical weapons, and built high-powered production facilities for a new group of CWA (organophosphorous V-gases: sarin and then soman). Naturally, these successes of the domestic industry could not be possible without the existence of a powerful chemical and industrial base and advanced research concepts represented by a great number of scientific research institutes and organizations that were based on the fundamental work of domestic scientists such as A.E. Arbuzov, P.P. Shorygin, N.D. Zelinsky, A.N. Nesmeyanov, K.A. Kocheshkov, K.A. Andrianov, I.L. Knunyants, etc.

Detailed research into the structure of some natural poisons with especially high toxicity brought chemists to the conclusion that many of them were proteinaceous in nature and a huge molecule, built of twenty different building blocks—amino acids connected with peptide bonds in which the amino group of one acid bonds with the carboxyl group of another. Proteins are polymers made of up chains of repeating units with different chain size, shape, charge and chemical reactivity, and they display characteristic properties. To ascertain the correct order of the positioning of amino acids in proteins is difficult. It is significant that Emil Fischer, mentioned above in connection with optical isomerism of sugars, did not only develop the conception of the structure of proteinaceous molecules but also stated an important hypothesis suggesting that proteinaceous molecules could possess both chemical and biological individuality owing to the ability to form countless numbers of isomers. This proposition is one of fundamental conceptions of present-day molecular biology. The distinguished English chemist Frederick Sanger required eight years of laborious work to synthesize the somewhat simple proteinaceous hormone, insulin, consisting of approximately 50 amino acids, located between two interrelated polypeptide bonds. In 1953, the exact structure of insulin and then larger molecules (the nucleic acids carrying the hereditary information in genes) was determined. In both 1958 and 1980, Sanger was awarded the Nobel Prize in the same category (chemistry). Marie Curie (chemistry and physics), John Bardeen (physics, 1956 and 1972) and Linus Pauling (chemistry and peace) also received two awards.

Such attention to the work of Sanger is not without merit so long as further successes in the synthesis of various protein derivatives will be connected with the search and development of new methods (appreciably different from the classic) for the synthesis of polypeptide chains. Methods differ both from the point of view of intensification and selectivity in bonding amino acids to each other in precise order and with great selectivity to build a desired isomer from among a huge number of possibilities. Biotechnology signifies extraordinary progress in this direction. Using specific strains of bacteria, other elementary organisms or enzymes allows synthetic production of the most complicated natural compounds and production of unique stereo and optical isomers.

We have tried to present the facts logically based on the evolution of events. The history of science as a whole and the history of the chemistry of physiologically active compounds specifically helps scientists to recreate a logical unity of knowledge with the integration of current processes and tendencies. History is necessary to better comprehend the changes taking place in order to estimate the correct role of any concept within the most complicated developing system of knowledge. It is natural that there are also a number of self-restraints in the chosen approach to the chemistry of poisons in consideration of its history. First of all, we did not attempt to account for all known historical facts regarding the application of poisons, and did not consider or systematize the reasoning behind the progression in the use of poisons. In contrast to German toxicologist Lewis Lewin (*Poisons in World History*, 1920) or the popular science statement of I.D. Gadaskina and N.A. Tolokontseva (*Poisons Yesterday and Today: Sketches on the History of Poisons*, Nauka series "From Molecule up to Organism," 1988), we mentioned the most typical (in our opinion) chemical and biological structures and new features of reception and application of PhAS in their historical evolution. We appropriately did not mention questions connected with disagreements among supporters of different conceptions, various theories, scientific hypotheses and propositions. We tried to present unbiased facts uniting the logic of the scientific evolution of the chemistry of poisons with some important events in its long and complicated history and to comprehend perspectives of this branch of knowledge based on concrete examples.

Chapter 5

Poisons and Elementary Bases of Toxicology

In order to determine the structure of a substance in the modern chemistry of natural physiological active compounds, a complex of different methods of analysis are used that are sometimes very labour intensive, difficult and time consuming, because individual or even classes of natural substances and, in particular, highly toxic poisons, have a complicated structure. The structure of such compounds is ascertained, as a rule, on the basis of high-resolution mass spectral analysis, nuclear magnetic resonance (NMR), IR- and UV-spectra chromatography of various carriers, mathematical data processing of diffraction of X-rays, dialysis, electrophoresis and other physical and chemical methods along with widely-used classical methods of chemical analysis. Generalization of the whole complex of the received data with subsequent experimental chemical evaluation of the hypothetical structure allows consideration of the theoretical structures as true ones. In spite of such powerful analytical "weapons," chemists have not yet determined the structures of many natural poisons—in particular, toxins. They are products of vital activity of some bacteria, the toxins of snake poisons and even some plant poisons. The difficulty lies in their complicated structure, the mainly albuminous structure of these poisons, their huge molecular weight and the uncountable number of possible stereo and optical isomers. The best known and typical natural and synthetic poisons of the beginning of the twenty-first century are shown below (see Table 1). The main criterion for the inclusion of a substance in the table was its minimum fatal dose. Substances with a rather low toxicity fall later in the table. These poisons induce other, specifically expressed physiological effects (infringement of mental status, irritation, etc.) in doses close to those of the most highly toxic poisons, and that's why they are the most interesting.

Let us also point out that poisons in the table from the first to the sixth (inclusive) have a polypeptide (protein) structure, and the seventh and later are not protein structures. Before we proceed to a detailed consideration of the compounds given in the table, we briefly take a look at modern conceptions of the character of action of poisons. Once in an organism, poisons enter the bloodstream and spread throughout an organism. They distribute unevenly to organs, tissues, and cells, depending on their structure. A number of poisons have an immediate local effect (for example, irritating, stinging, cauterizing, etc.).

Table1. The strongest poisons at the beginning of the twenty-first century

No.	Poison name	Min. lethal dose, mg/kg	Source	Common formula or state	Molecular weight
1	Botulinium toxin (type A)	0.00000003	bacteria *Clostridium Botulinum*	crystals	150000
2	Tetanus toxin	0.0000001	bacteria *Clostridium Tetani*	crystals	100000
3	Ricin	0.00002**	plant *Ricinus communis*	crystals	62057
4	Diphtherial toxin	0.0003	bacteria *Cory nebacterium diphtheriae*	—	72000
5	Neurotoxin of cobra	0.0003	snake *Naja naja*	dry poison	—
6	Crotalotoxin (dry poison)	0.0012	pit-viper *Crotalus atrox*	$C_{17}H_{26}O_{10} \cdot 0.5\ H_2O$	399
7	Palytoxin	0.00015	bacteria *Palytoa toxica*	crystals	2680
8	Batrachotoxin	0.002**	frog *Phyllobates Aurotaenia*	$C_{31}H_{42}N_2O_6$	538
9	Saxytoxin	0.0034**	oyster *Gonyaulax catenella*	$C_{10}H_{17}N_7O_4$ 2 HCl	372
10	Tetrodotoxin or Tarichotoxin	0.008	fish *Sphoeroidas rubripes* or newt *Taricha torosa*	$C_{11}H_{17}N_3O_8$	319
11	Ethoxy methyl phosphoryltiocholin e (V-gases)	0.03**	synthetic	$C_7H_{18}PSNO_2$	211
12	Bufotoxin	0.3***	toad Bufo vulgaris	$C_{40}H_{60}N_4O_{10}$	757
13	O-isopropylmethyl flourphosphonate (sarin)	0.4**	synthetic	$C_4H_{10}PO_2F$	140
14	Curare	0.5	plant *Chondodendron tomentosum*	d-tubocurarin chloride $C_{38}H_{44}N_2O_6Cl_2$	696
15	Strychnin	0.5	plant *Strychnos nux-vomica*	$C_{21}H_{22}N_2O_2$	334

No.	Poison name	Min. lethal dose, mg/kg	Source	Common formula or state	Molecular weight
16	Anisatine (alkaloid sort of aconitine)	0.7**	seeds *Illicium anisatum L.*	$C_{15}H_{20}O_8$	328
17	Muscarine	1.1***	fungus fly-agaric *Amanita muscaria*	$C_9H_{20}NO_2Cl$	210
18	Samandarine (Salamandarine)	1.5	lizard *Salamandra maculosa*	$C_{19}H_{23}NO_2$	397
19	Diisopropyl fluor-phosphate (DFP)	3	synthetic	$C_6H_{14}PO_3F$	184
20	Cyanic sodium	10	synthetic	NaCN	49
21	Diethylamide lysergic acid (LSD-25) psychotomimetic	46** (0.2–0.3)+	Alkaloid rye, maize spurs	$C_{20}H_{25}N_3O$	323
22	3-quinuclidinyl benzilate (BZ) psychotomimetic	>50** (0.01)+	synthetic	$C_{21}H_{23}NO_3$	336
23	*o*-chlorobenzilidene-malonodinitrile (CS) sternite	(0.001–0.005)+	synthetic	$C_{10}H_5N_2Cl$	188,5

Note: the minimum lethal dose in all cases is on mice, intraperitoneal.
* guinea pig;
** LD_{50} on cats, intravenously; *** LD_{50} on mice;
\+ a threshold dose in mg/kg or threshold concentration in mg/l of air for humans.

Some poisons—for example, yperite—have a latent period of action and at the moment of introduction into an organism they do not show their properties. Another group of poisons have a localized action. They can be identified according to this sign, and if this obvious trait is visible the poison represents a somewhat small danger to the human. The majority of poisons at the moment of entering an organism do not reveal their presence, and just after entering the bloodstream, their transport to the vital centers and interactions with them display their nature. The method of action of a poison takes place at the cellular and molecular level of the structures of an organism and, therefore, it is inseparably linked with the success of biochemistry and the defenses of the molecular and cellular mechanisms of an organism to maintain its vital activities. The determination of the chemical essence of processes taking place during metabolism, detection of separate elements of subtle biochemical processes and detection of their importance and volume of "contribution" to the general life support of an organism allows an understanding of why some poisons in the most insignificant doses express their biological activity. It is connected with the highest selectivity of their action on concrete points of enzymes and substances providing the life-sustaining ability of an organism. At the present time, there are several known groups of poisons, each of which consists of several compounds that affect certain enzymes of an organism. Modern treatment based on toxicology is most fully stated by S.A. Kutcenco (2004), professor at the St. Petersburg Army Medical Academy. The greatest successes are obtained by studying the actions of poisons upon excitation (nerve impulse) of the nervous system from one axon (nerve cell), through the synapse, to another axon, and from the final axon to the functioning cell of an effector organ (muscle). The process of the transfer of excitation in the areas of contact is realized chemically through the mediator (intermediary) acetylcholine or, in some cases, through adrenaline. The principal circuit of the synaptic structure is shown in Figure 1.

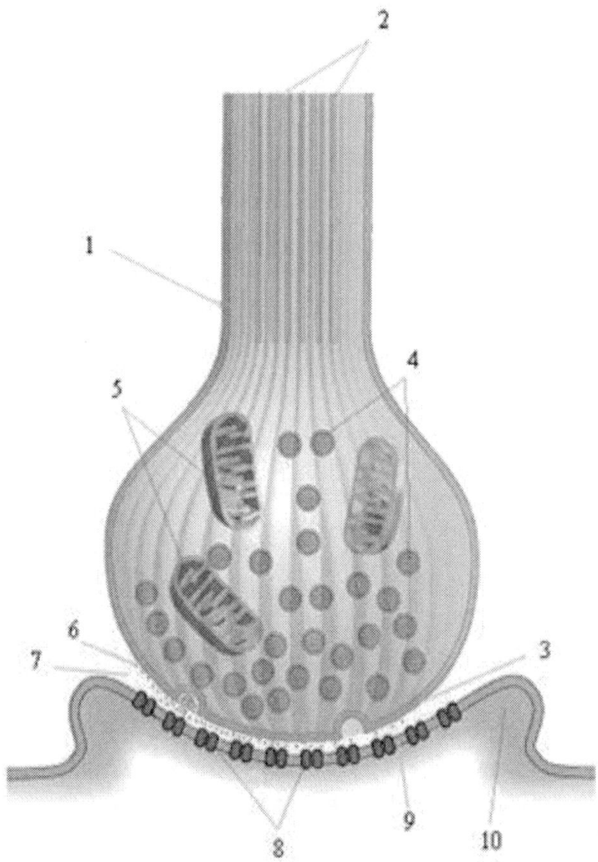

1 – axon; 2 – microtubules; 3 – presynaptic membrane; 4 – vesicles with mediator (synaptic vesicles); 5 – mitochondrions; 6 – mediator; 7 – synaptic cleft; 8 – receptors; 9 – postsynaptic membrane; 10 – dendrite.

Figure 1. The principal circuit of a synapse.

Many toxicologists and pharmacologists consider it convenient to describe the action of the mediator in the synapse or nerve-muscle combination, such as in nicotine, muscarin or curare. This historically developed differentiation in the features and poisoning symptoms, based on the character of alkaloid action (nicotine, muscarine and curare), also proves to be true today based on the lastest research of toxicologists.

The poisonous action of nicotine is characterized by contraction and spasms of skeletal muscles and a decrease in muscle power (the mentally ill have an increase in muscle power). It affects the central nervous system in the form of sleeplessness, headaches, nightmares, and initial time stimulation with the subsequent depression of the sympathetic and parasympathetic nervous systems. The action of muscarin is characterized by a display of gastroenteric symptoms (loss of appetite, nausea, spasmolytic pains in the stomach, vomiting, and diarrhea), increased perspiring and salivation (excretion of mucous), miosis (pupil constriction), malfunction of vision, bronchospasm, frequent urination, cardiac arrhythmias, and drop in blood pressure. The action of curare action is characterized by relaxation of skeletal and smooth muscles, immobilization, subsequent respiratory arrest because of paralysis of respiratory muscles, and death. The first signs of curare intoxication are drooping eyelids, drowsiness, loss of speech, and paralysis of cervical muscles. Then it affects the extremeties, muscles of the diaphragm and intercostal muscles, which lead to insufficiency and subsequent respiratory arrest. By the way, the fastest and the most effective experimental method of curare activity detection is the "falling rabbit head" test in which, after injection of the test compound into an eye vein of a rabbit, the animal cannot lift its chin and hold its head in a neutral position from 2.5 to 5 minutes. The method of action and point of application of a poison on a nerve cell (neuron) vary. Some directly attack the axon, blocking transfer of nerve impulses (tetrodotoxin); others neutralize the release of acetylcholine at the end of the axon (botulinium toxin); a third type breaks the contact between acetylcholine and muscles (curare); and a fourth type blocks the decomposition of acetylcholine (sarin, V-gases). Methods and points of action are shown in Figure 2.

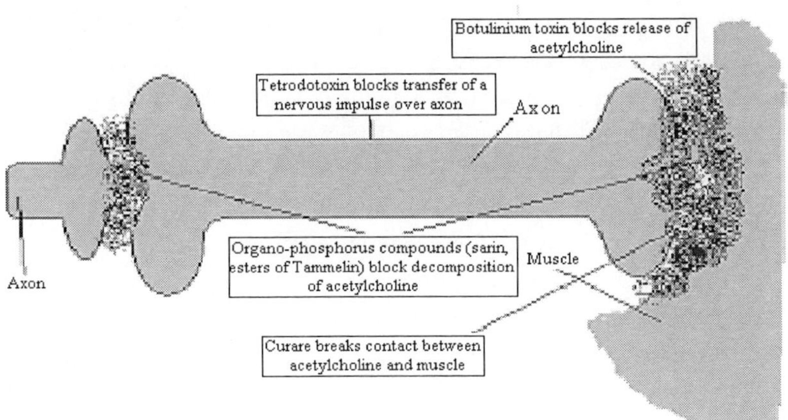

Figure 2. Method and location of action of some poisons (according to I.L. Knunyantc and R. Kostyanovsky).

The action of acetylcholine (acetylcholine in connections between the nerve termination and skeletal muscle and between preganglionic and postganglionic nerve fibres) is similar to the action of nicotine; acetylcholine action on the endings of the postganglionic parasympathetic compound is similar to the action of muscarine. In the latter case, the blocking agent is atropine. It is thought that atropine approaches receptor parts, blocking them from acetylcholine, and thus it is an antagonist with the muscarine-like action of acetylcholine. It causes mydriasis (dilation of the pupils of the eye), the opposite effect of the action of muscarine; however, atropine itself has pharmacological action, for example, on the central nervous system.

In biology, the term "receptor" describes the structures directly participating in perception and transfer of biological signals and connecting selectively with foreign compounds other than endogenous ligands (neuromediators, hormones, and substratum). In toxicology (as well as in pharmacology), the term "receptor" means any structural element of a biological system with which a toxin (drug) chemically interacts. This was introduced in biochemistry at the beginning of the twentieth century by Paul Ehrlich. Selective receptors of cellular membranes are the proteins integrated in the lipid bilayers with hydrophobic and hydrophilic parts. The hydrophobic part of α-spiral proteins provides their strong connection with a membrane. The hydrophilic part is outside the lipidic bilayer. Indeed, that fragment of protein provides a connection with the ligand that forms the receptor area. Below is a discussion of the main types of selective receptors, including those that:

- form ionic channels
- are connected with G-proteins
- have tyrosine kinesis activity
- form interreceptors networks

1. Receptors forming ionic channels. These receptors participate in the transfer of nerve impulses in the central nervous system and at the periphery. Usually, receptors of that type consist of several subunits penetrating the entire thickness of a biological membrane. One to two of these subunits represent the receptor area connected with the ligand. Other subunits, after the interaction of receptor areas with ligands, change their conformation and thereby participate in the formation of the ionic channel. The nicotinic acetylcholine (N-cholinergic) receptor, GABA-ergic, and glutamate receptors relate to channel formation. The first mentioned is the channel for Na^+; latter two for Cl^- ions. The majority of the substances affecting these receptors is known—for example, curarine, nicotine, anabasine (affecting cholinergic receptors), bicyclophosphates, norbornane, pyrotoxininyn (affecting GABA receptors), and strychnne (affecting lycine receptors). It is possible to place among them the same group of receptors of Na^+ -, K^+ -, Ca^{2+}, channels of excitable membranes for which endogeneous chemical agonists have not yet been found. Nevertheless, ionic channels possibly have a receptor area of linkage of highly toxic poisons of an animal origin, such as tetrodotoxin, saxytoxin, batrachotoxin, etc. The first studied channel-forming receptors were the nicotinic acetylcholine receptors. These receptors consist of four types of subunits from which the acetylcholine-connecting α-subunit twice presents in the receptor. As it supposed, all subunits in the process of evolution have arisen from one predecessor. The close sequence of amino acids in their molecules is evidence of it. The last represents the transmembrane α-spiral consisting of 20–25 amino acids. For all subunits, the method for fixing in the lipid bilayer is also identical.

2. Receptors connected with G-proteins. This special variant of regulatory signal transfer is presented by the interactive mechanism of endogenous ligands with receptors associated with G-proteins (regulatory proteins). In that case, the signals caused by ligand action lead to conformational changes in the receptor protein. They are transferred to binding proteins which, in turn, have already been stimulating or oppressing a certain system as a whole. Binding proteins during a signal transmission link a molecule, guanosinetriphosphate (GTP), and split it into guanosinediphosphate and phosphate (the names GTP-ase and G-proteins are taken from this term). In particular, muscarinic cholinergic receptors (M-cholinergic receptors), α- and β-adrenoreceptors, etc. are related to a number of receptors of this type. Muscarinergic and adrenergic receptors are formed by the protein molecule fixed in a cellular membrane by means of seven transmembrane parts of a peptide α-spiral. Both receptors, taking into account the sequence of amino acids, are rather close, indicating the closeness of their evolutionary development. It is supposed that various types of α- and β-adrenoreceptors, M-cholinergic receptors, dopamine, serotonergic, histaminergic receptors, and a number of other receptor structures represent the subtypes of a certain initial formation differing with insignificant features of tertiary structure, conformation, and linkages with lipid membranes. The complex of G-proteins consists of three subunits. The greatest, with a molecular weight of 40,000, is called the α-subunit. It contains in the catalytic centre a site of selective GTP linkage and during activation acts as GTP-ase. On one hand, the α-subunit is interfaced with the membranous receptor protein; on another, with a molecule of adenylate cyclase. The β-subunit has a molecular weight of approximately 35,000 and possibly begins the splitting process of GTP, disconnecting from a complex of G-proteins. There is practically nothing known about function of the smallest γ-subunit (molecular weight of approximately 10,000). The functioning of a signal transmission system by means of G-proteins is best studied with the example of the β-adrenoreceptors. At present, most substances with synthetic and natural origins selectively interacting with receptors of any given type are known. Among them are numerous medical products (affecting cholinergic, catecholaminergic and serotonenergic synapses), intoxication with which develops at receptors during excitation (proof of activation) and blockade (proof of suppression). Many such substances (lysergic diethylamide acid, psilocin, psilocybin, bufotenine, mescaline, quinuclidinyl benzilate [BZ], etc.) have various psychoactivity.

3. Receptors with tyrosine kinase activity. In particular, insulin and growth hormone concern these receptors, which consist of one or two albuminous subunits, fixed in a lipid bilayer with the help of the peptide α-spyral. The receptor molecule partially enters a cell after interaction with the ligand. At the same time, the tyrosine kinase activity of the special receptor subunit or enzyme is closely connected with it. The activating signal of the processes leading to activation of a cell is phosphorilation of endocellular proteins (of a molecule of tyrosine).

Toxicants selectively affecting this type of receptor are not yet known.

4. Receptors forming interreceptors networks. Unlike other membrane binding receptors, a linkage with the ligand in this case does not lead directly to a signal transmission of the effector system. The process of perception of a signal is connected with formation of interreceptor networks on the surface of cells. The best way to study the Fc-fragment (fragment crystalline) of antibodies (immunoglobulin) is with this group of receptors. These receptors represent aggregates of two or more aluminous subunits whose molecular weight is approximately 30,000–50,000.

Selective linkage of a toxicant with receptors of one type is typical only for a very small number of highly toxic compounds (for example, some phosphor organic compounds, botulinium toxin, saxytoxin, tetrodotoxin, amanitine, and muscarine). Often, the substance has a roughly identical affinity for several receptors, interaction with which leads an unavoidable biological effect (a profile of toxic reactions). Therefore, variations in the severity levels of the manifestation of intoxication of the same substance are caused not only by an increase in the quantity of one type of receptor that has come into contact with the toxicant, but also by an increase in the spectrum of interacting receptors. For this reason, even though the manifestation of intoxication is often known, we cannot precisely define a toxin's mechanism of action. The information above concerns toxins with various mechanisms of action, including those influencing the neurotransmitter system.

In the determination of original compounds, their spatial structure and other properties of receptor sites; the properties of enzyme and mediator complexes; those of enzymes and poisons; and many other peculiarities of structure and mechanism of poisons' interaction with binding sites in an organism; will favor the development not only of effective antidotes, which is important in itself, but will also pave the way for the synthesis of new medical products with high precision in binding sites.

On the whole, all of the above-stated qualitatively expressed physiological actions—separately or in combination with each other—act as the characteristic of most, but not all, biologically active compounds. A significant number of synthetically produced poisons affect other sites and links of the fine biochemical processes connected not only with the transfer of a nerve impulse, but also with other no less important functions of metabolism of an organism (blood oxygenation, substitution of a metabolite with an antimetabolite, reproduction abnormality, mutation, etc.). An antimetabolite is any substance, usually similar to a metabolite, that enters a metabolic process in place of a metabolite and either disturbs or stops it. Chemical substances causing hereditary mutations are called mutagenics, and they are toxic compounds. A number of poisons, including toxic agents (yperite, sarin and similar substances) have mutagenic properties.

The character and degree of a poison's toxic action depends basically on the role that the affected system plays in organism, and on the ability of the latter to form stable compounds with the poison connected with the possibility of effective restoration of this system or rapid creation of a new one by an organism, instead of becoming disabled. It is difficult to reproduce in a laboratory the processes proceeding in an organism, and their essence has not yet been determined. The reaction of an organism to poison depends on many factors noted above, and on the character and structure of the poison, the method of its injection and its condition. It is well known that the susceptibility to poisons varies among individuals even in the same kind of animal, and the idiosyncrasy phenomenon (an organism's hypersensitivity to some chemical substances) under the influence of poisons has been experimentally confirmed during human research by scientists in different countries. For example, results of yperite tests are the following: hypersensitivity, 4.9%; normal sensitivity, 47%; increased resistibility, 41.9%; high resistibility, 6.2%. Also, it has been noted that yperite's effects on an organism are much weaker at the same concentration in winter. Thus, the individuality of a live organism complicates the establishment of general laws. Data obtained from different kinds of animals cannot be transferred without essential corrections for humans, and a method of correlating a poison's dosage per kg of animal weight accepted by physiologists and toxicologists is not always well grounded. It explains the frequent contradiction of the toxicological characteristic of this or that poison and, for this reason, such figures should be considered approximate. The basic action of poisons on an organism is in close connection with their composition and structure, but there is not sufficient material for the establishment of a general law. A lot of established laws are typical only for a closed group of the described compounds, while substances close in composition and structure do not submit to these laws and there are numerous examples proving it. In spite of the huge body of experimental work undertaken by toxicologists and pharmacologists that has solved a number of problems and established some laws, the solution to the major problem (establishment of the connection and the general laws between the physiological action and the structure of the chemical compound) in the chemistry of poisons can be found only with further advanced and comprehensive research into the endocellular mechanisms of vital activity at the molecular level. Numerous and various synthesis analogues, homologs and compounds related to poisons, studying their biological activity, establishment and specification of their structure and binding sites are subordinate to the solution of this problem.

It is expected that the use of immunogenetic achievements and new immunology (sciences that reemerged after 1945 from Mendel's classical genetics and Pasteur's immunology) will initiate a considerable contribution in explanation of the molecular and endocellular answers to the puzzle of an organism's reaction to the intrusion of toxins. Prospects of these sciences are grandiose and amusing, as stated by the passionate propagandist of immunology, R.V. Petrov, in *Conversations about New Immunology*.

Specific poisons or their groups specified in the table in the beginning of the chapter and, where possible, the basic results in the establishment of laws and the interconnection between physiological activity and structure will be discussed in subsequent chapters.

Chapter 6

Muscarine

From time immemorial, fly agaric, containing the alkaloid muscarine, has been used by many peoples and tribes for various purposes, including treatment of spinal and encephalic illnesses, psychosis and heart conditions. Numerous cases of fly agaric poisonings have been described, and the symptoms are so typical (see chapter 5) that a particular set of poisoning signs are now characterized as "muscarine activity," and substances, including synthetics, having such "muscarine" activity are united under the general term "muscarine-like compounds." The first attempts to extract muscarine took place in 1811 and in 1869. Schmideberg and Koppe published the first fundamental work about muscarine.

For the first time, an alkaloid was obtained in a water-alcohol extract from *Amanita muscaria*, a mushroom widely known as red fly agaric throughout Europe, northern Asia, southern Africa, and North and South America. The quantity of muscarine in fly agaric depends on the area, climate, age and time of vegetation, ranging from 0.0002–0.0003%.

Along with muscarine—the classical alkaloid of red fly agaric (*Amanita muscaria*) in the tuber-like fly agarics of the *Amanita* type—there is a variety of other poisons, including hallucinogens. Extracts or broths were used by shamans of the Far East, Alaska and Chukci Peninsula. It is notable that, in the early days of its use, the substance was released in the urine of an organism with practically no changes and, with a view of economy, was reused.

Insignificant quantity, the presence of other alkaloids and the imperfection of extraction methods of those times all complicated the "muscarine problem" and caused many disputes and contradictions. Erich Harnack allocated a number of chloroaurates with fractioned recrystallization; he also obtained choline and a substance to which he attributed the formula $C_5H_{11}AuCl_4NO_2$. He named this product muscarine and subsequently suggested the structure $(CH_3)_3N\text{-}CH_2\text{-}CH(OH)_2$ (I). Attempts were made to confirm this structure by synthesis. So-called "synthetic muscarine" has been synthesised from choline by the action of nitric acid. It is considered be identical to natural muscarine. However, synthetic muscarine showed curare-like activity, whereas natural did not demonstrate such action. Much later, Arthur James Ewins, having reconsidered the technique of producing synthetic muscarine, came to the conclusion that the product extracted by Harnack was choline ether of nitrogenous acid: $(CH_3)_3N\text{-}CH_2\text{-}CH_2\text{-}ONO$ (II). In 1922, Harold King extracted muscarine almost in the pure state, using its solubility in absolute alcohol and ability to form a sediment under the influence of an alcohol solution of a sublimate. Fritz Kögl started his work of determining the structure of muscarine in 1928. Though the presence of aldehyde groups was denied, it was known that muscarine chloride demonstrates reactions typical of the aldehyde groups; the presence of hydroxyl groups was proven by the formation of a benzoyl derivative. Splitting in accordance with Hoffmann yielded two products: trimethylamine and α, β-dioxyvaleric acid, which sparked many hypotheses concerning structure of muscarine. Having taken into consideration all of these data, Kögl et al. found that muscarine chloride should be quaternary ammonium salt having one of two structures: III or IV

```
CH3-CH2-CH-CH-CH=O                          CH3-CH2-CH-CH-CH=O
          |   |                                       |   |
         OH  N+(CH3)3Cl-      III       Cl- (CH3)3N+   OH              IV
```

Kögl considered the most probable structure to be III. However, synthetic racemate appeared to be 40,000 times less active than muscarine; therefore, the aldehyde structure did not receive recognition. Moreover, betaine aldehyde V and a number of the related compounds synthesized earlier had a nicotine-curare-like action, which dramatically differs from the action of muscarine.

$$(CH_3)_3N\text{-}CH_2\text{-}CH{=}O \qquad \text{V}$$

Fourneau et al. synthesized derivatives of dioxolane VI, having a high physiological activity; however, the character of action of these compounds differed from that of muscarine.

```
CH2-CH-CH2-N+(CH3)3 Cl-
|    |
O    O
 \  /
 CH-CH3                    VI
```

Other authors offered the alkoxymethylammonium structure (VII) for muscarine.

```
CH3-CH2-CH-CH-CH2-O-N+(CH3)3 Cl-
         |   |
        HO   OH                          VII
```

Comparison of all data led researchers to the thinking that the reason for all errors was the heterogeneity of the extracted fractions of muscarine. Thus, the problem was determined to be related to having enough pure muscarine. For the first time, pure muscarine was extracted in 1954 by C.H. Eugster and P. Waser in a quantity of 260 mg from 1240 kg of fresh fly agaric in the form of muscarine chloride with the gross formula $C_9H_{20}O_2NCl$. They did not find in the structure of the extracted product either aldehyde or a trimethylamine group, but confirmed the quaternary character of nitrogen. Later, Balenovich et al., using chromatography on a column with cellulose, allocated the base whose homogeneity was proven by toxicological control tests and chromatography. Kuehl, Lebel and Richter (1955) extracted muscarine preliminary from resin JRC-50, and then purified it with chromatography on cellulose. Kögl, after unsuccessful attempts to extract muscarine by crystallization with Reyneke salts, extracted it with chromatography on norite.

Thus, in four laboratories, almost identical samples of muscarine chloride were extracted, which proved the analysis and properties.

Eugster et al. made a great contribution to the establishment of the structure of muscarine. They showed that the second oxygen atom is in a tetrahydrofuran ring. Eugster and Waser, for the determination of the structure of muscarine, applied catalytic oxidation, which played a significant role in the definition of its stereoisomer structure. Oxidation of muscarine chloride yields oxoderivatives—muscarones—which under IR spectra resembles spectra cyclopentanone; consequently, muscarine hydroxyl should be in a tetrahydrofuran ring. In accordance with Hoffmann's splitting, Kögl et al. isolated trimethylamine. Spectral bonds have been found in an infra-red spectrum of muscarine iodide for a hydroxyl group (3300 and 1380 cm^{-1}), quaternary ammonium group (1495 cm^{-1}) and tetrahydrofuran (1079 cm^{-1}), while bonds with a carbonyl group (1600 and 1830 cm^{-1}) were absent.

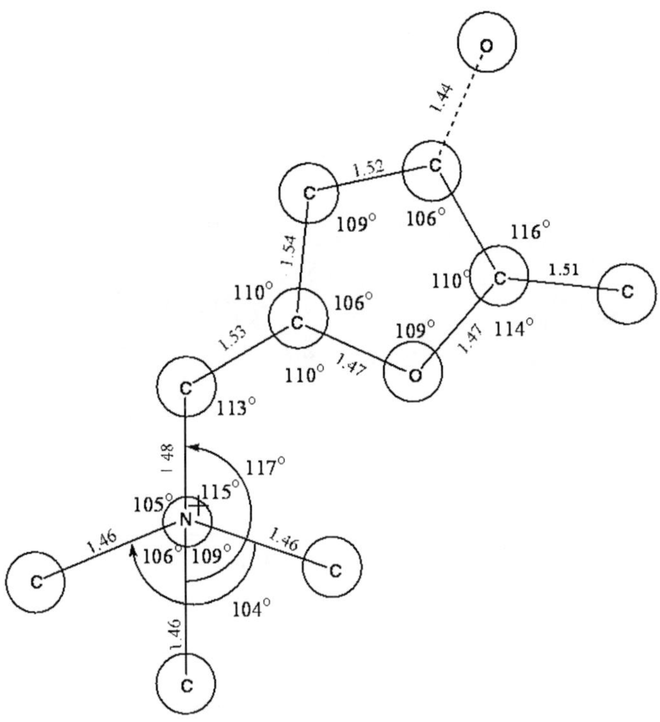

Figure 3. Lengths of bonds and valency angle in a muscarine ion.

The final muscarine structure was proven by Jellinek with X-ray analysis of muscarine iodide crystals. Thus, the true structure of muscarine can be most precisely shown in Figure 3, and its possible conformations in Figure 4. Owing to three non-symmetric atoms of carbon, there are four possible racemates or, accordingly, eight optically active forms. Under the arrangement, racemates were given following names and configurations (see Figure 5).

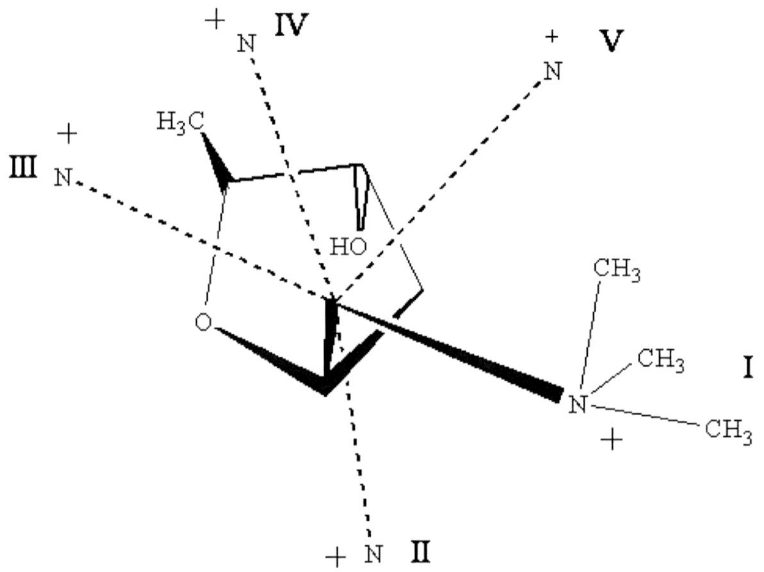

Figure 4. Some possible muscarine conformations owing to rotation of lateral methylenetrimethylammonium chains (positions I–V).

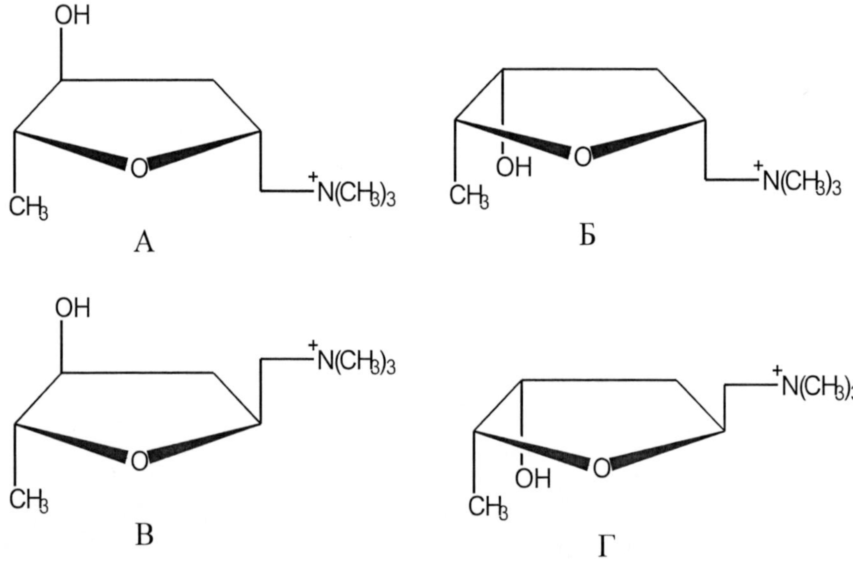

Figure 5. Muscarine and its stereoisomers: A—muscarine; B—epimuscarine; C—allomuscarine; D—epiallomuscarine.

A number of muscarine synthesises and its stereoisomers followed the final establishment of its structure. The most convincing should be identified as the synthesis carried out by E. Hardegger et al.

This graceful method (see Figure 6) provided an opportunity to obtain both natural muscarine and its optical antipode, which does not appear in nature. Arabinosa is the initial raw material that transforms into glucosamine acid (I); this acid at diazotization yields hitaric acid, which converts to dimethylamide (II), and then into threetosilate (III).

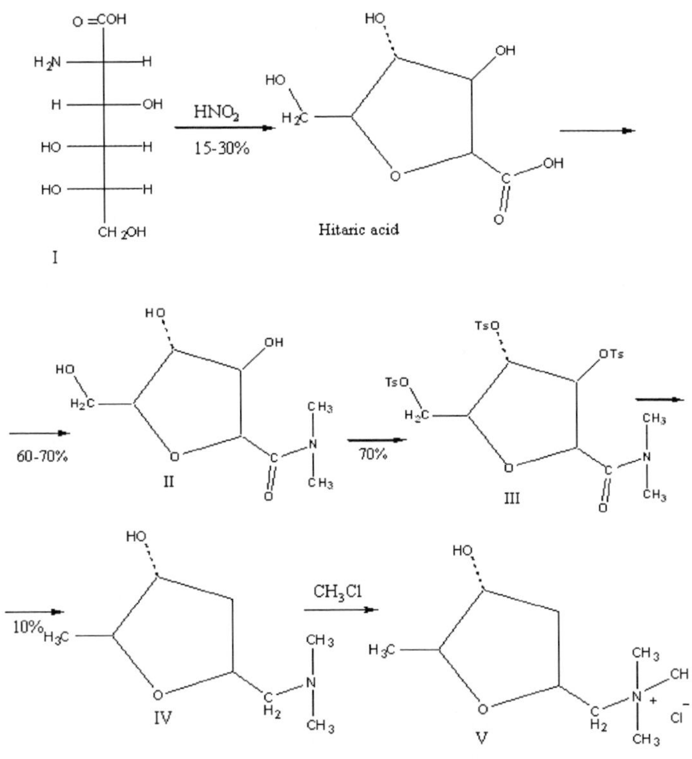

Figure 6. Muscarine chloride synthesis through hitaric acid.

Boiling the latter in tetrahydrofuran in the presence of lithium aluminum hydride, it converts to normuscarine (IV). Normuscarine with methyl chloride treatment yields muscarine chloride (V) with the general yeild of 0.6–1.4% (in glucosamine acid). It is necessary to notice that natural L (+)-muscarine was derived from L-glucosamine acid, and from D-glucosamine acid, D(-)-muscarine, an antipode of natural alkaloid. Racemic DL-muscarine was synthesized. Chromatography on powdery cellulose by washing with a mix of butanol-alcohol-water in the ratio 5:5:2 divided it into optical antipodes; at the same time, R_f of 132 fractions was defined. Racemic muscarine is three times less physiologically active than the substance in its natural form, and D(-)-muscarine is 20 times less active than its antipode.

Certainly, this method of muscarine synthesis has no preparative value, but it is very important in understanding the configurations of asymmetrical carbon atoms in a tetrahydrofuran ring; now it is supposed that natural muscarine has a configuration of 2S, 3R, 5S, i.e., it meets L-hitaric acid and its antipode meets 2R, 3S, 5R; i.e., it corresponds to D-hitaric acid.

Another method was offered by H. Corrodi et al. (see Figure 7). During the action of silver carbonate in a mixture of ethyl ester of iodpropionic acid (I) and diethyl ester of malic acid (II), triether (III) forms. Further, it cyclizates with sodium ethylate in 2-methyl-4,5-dicarboethoxy-tetrahydrofuran-3-one (IV).

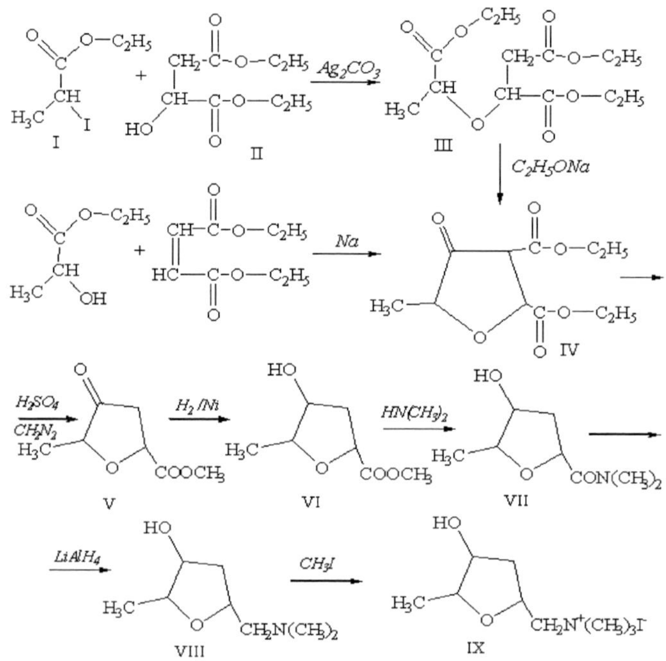

Figure 7. Muscarine synthesis in accordance with Corrodi.

(The same product can be obtained with condensation of ethyl ester of 2-oxypropionic acid with diethyl ester of maleic acid in the presence of sodium). Sulphuric acid treatment with the following methylation gives methyl ester of 2-methyl-tetrahydrofuran-3-one-5-carbonic acid (V). Hydrogenation of this methyl ester in the presence of Raney nickel yields 2-methyl-3-hydroxy-5-carbomethoxy- tetrahydrofuran (VI), which converts in appropriate amide (VII) with the action of dimethylamine. Reduction of this amide with lithium aluminum hydride yields a mix of stereoisomers of 2-methyl-3-hydroxy-5-dimethylamino-methyl tetrahydrofuran (VIII); with the action of methyl iodide, a mix of stereoisomeric iodmethylates (muscarine iodide) (IX) is formed. The action of silver chloride on this mix renders a mix of muscarine chloride stereoisomers. At first, the authors supposed that they produced muscarine and its stereoisomers. Later, they came to the conclusion that they received a small amount of muscarine or none at all, and that the extended crystal isomer had an allo-configuration. Criticizing this work, Eugster noticed that the authors "did not provide the strict proof of that configuration, and boiling temperatures of norbase and allomuscarone, as well as many other physical constants, hardly connected with the offered structure."

Kögl et al. offered their own method of muscarine synthesis (see Figure 8), starting from epichlorohydrin and sodium acetoacetic ether. At condensation of these compounds, α-acetyl-δ-chloromethyl-γ-valerolacton forms smoothly. At its heating with trimethylamine at 150°C, quaternary salt 5-trimethylammoniummethyl-3-acetyl-tetrahydrofuran-2-one formed; further, this product after chlorination was hydrolyzed with 20% hydrochloric acid at 100°C to 2-hydroxy-4-chloro-5-ketohexyl-trimethylimmonium chloride; chlorine was saponified with silver acetate or calcium carbonate, and a ketogroup was hydrogenated over Raney nickel or reduced with sodium borohydride to hydroxyl.

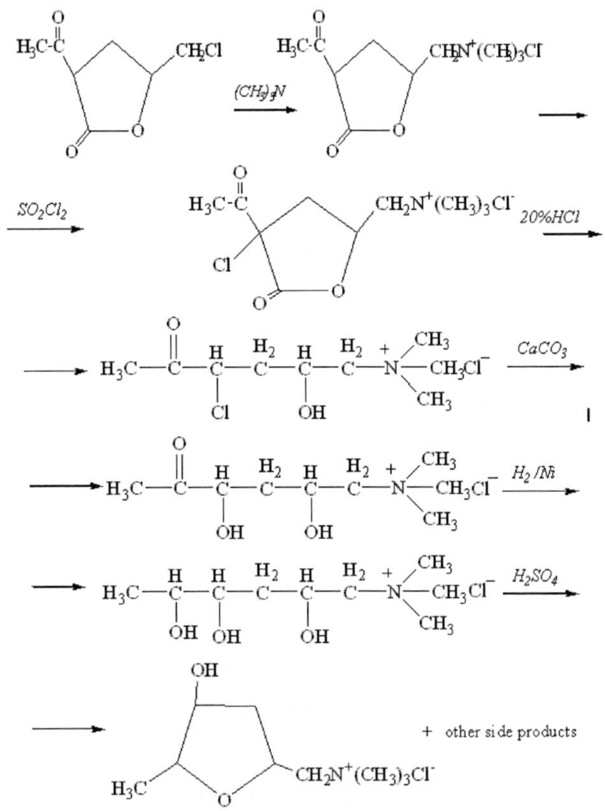

Figure 8. Muscarine synthesis in accordance with Kögl.

The resulting triol was cyclizated with concentrated sulphuric acid. During an attempt to purify the final product on columns with cellulose, the presence of many structurally various impurities in it was established. Neither muscarine nor its impurities were extracted in the pure state. Eugster considered that “the published data with the synthesis description do not seem convincing enough.”

In 1958, Matsumoto offered the mix synthesis scheme of DL-muscarine and DL-allomuscarine starting with β-butylenemalonic acid (see Figure 9); its diethyl ester of performic acid oxidation and the subsequent treatment with ammonia yieldss diamide *erythro*-2,3-butyleneglycolmalonic acid, which with bromine treatment gives appropriate bromlacton, and the last converts into diamide 3-hydroxy-2-methyl-tetrahydrofuran-5,5-dicarbonic acid; diamide saponification with caustic soda gives appropriate diacid, which decarboxylated in a vacuum at 180°C. The mix of stereoisomeric 3-hydroxy-2-methyl-tetrahydrofuran-5-carbonic acids (α-form m.p. 143–145°C and β-form m.p. 109–111°C) is formed. With diazomethane action, they convert to methyl esters which, with dimethylamine, form appropriate dimethylamide. Dimethylamide is reduced with lithium aluminum hydride. The formed 2-methyl-3-hydroxy-5-dimethylaminomethyltetrahydrofuran is treated with methyl iodide; iodide converts in chloride with the action of chloride caesium.

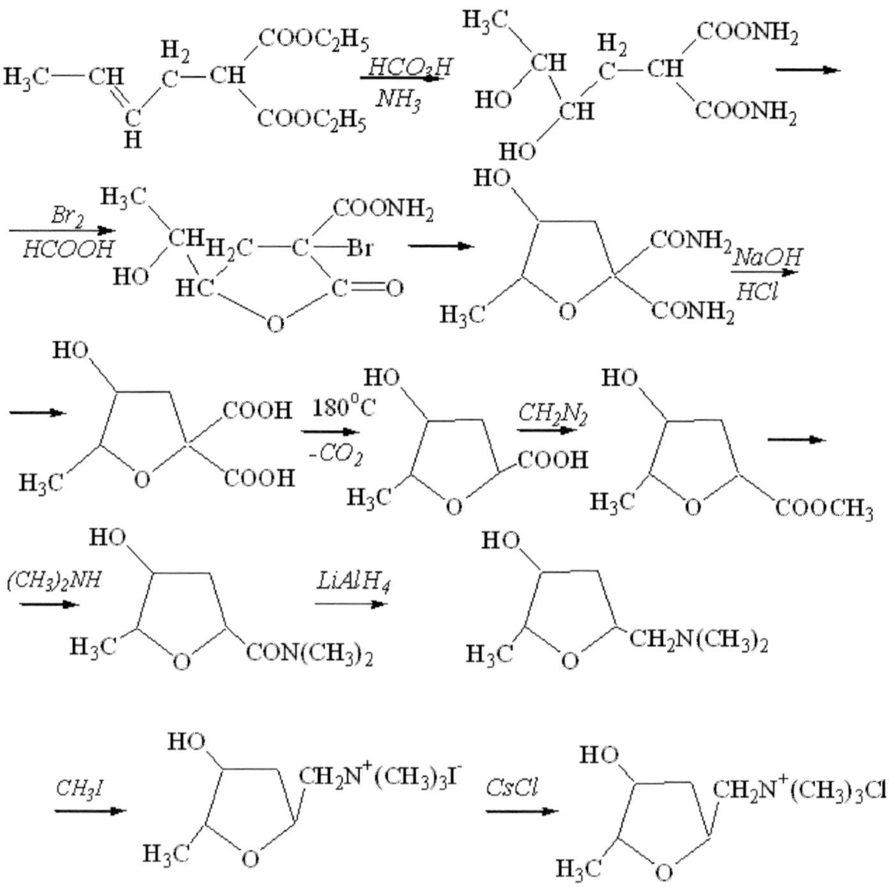

Figure 9. Muscarine and allomuscarine synthesis in accordance with Matsumoto.

Eugster et al. made the most essential contribution to the synthesis of all muscarine isomers in 1957–1958. Glucose condensation with acetoacetic ester gives an ethyl ester of 2-methyl-5-tetraoxybutyl-furan-3-carbonic acid (see Figure 10). This ester, being oxidised to 2-methyl-3-carbethoxy-furan-5-aldehyde, further to dimethyl formamide and the action of a formic acid mix, transforms the aldehyde group into dimethylaminomethyl. The obtained 2-methyl-5-dimethylaminomethyl-furan-3-carbonic acid, with the action of hydrazine, converts to hydrazide which, under diazotization, yields azide. Azide, under the action of benzyl alcohol, yields urethane which, being hydrolyzed with hydrochloric acid, produces 2-methyl-2,3-dihydro-5-dimethylaminomethyl-furan-3-one.

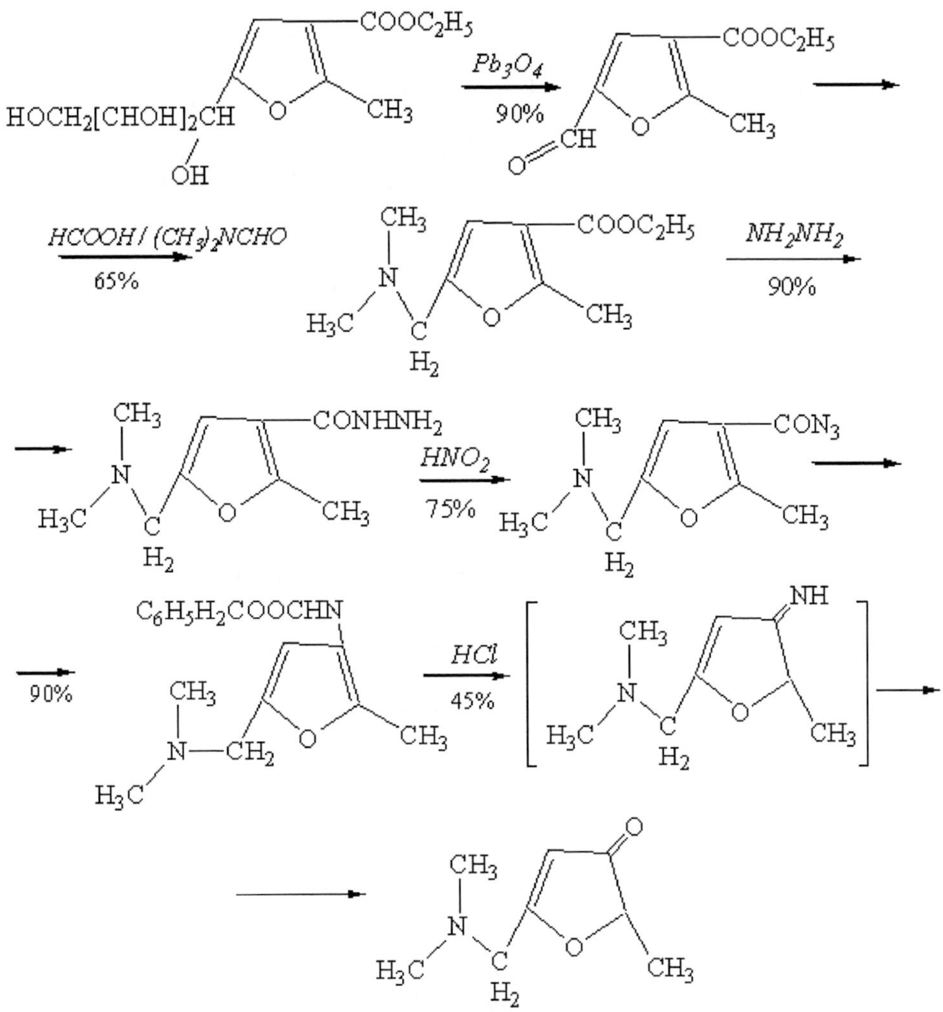

Figure 10. Muscarine synthesis in accordance with Eugster

This product was to Eugster a key compound for the synthesis of all muscarine and muscarone stereoisomers (see Figure 11). Depending on the reduction method, a mix of stereoisomers appeared and the ratio of components was unequal. In conclusion, Eugster noticed that "yields are insignificant at all stages and, in general, apparently, do not strongly differ from muscarine yield obtained through hitaric acid."

In the beginning of the 1960s, a number of works devoted to the synthesis and study of properties of substances close in structure to muscarine were published. Gryszkiewicz-Trochimowski synthesized a structural muscarine isomer and noticed that it did not have any physiological activity. Eugster offered a method for synthesizing thiomuscarine (instead of tetrahydrofuran cycle, tetrahydrothiophen) and desmethylmuscarine. Corrodi described methylmuscarine synthesis and Kiss synthesized a number of dionium derivatives of tetrahydrofuran. Thus, it is necessary to say that until the middle of the 1960s a method for synthesizing muscarine and its isomers, despite the huge amount of work done in this direction, was absent.

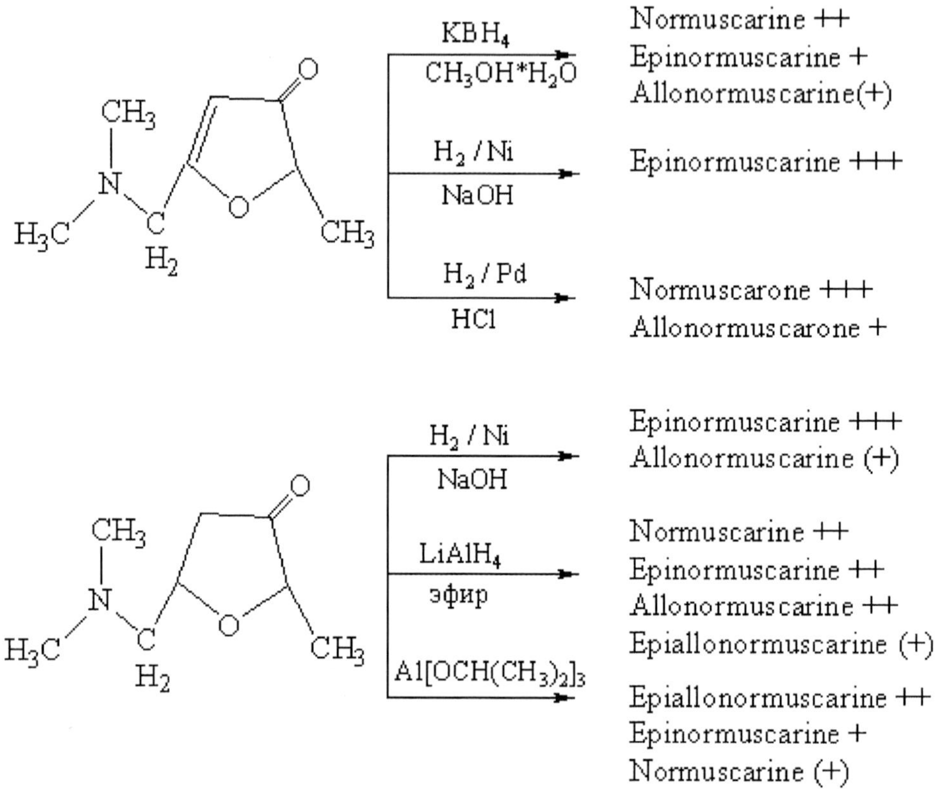

Figure 11. Reception of normuscarine stereoisomers in accordance with Eugster (plus sign indicates an estimate of the relative content of stereoisomers in a mix).

A significant contribution to the synthesis of muscarine and the study of the properties of muscarine and muscarine-like compounds was made by Russian chemists in the subsequent years. Under the guidance of V.V. Smirnov (one of the brilliant chemists and pupils of I.L. Knunyants, the translator of K.K. Ingold's works, and one of the authors of additions to B. Sonders's monograph, *Chemistry and Toxicology of Phosphorus and Fluorine Organic Compounds*), F.V. Mudry, editor and author, offered a new way to produce a mix of muscarine stereoisomers and its sulphonium analogue on the basis of 4-chlorohexene-1-ol-5. This method, to a certain extent, has none of the disadvantages of the methods described above, and can be used for the synthesis of other muscarine-like compounds (see Figure 12). High yields at all stages of the synthesis of muscarine stereoisomers allows a final yield of about 50%. Iodination reaction of unsaturated diol is a key stage of the process, which allows the combination of both formation of tetrahydrofuran cycle and the presence of necessary substituents in required positions of this cycle in one stage. Initial 4-chlorohexene-1-ol-5 is somewhat readily accessible and it is produced with methods of ester condensation from acetoacetic ether. The latter is converted in α-chloro-α-allylacetoacetic ether, saponified to 4-chlorohexene-1-on-5 and reduced with lithium aluminum hydride in standard conditions.

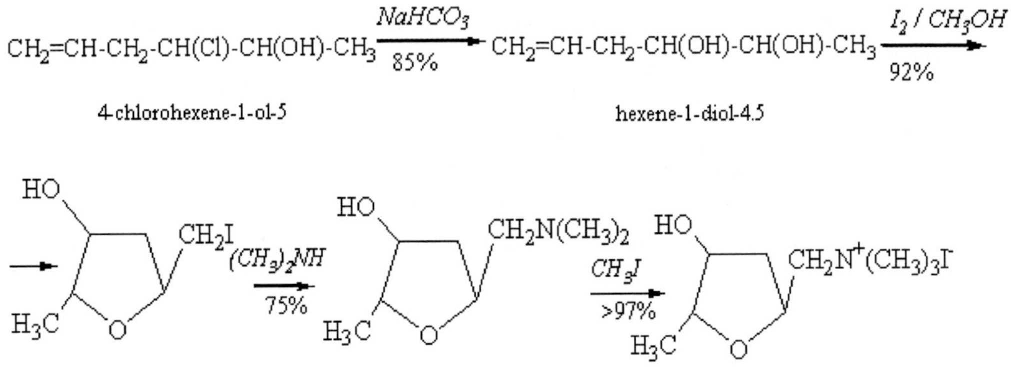

Figure 12. Scheme of preparative synthesis of a mix of muscarine stereoisomers.

Hexene-1-diol-4,5, obtained by saponification of appropriate chloride, obviously, represents a mix of treo and eritro forms. Names of these stereisomeric forms became common because of the similarity and analogy with asymmetrical centers in sugars, i.e., treosa and eritrosa:

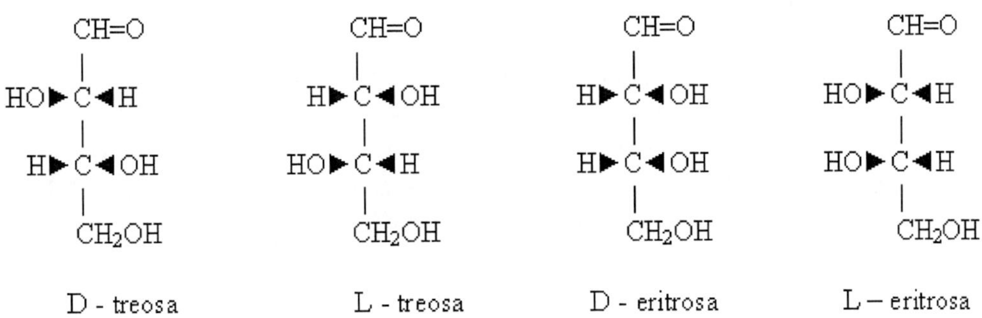

Reaction of cycle formation also is not stereospecific in this connection; the obtained muscarine iodide is a mix of all four stereoisomers: epiallomuscarine, muscarine, allomuscarine and epimuscarine (see Figure 5). This conclusion is proven with a number of direct and indirect indicators:

- Synthesized norbase has a wide interval of boiling temperature, i.e., 60–90°C (0.003mm); it can be divided with fractional distillation, as in a vacuum and at this temperature range four accurately expressed intervals were observed: 60–64, 68–70, 75–79, and 86–89°C. Initial iodmethylderivative of tetrahydrofuran boils at a much narrower temperature interval of 100–105°C (0.01mm), which can be explained with the absence intermolecular (3415sm^{-1}) and intramolecular (3230sm^{-1}) hydrogen bonds, causing *cis-* and *trans*-arrangement of hydroxyl and dimethylaminomethyl groups in norbase. In the IR spectrum, a mix of norbase stereoisomer strips characterizing these hydrogen bonds are accurately visible at 3415sm^{-1} and 3230sm^{-1}.

- The melting point of the received muscarine iodide stereoisomer mix differs from the melting point of each stereoisomer.
- Cromatography of synthesized muscarine iodide in a thin layer on silica gel CSC confirms the presence of all of four stereoisomers, and values R_f are either very close or completely coincide with the literary data of Hardegger.
- A thioanalog of normuscarine (2-methyl-3-hydroxy-5-methylthiomethyl-tetrahydro-furan) synthesized by us and boiled in a narrower range of temperatures (111–116°C, 2mm) than normuscarine and in its IR spectrum; only one strip of a hydroxyl group (3376sm^{-1}) predictably was present, and strips typical for intramolecular hydrogen bonds were absent.
- Synthesized muscarine iodide and iodmethylate of its thioanalog showed clearly expressed muscarine action (fall in blood pressure, salivation, miosis, vomiting, frequent urination, etc.). Predictably, muscarine iodide toxicity was more than 10 times lower than natural L (+)-muscarine, which was explained by the presence in a mix of DL-muscarine iodide racemate (which, as it is known, is three times less toxic than natural) and another three racemates that are its stereoisomers (allo-, epi-, epiallo-); it is known that each of these are even less toxic than racemate of DL-muscarine iodide.

It is necessary to especially empasize that the thioanalog of normuscarine mentioned above has a strong, saturated and pronounced smell of newly-cut mushrooms (normuscarine has a weak amine smell). This allows the assumption that thioanalog and normuscarine are related products of metabolism and to a greater or lesser extent can be present in the highest basidial mushrooms (fly agaric, cep, milk mushroom, deadly amanita etc.).

The work of Italian researchers extracted and identified all eight muscarine enantiomers in 1991 by asymmetric reduction of *cis*- and *trans*-2-methyl-5-iodomethyl-tetrahydro-furanone-3, catalyzed with 3α,20β-hydroxysteroid dehydrogenase from *Streptomyces hydrogenans* (20 β-HSDH) and 3β,17β-hydroxysteroid dehydrogenase from *Pseudomonas testosteroni* (β-HSDH); the further reception of intermediate and final products with typical chemical methods is rather persuasive. Use of the above-stated enzymes earlier only for reduction of natural products (steroids) was effective enough even for synthetic products of *cis*- and *trans*-2-methyl-5-iodomethyl-tetrahydrofuranone-3 type. It is interesting that Italian scientists, as well as we, used as the basic intermediate product 2-methyl-5-iodomethyl-tetrahydrofuranol-3, but in contrast to us it was not its racemic mix of four stereoisomers (our data: B.P. 100–105°C at 0.01mm); rather, they used eight appropriate enantiomers (Italian data for each enantiomer is B.P. 110°C at 0.5mm). And though the boiling points of iodomethylderivatives are close, unfortunately, there are no other constants (n_D^{20}; d_4^{20}, etc.) of this compound in the experiment or the appropriate tertiary amine, which does not allow a full comparison with our similar data. Let us point out that from 1970 to 2008, not one from more than 20 publications about muscarine synthesis was as simple and available as ours. J. Hartung and R. Kneuer used our principle of tetrahydrofuran cycle construction with substituents in the required position by haloidocyclization reaction (called "alkoxyl radical cyclizations"), but instead of iodine they used $BrCCl_3$ with reception of appropriate bromomethylderivative of tetrahydrofuran, and instead of 4-chlorohexene-1-ol-5 used its derivative. D.W. Knight and E.R. Staples had already used the term "iodocyclization" and applied the same approach to another substituted ene-diol, at the same time noting the efficiency and simplicity of this four-stage method. However, no one work has made reference to our research. Let us note the eight-stage stereoselective synthesis of (+) muscarine iodide developed by J. Boukouvalas and I. Radu, with a general yield of 20% from commercially accessible (S) γ-hydroxymethyl-γ-butyrolactone. The reaction of cycloaddition of aldehydes and allyl silanes results in the formation of appropriate di-, three- and tetrasubstitution of the tetrahydrofuran cycle, which is finally used to yeild (-) allomuscarine and (+) epimuscarine with a practically small yield (less than 3%).

Under the guidance of V.V. Smirnov, several hundred ammonium and sulphonium compounds were synthesized and their properties researched for structural features related to muscarine, mainly oxygen-containing heterocyclic structure types such as the following:

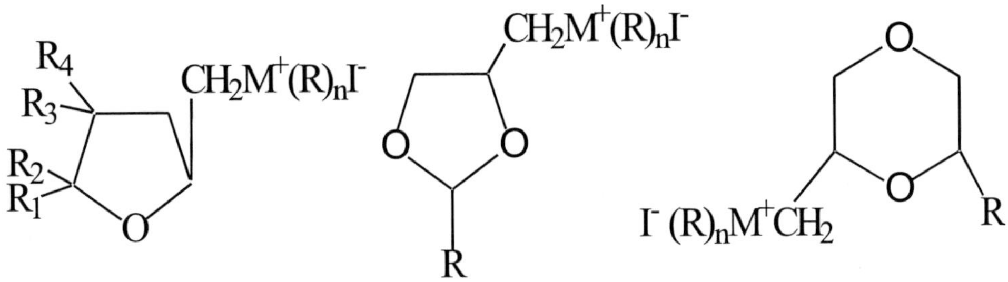

This work allows the introduction of certain corrections in the conclusions of P. Waser in the fundamental review of 1962 concerning the mechanism of toxic action and influence of molecule structure and confirmation of the activity of muscarine-like compounds. In a molecule of a muscarine-like compound for display of high physiological activity, the presence of three pharmacophore groups (trimethylammonium and two nucleophilics [mainly oxygen] in ether or carbonyl and hydroxyl groups) is necessary. In accordance with Waser, the cationic trimethylammonium group links with the anionic site of the receptor surface, showing no specific muscarine or nicotinic action. An electrostatic link is responsible, mainly, for fixing and general cholinomimetic activity of the molecule. The loss of methylene bonding or inclusion of an ammonium group in a cycle dramatically reduces activity. During consideration of various radicals' (directly connected with an atom of nitrogen) influence on physiological activity, it is necessary to notice that aside from the inductive influence of the substitute, a methyl replacement on a "heavier" radical leads to a considerable decrease in activity in all cases. Researchers explain that fact as the appearance of spatial difficulties during the cationic end molecule attack on the anionic receptor centre. Proceeding from this, attempts to increase the activity and, in particular, the toxicity of muscarine-like compounds by replacement of methyl by other radicals at the nitrogen atom are limited in perspective. But replacement of positively-charged nitrogen by other positively-charged elements represents a certain interest. It is necessary to underline that the area of effective PhAS and medical products synthesis based on the replacement of one heteroatom with another while preserving another part of the molecule's structure is far-reaching enough and has been used for a long time by researchers. Considerable interest from this point of view is represented by replacement of the nitrogen atom with a sulphur atom. Organic sulphur compounds occupy one of the leading places among PhAS and medical products for various prescriptions. Research of new sulphur-containing structures has intensively proceeded, and a 2007 review in the scientists' monograph of the Yaroslavl State Technical University testifies to it. In L.E. Craig's review, it is noted that a decrease of curare-like activity is observed as follows:

$$(CH_3)_4N^+ > (CH_3)_3S^+ > (CH_3)\ _4P^+ > (CH_3)\ _4As^+ > (CH_3)\ _4Sb^+.$$

Similar works of research for muscarine-like compounds have been absent, while in a number of works the important role of the onium group's positive charge for display of physiological activity was noted. It is known that with a replacement of a quaternary nitrogen atom by a positively-charged sulphur atom, sometimes not only preservation of but an increase in the toxicity of some compounds is observed; for example:

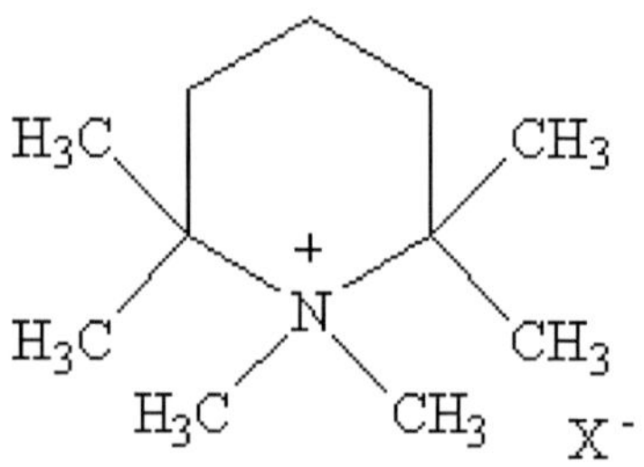

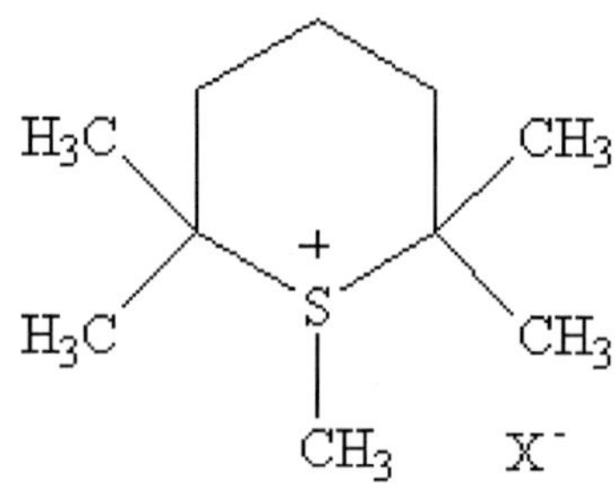

LD_{50} = 11,0 mg/kg (mice, i/p) LD_{50}= 6,5 mg/kg (mice, i/p)

It is also necessary to clarify that, in the case of sulphonium compounds, spatial difficulties from the radicals present in a positively-charged sulphur atom at the anionic receptor site attack will not play so essential a role, because the covalent radius of the sulphur atom is much larger than the radius of the nitrogen atom (see Figure 13).

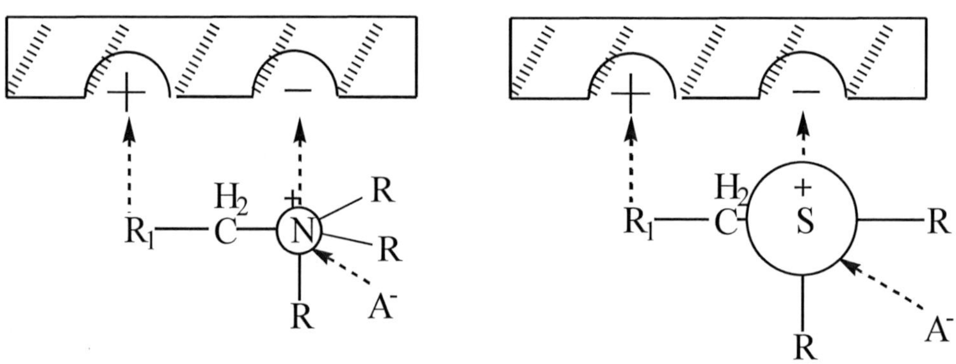

Figure 13. Scheme of interaction of onium structures (receptor).

On the other hand, it is necessary to consider the features of an electronic structure of the sulphur atom and, first of all, the presence in it of somewhat accessible 3d-orbitals, which should cause the appearance of pecularities in behavior of such cations and, in particular, their acceptor properties. The positive charge of a sulphonium atom at the expense of a 3d-orbital resonance is significantly "spread" on the next primary, a radical substitutes, and a "sulphonium cation-receptor" complex is formed because of the somewhat large volume; besides, it appears to be vulnerable to attack from other anions (Figure 13). This results not only in bond weakening in the complex, but also should promote destruction of the complex at the expense of competitive interaction with participation of other anions or anionic sites. This position was proven and confirmed in A.A. Sosunov's dissertation, also done under the guidance of V.V. Smirnov. He examined some features of trialkylsulphonium compounds' reactivity on an example of the interaction of the latter with the active centers of butyryl- and acetyl-choline esterases. In terms of structural features and bond formation with the participation of a sulphur atom's 3d-orbitals, for an exception or substantial discharge of hyperconjugation with the participation of its 3d-orbitals, thereby increasing the effective charge on an onium sulphur atom, it is necessary either to: (I) maximize the possible exception of hydrogen atoms present in neighbouring sulphonium centre carbon atoms, for example:

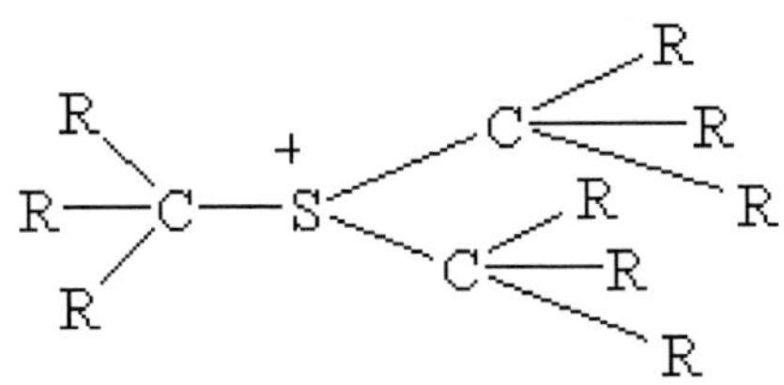

I

or (II) include a positively-charged sulphur atom in bicyclical structures, for example, in one of the following:

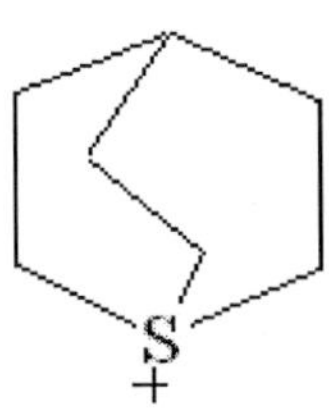

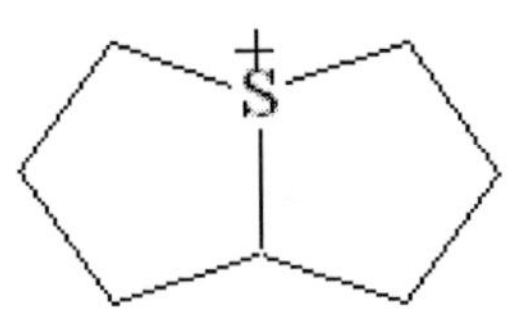

II

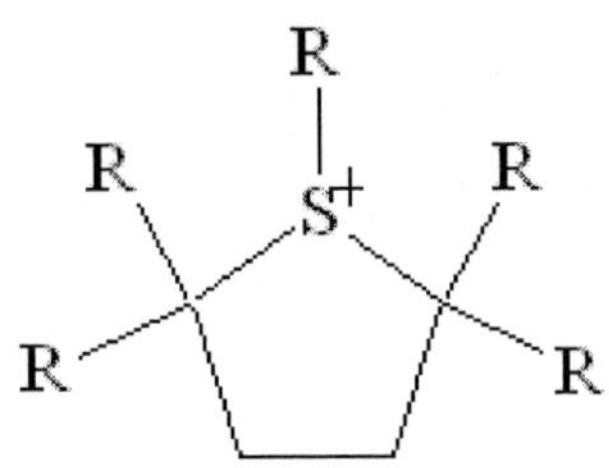

III

In the case of (II), along with a possible limitation of close access of another competing anion to a sulphur atom, an atom's possibility to gain a biassociated character with nearby carbon atoms deriving from features of the 3d-orbitals' structure essentially becomes limited, and consequently it should promote an increase in the effective charge of a sulphonium ion. Taking into account that a variant (I) of sulphonium cation construction is difficult to realize and also probably because of steric obstacles, the effective access to the anionic part of a receptor will be difficult. The optimum decision, as usual, is a golden mean. In particular, for an increase in the effective charge of sulphur atom, we successfully used 2,2,5,5-tetramethyltetrahydrothiophen (III), including positive sides of both variants (I) and (II). This product by reaction with iodomethylderivatives of various compounds smoothly led to appropriate sulphonium salts of the following type:

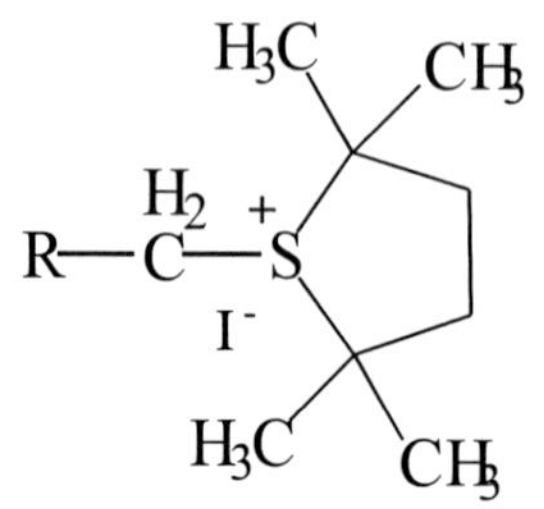

After examination of the role and features of cationic groups, let us estimate the functions of oxygen and distribution of electronic density in a ring. These functions undoubtedly play a main role in the appearance of muscarinic or nicotinic activity. For the appearance of such activities, electron donors—both ether and/or carbonyl oxygen atoms—can form hydrogen bonds with a receptor. Steric obstacles preventing the formation of an "ether oxygen-receptor" or replacement of oxygen by fewer electron-donor atoms (for example, sulphur as in the thiomuscarine cycle of Eugster) reduce the activity of muscarine-like compounds. Transposition of hydroxyl groups for this effect is also important. But even steric obstacles created by the large-size phenyl group at carbon-3, or acyliration of hydroxyl, do not influence activity (in some active furane derivatives the hydroxyl group is absent). These facts specify inconclusively that the role of the hydroxyl group may be only a potential.

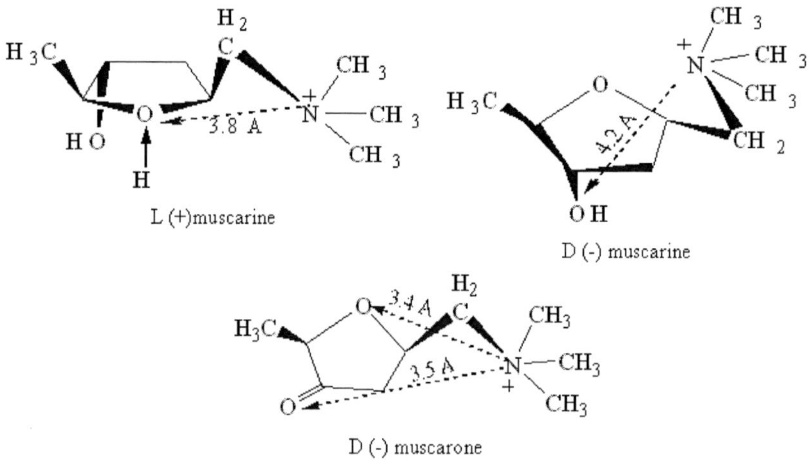

Figure 14. "Elongated" conformation of L (+)-muscarine and "curved" conformation of D (-)-muscarine and D (-)-muscarone, explaining their muscarinic action.

On the contrary, the appearance of steric obstacles preventing the formation of a hydrogen bond with ether oxygen in muscarone or a reduction in the electronegativity of the heteroatom cycle in thiomuscarone do not lead to a dramatic change in muscarinic activity. In these compounds, a hydrogen bond can be achieved by the oxygen of carbonyl groups. Thus, to meet the same "muscarine receptor," muscarine and muscarone should have various conformations with distances of approximately four angstroms between the cationic centre and nucleophilic oxygen function (see Figure 14).

In conclusion, Waser underlines that "maximal muscarine action of muscarine-like compounds depends mainly on cationic nitrogen with three methyl groups and nucleophilic groups (ether or carbonyl oxygen) at a distance of four angstroms." The given conclusion is made by the author on the basis of examination of the muscarinic activity of a large group of compounds. The basic classes of these connections, supplemented with structures, synthesized and examined under the guidance of V.V. Smirnov, are shown below in Table 2.

Table 2. Comparative muscarine activity of some heterocyclic compounds

No.	Compound	Relative activity, reducing blood pressure in relative units (cats) Acetylcholine activity = 1
1	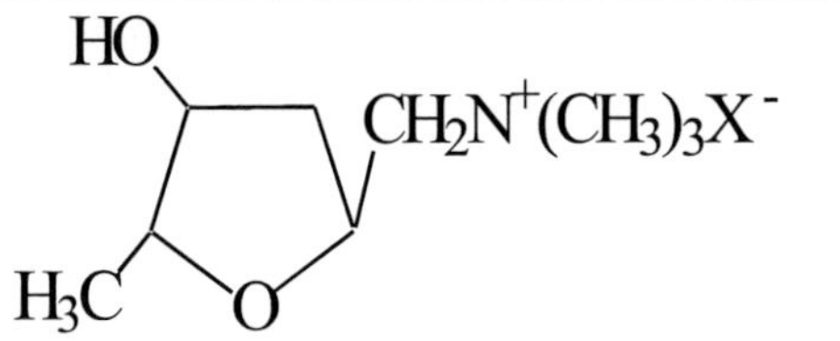 L (+)-muscarine DL – muscarine Racemic mix of muscarine stereisomers	0.5 1.5 15–20
2	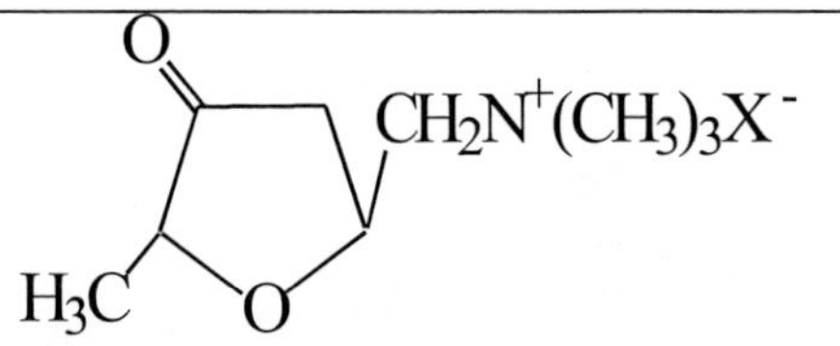 D(-)-muscarone	0.5–0.8
3	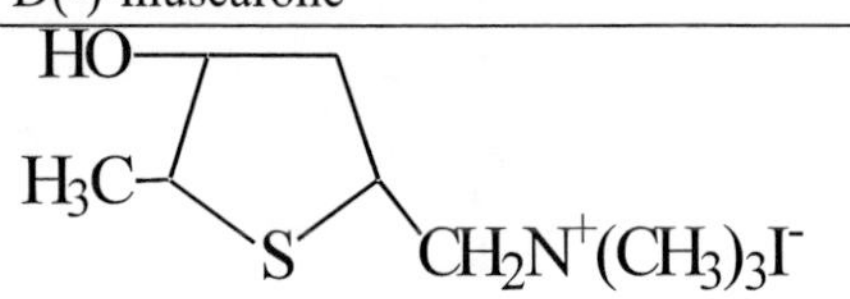	2000
4	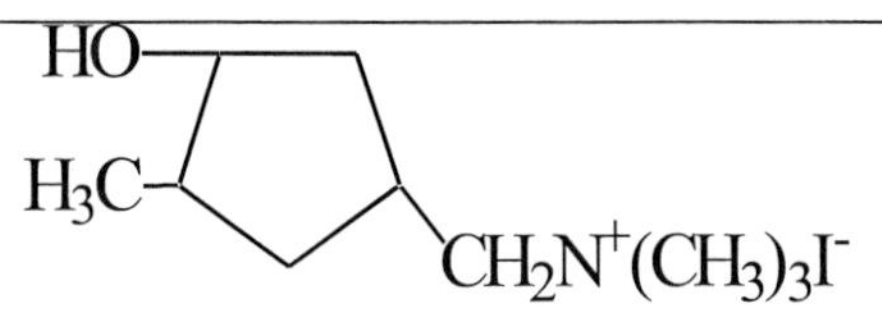	10–15
5	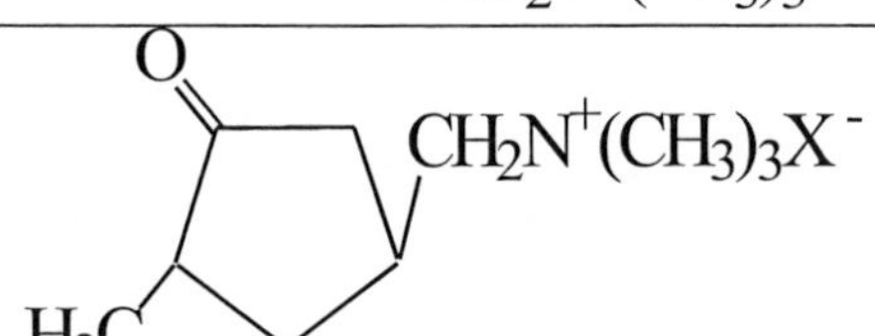	20–50

Table 2. (Continued)

No.	Compound	Relative activity, reducing blood pressure in relative units (cats) Acetylcholine activity = 1
6	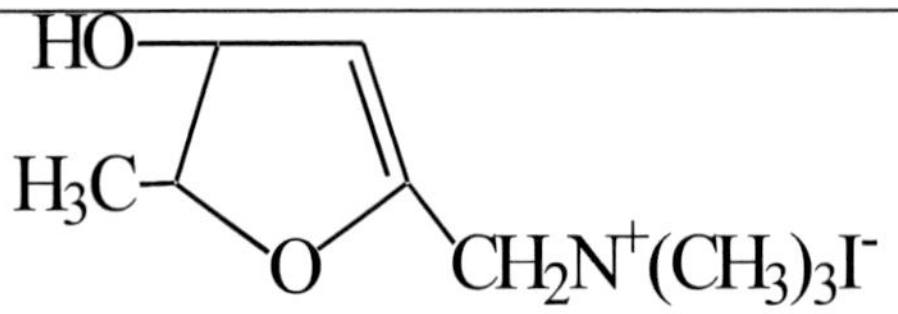	1.2
7	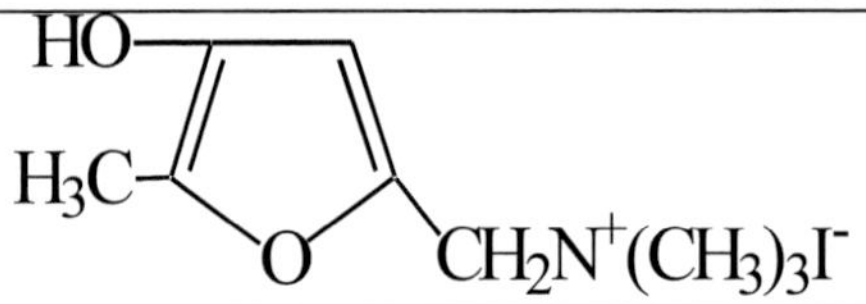	1–3
8	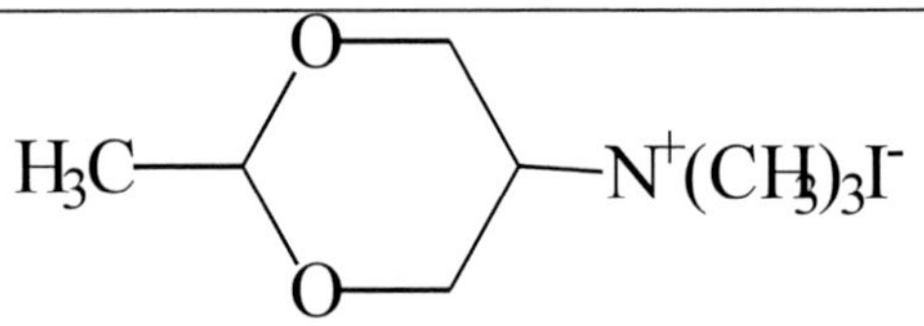	200
9	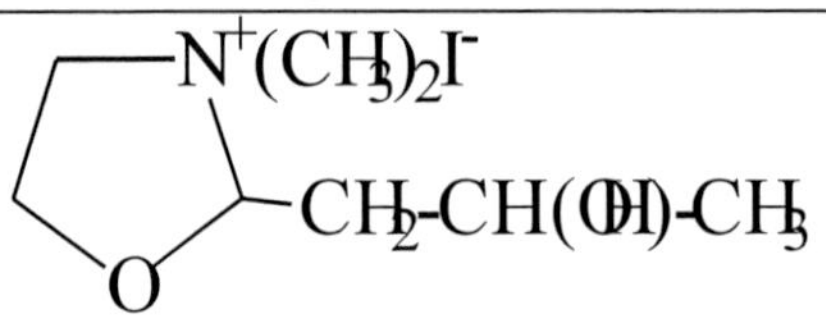	1000
10	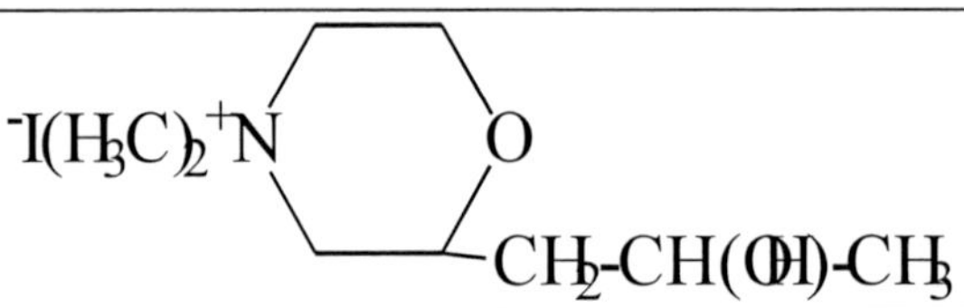	1000
11	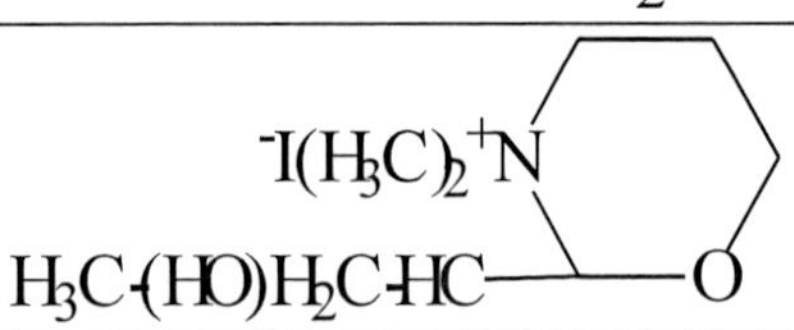	1000
12	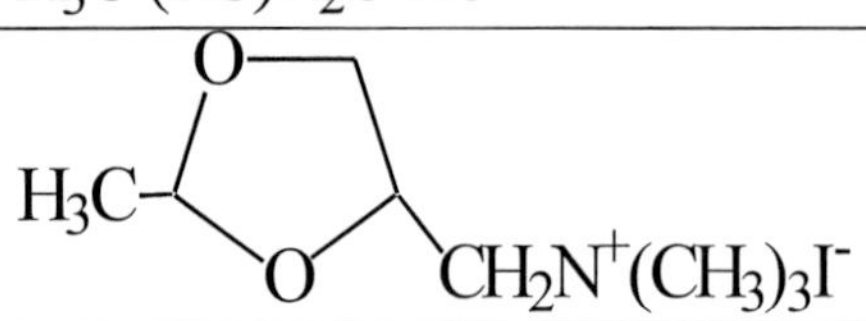	2
13	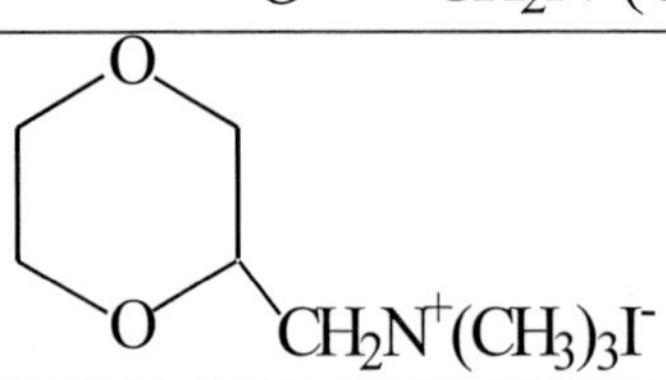	1 (dogs)

No.	Compound	Relative activity, reducing blood pressure in relative units (cats) Acetylcholine activity = 1
14	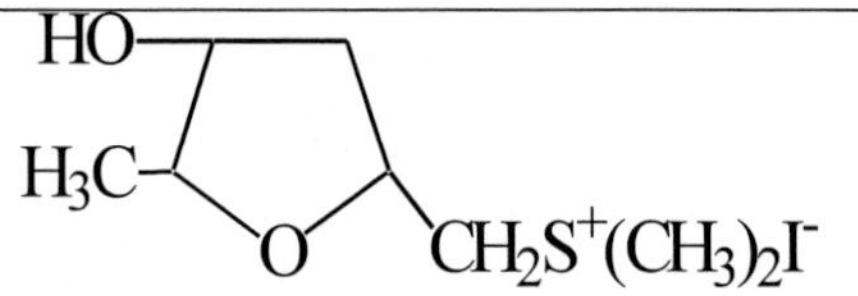	25
15	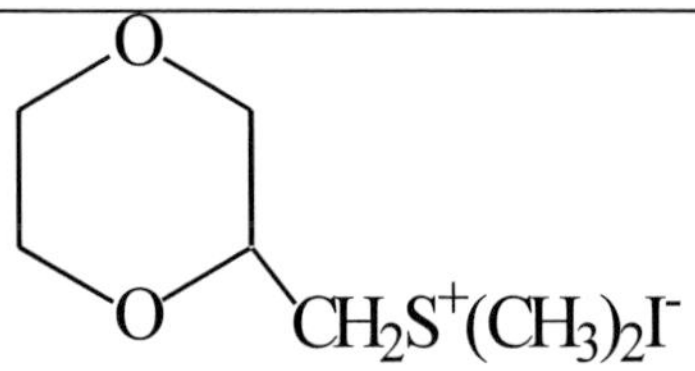	50
16	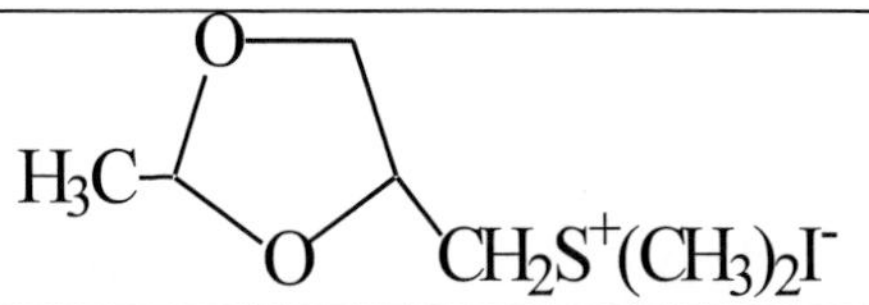	30
17	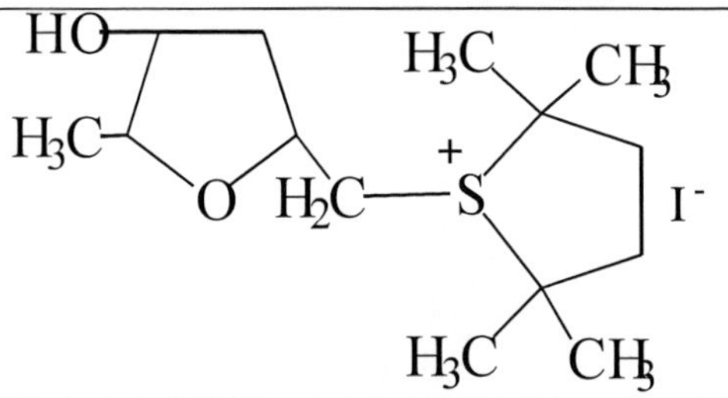	1

Note:

1. All sulphonium compounds were tested on dogs, intravenously;
2. All compounds, except where noted, were tested in a type of racemic mix of stereoisomers.

It is necessary to underline that each of the specified types of compounds was examined with the diversified substitutes both in a cycle and with an onium group. Muscarine activity of 1,4-dioxane derivatives was first noted by Fourneau after the publication of P. Waser's review. A detailed examination of trimethylammoniummethylene-1,4-dioxane (Table 2, product 13) was carried out by R.A. Ivanova and G.A. Patrushev in the USSR. The minimum fatal dose of the substance for dogs is 0.1mg/kg intravenously and 1mg/kg intramuscularly. A clinical picture of a poisoning is characterized mainly by muscarine-like symptoms with some nicotine- and curare-like features. Definitive importance in the development and outcome of intoxication belongs to dysfunction of respiratory apparatus and blood circulation, which are connected mainly with the blocking effect of the substance in neuromuscular synapses of the respiratory and heart muscles; the important, main role is assigned to stimulating the influence of a substance on M-cholinereactive systems of nerves in the bronchi and heart.

A similar examination of a greater quantity of 1,4-dioxane derivatives has shown, that, as well as in the case of other oxygen-containing heterocycles, replacement of methyl with "heavier" radicals at the ammonium atom leads to a dramatic decrease in activity in all cases.

This result also followed expectations, and the somewhat high M-cholinemimetic activity of other onium compounds—in particular, sulphonium—was established for the first time. In this case, the somewhat high activity is noted for compounds having such radicals at the positively-charged sulphur atom which, as predicted by us, allows both certain spatial shielding of the formed complex of the oniom molecule's centre and the anionic part of the receptor as well as the greatest possible effective positive charge on the sulphur atom due to an exception or reduction in the 3d-orbitals' influence. With the insertion of substitutes in various positions of the dioxane cycle (methyl, ethyl, hydroxymethyl, alkoxymethyl, haloidomethyl, etc.)—including positions 2,6—the physiological activity of appropriate compounds dramatically decreased, while among derivatives of tetrahydrofuran, the transition from desmethylmuscarine to muscarine is followed by a substantial increase in a hypotensive (lowering a blood pressure) effect:

Structure:

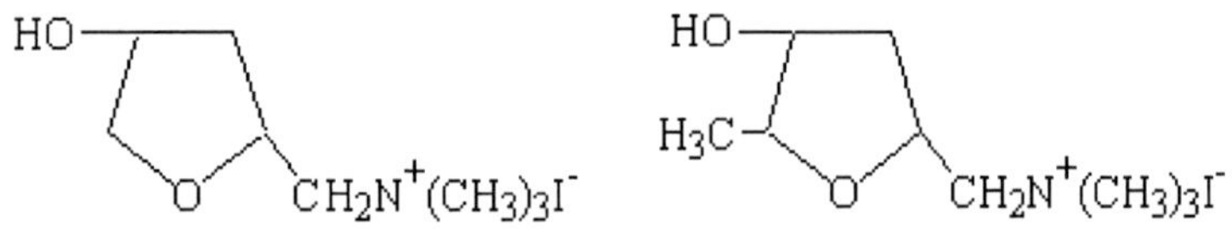

Hypotensive effect (cats, intravenously)	1,0mg/kg	0,003mg/kg

It is probable that in maintaining contact of a substance with a receptor, the role of the methyl group in the practically flat tetrahydrofuran cycle of muscarine is carried out by a fragment or the 1,4-dioxane cycle itself; as a rule, it appears in the most profitable energy form of an "armchair," and the equatorial position of the methylene center provides, as well as in case of L (+)-muscarine or D (-)-muscarone (see the scheme in Figure 14), a distance approximately equal to four angstroms between the onium centre and nucleophilic atoms of oxygen. And in this sense, both the fact of recurrence of the molecule and the character of the cycle (five or six members) play a certain role.

Taking into account that poisoning with substance 13 described above, as well as some other derivatives of 1,4-dioxane—with the exception of pronounced muscarinic actions—are followed by symptoms of nicotine- and curare actions, it is possible to suggest that part of the substance begins interaction with receptors of other types or includes a wider site of the same receptor. An interesting hypothesis about a four-centered structure (with rhombus corners) of a curare receptor was offered by R.S. Rybolovlev (see chapter 7).

Thus, taking into account the new data received after publication of the review of P. Waser, conclusions of the latter require correction; i.e., maximal muscarinic action of muscarine-like compounds depends, mainly, on two factors:

a) the presence of a cationic onium centre with corresponding substitutes, providing not only its unimpeded contact with the anionic part of receptor, but also the subsequent effective connection and defined steric obstacles of its rupture by another anion from an opposite side;

b) the presence of two nucleophilic groups (two ether oxygen, ether-carbonyl or ether oxygen-hydroxyl), located approximately equally-spaced from the cationic center of a substance at a distance of approximately four angstroms.

The presence of one such group generally is obligatory, and the role of the second, in the case of its absence (for example, carbochain—a cyclopentane analogue of muscarine or muscarone; in an analogue of muscarine or muscarone, where instead of a hydroxyl or oxogroup, correspondingly, one or two atoms of fluorine are found), can be compensated either by other groups or structural features of the molecule that are connected, apparently, with structural features such as, first of all, the steric structure of the field surrounding the anionic site of M-cholinereceptor, or the presence of various muscarine receptor structures. Since 1980 to the beginning of 2009, there has been a growth in the interest of researchers and in the number of articles in scientific publications (557 articles) on various aspects of the problems of the role, behavior and structure of M-cholinoreceptors in an organism. These research studies have revealed and established the presence of five subtypes of muscarine receptors (M_1–M_5), which are characterized by various types of interactions with ligands, once more underlining the complexity and ambiguity of their structure. The subtypes of M_1, M_3 and M_5 receptors are structurally similar; in turn, receptors of subtypes M_2 and M_4 are also structurally similar. This fact has found unexpected application in the working out of new approaches to the problem of pathogenesis by phosphour organic compound intoxication by S.N. Golikov's pupils. The estimation of the protective action of various activities of M-choline blockers from poisoning by phosphour organic compounds has shown that blockade of M_1-cholinoreceptors provides an antidotal effect of antagonists, and blockade of M_2-cholinoreceptors prevents it. The synthesized preparation, pentiphine, is an antagonist of M_4-cholinoreceptors; it contains a hydroxyl group structure and a positively charged nitrogen atom at the required distance, and is more effective than a standard antidote (atropine) for protection against sarin.

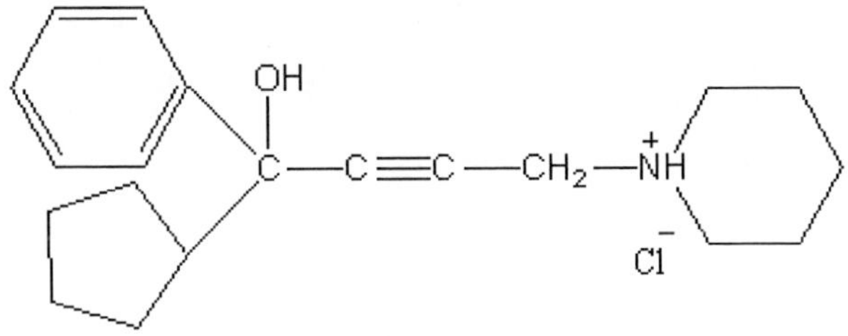

Pentiphine

Finally, the authors express hope that the conclusions (in many ways predicted by V.V. Smirnov who has since left this world) regarding the synthesis of muscarine-like compounds will not only help to define more exactly the spatial structure of M-cholinoreceptors, but also promote development and creation of new highly effective medicines for the prevention and treatment of many diseases and poisonings.

Chapter 7

Curare

In 1595, Sir Wallter Raleigh brought some paralyzing poison for arrows, called *curare* by natives of South America,to Europe. Only 200 years later, medical and chemical research studies of curare began, for several reasons. First of all, this poison was unknown to scientists of the Old World, as Indians carefully kept secret the method of preparation of curare and the kinds of plants used as its source. Curare as a poison was important for Indians, along with the mysterious ritual of its extraction and manufacturing as a means of barter with surrounding tribes and populations. Indians also widely used curare for internal consumption as a highly effective means of getting meat for food by hunting animals. It is known that Indians extracted the poison from plants of the *Strychnos* and *Chondrodendron* genera by "boiling" (evaporating) the juice of well-milled sprouts of these plants; readiness was characterized by the degree of bitterness. The extract was brought to a syrupy state and divided up into the three main kinds of tare accessible to them. The names of different sorts of curare came from the types of tare: para-, tubo- or bamboo-curare (in bamboo tubes); pot curare (in small earthenware pots); and gourd, calabash- or calebas-curare (in small gourds). As one would expect, these three main views of poison were not individual compounds but they were mixes of varied compositions including substances with no "personal" biological activity. Moreover, important differences in intoxicating effect were observed not only depending on the "sort" (packing) of curare, but samples of the same sort also had different intoxicating effects. In 1897, Rudolph Boehm systematized all of these data about curare and showed that all preparations of curare contain several alkaloids of two main types: quaternary ammonium bases (which demonstrate curare-like action) and inactive tertiary bases (amines). In 1904–1939, Reid Hunt and R.R. Renshaw published a series of articles about onium compounds and their effect on the autonomic nervous system. And at last, in 1935, Harold King isolated the first crystalline active alkaloid (d-tubocurarin chloride) from tubo curare, and in 1936 he was able to show that this alkaloid was a quaternary ammonium derivative of bis-benzyl tetrahydroisoquinoline:

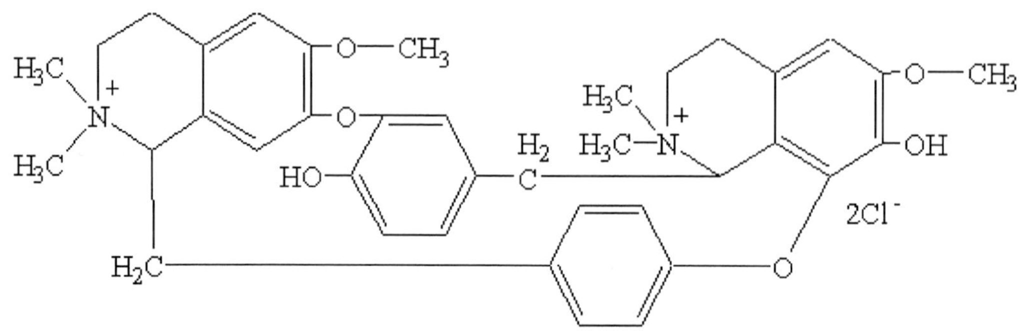

D-tubocurarin chloride

Its dose of 0.5 mg/kg caused full curare paralysis in frogs, while preparations of other types of curare caused a similar effect in doses of 2.5–5 mg/kg. King also showed a close interrelation of pot and tubo curare. At the same time, Heinrich Wieland and coworkers extracted a group of active quaternary alkaloids from pot curare and showed that it (pot curare) differed in chemical nature from other alkaloids of curare. Research studies of pot curare were much less intensive than research of tubo curare. In 1943, Oscar Wintersteiner and James Dutcher isolated d-tubocurarine chloride from South American *Chondrodendron tomentosum*. They provided a source of free active alkaloid and the possibility of preparation of its standard samples, which gave rise to an intensification and increase in the number of research studies in the field of chemistry and the physiological action of this sort of curare. Purification of this alkaloid was accompanied by isolation and identification with an extract of a homolog of curarine: d-hondocurarine, differing only by a change of position of the hydroxyl and methoxy group of the aromatic cycle of tetrahydroisoquinoline. D-hondocurarine is also four times more effective. Claude Bernard for the first time intensively studied the physiological aspects of the effect of curare poison on an organism. He indicated that curare develops a peripheral effect and prevents the sending of impulses from nerves to muscles in myoneural compounds (synapses). Bernard also demonstrated the possibility of therapeutic use of curare. Curare does not affect cardiac muscle. It is interesting that fugu toxin, causing an outwardly identical paralysis of skeletal muscles (part 9.2), affects both types of muscle cells but more slowly than nerve cells. The peripheral paralysis (result of the curare effect) progresses in strict order. The first symptoms of the curare poisoning are the following: drooping eyelids, sleepiness, loss of speech and paralysis of cervical muscles ("head falling" effect). Then, the extremities and muscles of the diaphragm are affected, and the human dies because of respiratory insufficiency. The route of administration of a poison into an organism is very important. The most effective in relatively comparative doses is intravenous administration, next intramuscular and then hypodermic administration. Finally, oral intake is absolutely ineffective. Curare does not kill irretrievably but only temporarily reduces reflexes, and paralysed muscle comes back to normal condition without visible negative consequences. This opens the door to the possible use of curare in therapy (in the case of neuromuscular abnormalities) and in surgery for relaxation of muscles. Anaesthetics only remove sensitivity to pain, but they do not cause the relaxation of muscles necessary for surgical intervention. Using both analgesics and muscle-relaxing drugs completely solves the problem of surgical narcosis. The medicinal properties of curare could not be used for a long time because of its inherent danger, as relaxation and paralysis of respiratory muscles inevitably causes respiratory arrest followed by death. An animal pierced by an arrow tipped with curare poison falls and lays helplessly immobilized until the respiratory muscles are paralyzed. The poison paralyzes only muscles and does not affect the brain, which was confirmed by Dr. Scott M. Smith's (University of Utah, U.S.) heroic experiment on himself, wherein he could describe all sensations and behavior of the poisoning process until the beginning of respiratory paralysis, at which time the experiment was stopped to save the doctor's life. A proposition about the peripheral effect of curare poison stated earlier was thus confirmed in a brutal way. A difference between dose sizes causing lasting curarization of an organism and doses causing a fatal outcome are somewhat small for d-tubocurarine, i.e., d-tubocurarine has rather low limit of safety that, along with ineffectiveness when taken orally, hampered its wide application in medicine, especially in surgery. Therefore, right after the discovery of the structure of d-tubocurarine (index "d" is used for designation of the dextrarotary isomer that yields the greatest curare effect), an intensive search for compounds with the curare effect and without the previously- mentioned disadvantages began. Daniel Bovet produced gallamine, the first synthetic curare. Diplazin, paramyon, decamethonium, hexamethonium, dithylinum, etc. had been put forward and then found application in the USSR. These and other synthetic agents are part of two classes of muscle relaxants: a) compounds with strong curariform effect (leptocurare), and b) compounds with ganglion-blocking action (pachycurare). The terms derive from *lepto* (thin, long) and *pachy* (thick). Muscle relaxants such as diplazin and paramyon possess competitive mixed action. Interval measuring between two ammonium groups shows that maximum curare effect is developed at a distance of 13–15 angstroms, and maximum ganglion blocking effect at a distance of 5–6 angstroms.

$$\begin{array}{r} (CH_3)_3N^+\text{-}CH_2\text{-}CH_2\text{-}CH_2 \\ | \\ (CH_3)_3N^+\text{-}CH_2\text{-}CH_2\text{-}CH_2 \end{array}$$

Hexamethonium

$$\begin{array}{r} (CH_3)_3N^+\text{-}(CH_2)_4\text{-}CH_2 \\ | \\ (CH_3)_3N^+\text{-}(CH_2)_4\text{-}CH_2 \end{array}$$

Decamethonium

$$\begin{array}{c} (CH_3)_3N^+\text{-}C_6H_4\text{-}CH\text{-}C_2H_5 \\ | \\ (CH_3)_3N^+\text{-}C_6H_4\text{-}CH\text{-}C_2H_5 \end{array}$$

Paramyon

$$\begin{array}{r} (CH_3)_3N^+\text{-}CH_2\text{-}CH_2\text{-}O\text{-}C(O)\text{-}CH_2 \\ | \\ (CH_3)_3N^+\text{-}CH_2\text{-}CH_2\text{-}O\text{-}C(O)\text{-}CH_2 \end{array}$$

Dithyline (Dicholine ester succinic acid)

The necessity for the presence of two onium centres in yielding a curare effect sparked a search for curariform compounds containing sulphonium, phosphonium and other hetero-atoms. All of them possessed marked curariform effect, but they were weaker than analogous ammonium compounds, all other things being equal. A decrease in curare effect is observed as follows: $(CH_3)_4N^+ > (CH_3)_3S^+ > (CH_3)_4P^+ > (CH_3)_4As^+ > (CH_3)_4Sb^+$. The effect of curare on neruromuscular conduction is caused by its ability to competitively replace acetylcholine in nicotine (N)-sensitive cholinoreceptors of a muscle fibre. But tubocurarine blocks the depolarization action of acetylcholine on the endplate. At the same time, curarization does not suppress the generation of acetylcholine in myoneural synapses. A model was suggested on the basis of a number of experiments according to which molecules of curare block receptors of acetylcholine and as a result break down a chain of stimulation of muscle cells. However, we cannot answer these centuries-old questions: Why do molecules of poison win in the fight for receptors (curare in this case)? How is the blocking of all cholinoreceptors completed in spite of the very small size of active dosages? Analyzing possible explanations of the efficiency of the curare effect, we will consider a group of processes occurring in the membrane of a muscle cell after the joining of acetylcholine to the cholinoreceptor. The opening of specific sodium and potassium channels and the transition of the membrane protein—namely, guanyl-cyclase—to the excited (activated) state are the most important among these processes in the first phase. Guanyl-cyclase catalyzes the transformation of GTP (guanosine triphosphate) into cyclic GMP (guanosine monophosphate). GMP stimulates the activity of endocellular enzymes that are responsible for contraction inside the muscle cell. It is necessary to "switch off" the action of acetylcholine attached to receptor in the second phase. This shut-down occurs simply enough: a cotton-like (as seen in electronic microscope images) substance is located a small distance from a cholinoreceptor. It contains an enzyme called acetylcholinesterase which destroys acetylcholine by cleavage of the ester bond. But first it is necessary to separate it from the receptor and to transform it into a solution for deleting unnecessary acetylcholine. The exit of sodium through channels evidently plays the major role in this process. The partial reduction in the concentration of sodium is equivalent to increasing the quantity of water and changing the constant physicochemical equilibrium along the lines of increased solubility of acetylcholine in the protoplasm of the synaptic cleft. It is possible to suppose that the probability of decay of a "receptor-acetylcholine" complex under the influence of molecular movement's increases precisely owes to the growth of solubility. Thus, the probability of acetylcholine meeting with choline esterase and its subsequent breakdown also grows. What will occur if a molecule of curare joins a cholinoreceptor? Even the lowest molecular weight of curareform compounds, i.e., dicholine ester of succinic acid (dithyline), is twice as large as a molecule of acetylcholine. Therefore, introduction of larger molecules into solution in spite of their chemical proximity to acetylcholine will lower the stability of hydrate shells of these molecules. The decrease can be so great that sodium leaving through channels will not be insufficient to return the system to a condition in which molecules of curare pass into solution. Cholinergic receptors can thus be disengaged, and activation of adenylate cyclase is completed. As a result, blocking mode occurs when a muscle cell is disconnected during overexcitation. It is fixed as an effect of the action of poison. The believability of this hypothetical model is proven by fact that toxicity correlates with the size of molecules among the broad range of curariform compounds.

In contrast to d-tubocurarine, decamethonium causes lasting depolarization in and around the endplate. Dicholine ethers of aliphatic dicarbonic acids also possess a depolarization effect; for example, dithyline selectively influences N-sensitive cholinereactive systems and do not influence muscarine (M)-sensitive cholinereceptors at all, and do not directly influence the CNS. In contrast to the interaction of muscarine (chapter 6) with the active centre of the enzyme, d-tubocurarine can and apparently does interact at once with two anionic areas of the receptor which are possibly are located on both sides of the esterase. But alkaloid shields the esterase area of the active centre, and the enzyme inactivates as a result. A possible interaction of d-tubocurarine with an enzyme is shown in Figure 15.

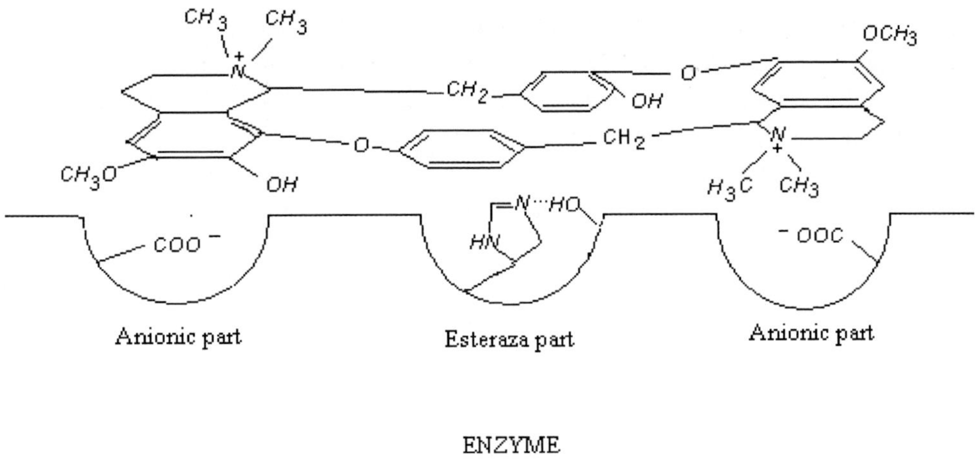

Figure 15. Interaction of d-tubocurarine with an enzyme.

The anionic area includes a free carboxyl group of bibasic amino acid residue, and the area includes a hydroxyl of serine amino acids activated by interaction with a histidine amino acid imidazole ring. Shields of the esterase area become simpler because of the flat structure of the d-tubocurarine molecule. Many research studies have concentrated especially on the interaction of curariform compounds with acetylcholine by N-receptors and M-receptors of the M_2 type in recent years. Professor Ulrike Holzgrabe and collaborators stated that 10 angstroms is a minimum necessary distance between positive charges. The size of appropriate peripheral small areas contacting a positive charge should be large and readily able to adapt to the spacial position of the aromatic skeleton with chains located between it: in the case of oxim-containing ethers, a distance of six carbon atoms is required, and in the case of amino compound chain, four carbon atoms are required for interaction of a pharmacophore conformation of the *S*-form.

Russian toxicologist R.S. Rybolovlev stated a number of laws when determining the interrelation of curare activity and the chemical structure of physiologically active compounds. It is shown through the example of dicholine esters of dicarbonic acids that the ability of the compounds mentioned above to stimulate sympathetic ganglia increases from low to high while the ability to block neuromuscular conduction on the contrary is more typical of dicholine ester of succinic acid and progressively decreases up to higher homologs. Substitution of methyl groups for the quarternary atom of nitrogen to hydrogen or ethyl, propyl and butyl radicals increases the curariform activity of derivatives of succinic and especially sebacic acids. Ester groups in the structure of dicholine esters of dicarbonic acids can promote the occurrence of stimulating action. It is typical only for compounds in which the structures of ester groups are separated from each other by a polymethylene chain of four to eight carbon atoms. The stimulating action on N-sensitive cholinergic receptors decreases with smaller chain length. Obviously, ester groups for their suitable spatial arrangement react with esteratic areas of cholinergic receptors, generating weak bonds as well as under the action of acetylcholine. A more strongly pronounced stimulation of cholinereactive systems occurs than when under the action of compounds of a group of decamethonium (without ester groups). But intensification of the blocking action is not observed. By substituting ester bonds for amide (-NH-C(O)-) or thio derivatives (-S-C(O)-) bonds, we can observe a typical subsiding of the blocking action of compounds on neruromuscular conduction.

Molecules of d-tubocurarine, being orientated on the surface of cholinergic receptors, can form a large quantity of Van der Waals bonds with it. That fact apparently translates into influence and duration of the curare effect. It is interesting that dicholine esters of dicarbonic acids and polymethene derivatives have two peaks of action by a 10-carbon bridge (about 14 angstroms) and by a 14- to 15-carbon bridge (20–22 angstroms) depending on the length of the carbon chain between ammonium cationic centres. The original four-centre structure of active centres of an enzyme with which physiologically active muscle relaxants react (see Figure 16) was suggested to unite these facts and to correlate them with receptor structure.

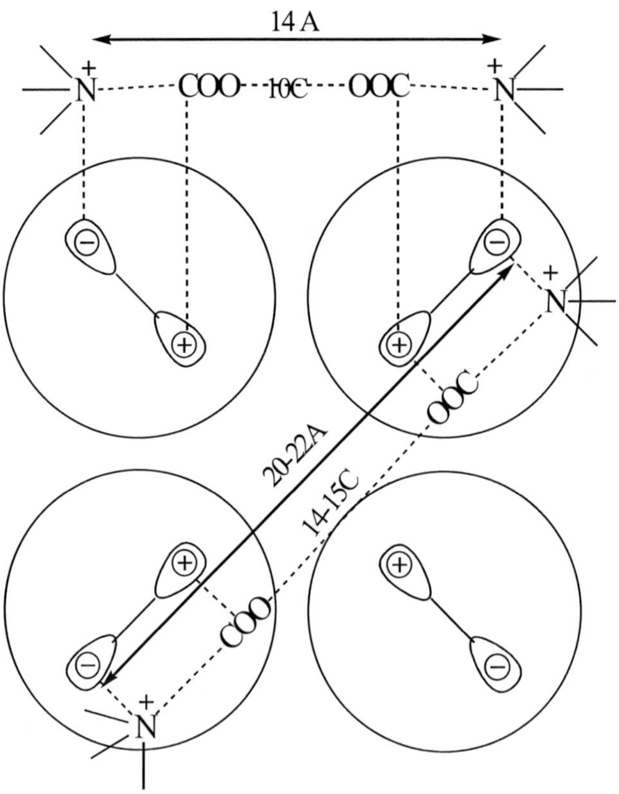

Figure 16. Hypothetical relative position of active centers of an enzyme.

Compounds with an anticholinesterase type of action (proserin) are antagonists of d-tubocurarine and other muscle relaxants, including agents with a competitive type of action. Anticholinesterase compounds do not display antagonism and in some cases even strengthen their blocking action in relation to depolarization agents. If it were feasible to register the curare effect of a number of muscle relaxants at least using an indirect method (influencing choline esterase), controlling the ganglioblocking effect was an unresolved problem until the 1970s. The first successes in this field are associated with the work of N.V. Khromov-Borisov and collaborators, who stated a hypothesis comprising a new principle of creation of medicines of controllable action. The heart of the hypothesis was that the medicinal compound comprising a sufficiently labile disulfide bond could be destroyed in an organism by using special agents. Agents can be injected from without and are capable of breaking up the -S-S- bond and stopping or considerably weakening the physiological effect. The background based on the use of specific properties of the -S-S- bond was completely corroborated. Muscle relaxant or ganglionic blocking agents containing labile -S-S- bonds, when influenced by a thiophilic agent (for example, sodium sulphite or another compound capable of breaking up a disulphide bond) cause a relief from physiological effect by direct inactivation of molecules of the medicinal substance. We can suppose that the use of this principle, when creating medicinal compounds (i.e., introduction of labile disulfide or, in general, introducing labile fragments into the structure of such a substance), will allow creation of various medicines with controllable action with the assumption that breaking up these labile fragments will cause the generation of products without physiological activity. In recent years, synthesis of a number of analogues and homologs of curarine and other amino- and diamino-containing structures were attempted. These structures can be used as inhibitors of acetylcholinesterase in connection with possibile therapy for Alzheimer's disease.

The "falling rabbit head" test, comprised of injecting a solution of a test compound into the animal's eye vein, is a classical method of determination of the curare effect. The ganglion-blocking action of chemical compounds is frequently estimated in experiments on narcotized cats by decreasing arterial pressure and reducing the tone of the third eyelid. Though these estimations are very frequent, experts also use other methods of research: the termination of muscle reaction to electricity, the dipping of nerve fibres or neuromuscular preparations into solutions of curariform compounds, etc.

The choline esterase activity of human blood is higher by several times than the activity of the blood of cats or rabbits. Therefore, humans need larger doses per kilogram of weight (for example, of dithyline) than such animals for an equivalent curare effect.

The first attempts at generalisation and systematization of data regarding the interrelation of action with the chemical structure of curare compounds led to interesting and, more importantly, fruitful conclusions. L.E. Craig systematised data about more than 1000 compounds demonstrating curareactivity in his fundamental review. He also showed that quaternary ammonium salts or bases are the most effective paralyzing compounds. Tertiary, secondary and other nitrogen-containing compounds are characterized by weak curare action that considerably increases when transforming them into quaternary compounds. Alkaloids of South American *Erytrina* (subspecies of *Erytrina Americana* Mill.) are a unique class of compounds for which such regularity is not characteristic. A tertiary atom of nitrogen is typical for two rings in these alkaloids, but they develop a full-blown curare effect. Transformation of such nitrogen into quaternary (quaternization) terminates curare activity.

Replacement of an alkyl group with an aryl group in a quaternary atom of nitrogen increases the curare effect. Benzyl groups often characterize the paralyzing effect of compounds. Their N-benzyl derivatives develop a stronger curare effect in salts of pyridine, strychnine, coniine and brucine. Bis-benzyl derivatives, specifically isoquinoline (alkaloid called curarine), have a clearly defined curare effect. The saturation value of a ring containing nitrogen (quaternary or any other atom of nitrogen) influences the intensity of curare action. Salts of piperidine, tetrahydroquinoline and tetrahydroisoquinoline have a stronger curare effect than equivalent salts of pyridine, quinoline and isoquinoline. Basically, all compounds that demonstrate a curare effect have nitrogen in a saturated ring. Methylation of two free hydroxyl groups in d-tubocurarine chloride strongly increases its paralyzing effect, while ethylation or introduction of butyl substituent neutralizes this effect. The efficiency of some calabash (calebas) curarines is stronger than the efficiency of d-tubocurarine. Calabash curarine itself paralyses frogs in doses of 0.12–0.16 mg/kg (d-tubocurarine, 0.5 mg/kg). Monobromine- and mononitro derivatives of calabash curare paralyse frogs in extremely low doses of 0.04 and 0.008 mg/kg, respectively. Gourd curare contains two groups of alkaloids ($C_{20}N_2$ and $C_{40}N_{2 \div 4}$ are suggested formulas of these groups). Alkaloids of the $C_{40}N_{2 \div 4}$ group demonstrably have the greatest toxicity. C-calebassin, C-curarine and toxiferines (C-toxiferine-1, C-dihydrotoxiferine) are among them. Toxiferines are the most toxic components of curarine. C-toxiferine-1 was separated in 1941 by Heinrich Wieland and Hans-Joachim Pistor; later, it was isolated from of products of decomposition of strychnine. C-toxiferine-1 is 5–10 times more toxic than aconitine. D-tubocurarine chloride is 10–100 times less toxic than C-toxiferine. Curarines do not decompose inside the gastrointestinal tract; they are only slowly resorbed and removed from an organism with urine. Therefore, meat and other products poisoned by and containing a small amount of curare can be eaten. C-toxiferine-1 has the following structure:

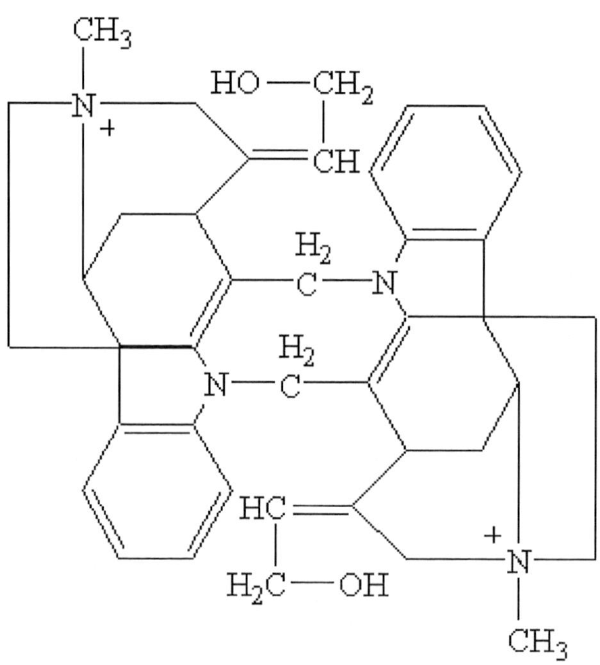

C-toxiferine-1 (hypothetical structure)

Some compounds not containing a quaternary atom but an atom of nitrogen (for example, α-glycerol esters) also develop a curare effect. For example, α-(*o*-tolil) glycerol ester (myanesin) *ortho*-$(CH_3)C_6H_4$-O-CH_2-CH(OH)-CH_2OH has LD_{50} with intraperitoneal administration of 1000 ± 56mg/kg. Thus, a mouse-paralyzing dose of PD_{50} with intraperitoneal administration is 325 ± 20mg/kg, i.e., the threshold of safety of LD_{50}/PD_{50} is sufficiently high and is equal to 3.07. Because of this, such compounds have a therapeutic value as paralyzing agents. Other compounds demonstrating a curare effect have been found and used in clinical practice in recent years. Diadonium, atracurium, anatruxonium, pyrocurine and other muscle relaxants and their effects are discussed in the monograph of D.A. Kharkevich, a recognised authority in this field.

Chapter 8

Strongest Nonprotein Poisons

Nature conceals an inexhaustible source of physiologically active substances. In the course of evolution and the centuries-old struggle for existence, flora and fauna developed extremely toxic substances that are threatening to humans. The variety of natural poisons is also the result of evolution, and the indefatigable searches of new toxic structures to crush the enemy met with resistance. At the same time, in estimating an immeasurable number of all natural poisons, it is possible to notice features of similarity among them. This means that in the process of development, some stages were repeated and duplicated, and after two distinct and distant species were established, they acquired the same weapon (for example, fugu fish [pufferfish] and the Californian newt have tetrodotoxin). The human is the one unique biological species that is capable of learning the secrets of poisons. We have not yet completely comprehended the secret recipes of synthesis in the natural laboratory, but their solution is close at hand. From the point of view of evolution, poisons have been playing a progressive role in the development of flora and fauna—they determined some defining characteristics of separate species, intensified strategies in the struggle for existence, stimulated the development of protective mechanisms, and gave rise to the formulation of antidotes. Unreceptive species became immune to the action of some poisons. By learning the secrets of the structures of natural physiologically active substances, chemists are able to synthesize them and research the fragments and close analogues of these structures, thereby determining not only the origin of the nature and metabolism of these substances but also collecting data on the interconnection between the effect of action and chemical structure.

The strongest nonprotein poisons can be divided into two groups: a) natural poisons and b) their artificial analogues, homologs and synthetic substances shown to have a similar effect. By examining the properties of the strongest poisons known by the end of the twentieth century (see table 1), it is possible to note the law mentioned earlier: an increase in toxicity, as a rule, is connected with an increase in molecular weight. This law was noted by many toxicologists, including Russian professor at Moscow State University, N.I. Kobozev, but N.S. Antonov (in the development of chemistry and technology of chemical warfare agents) came to an essential conclusion about the existence of limited values of minimum lethal doses of substances of a certain molecular weight. This conclusion, along with political, economic and other bases, promoted the conclusion of the 1993 Convention regarding the prohibition of chemical weapons. Further, the most interesting physiologically active and highly toxic substances have been studied in the disciplines of science, history and toxicology in order to increase their molecular weight and toxicity. The description of muscarine and curare as substances most known historically and most important for understanding the mechanism of interaction of poisons with receptors and organism enzymes have been discussed in the previous chapters. Natural nonprotein poisons have both plant (alkaloids) and animal origins.

8.1. Alcaloids

Examination of this group of substances appeared in the twentieth century as a separate branch of science; we will discuss only the most important for a modern understanding of poisons' influence mechanisms. One of the key "classical" alkaloids is nicotine—(3-methylpyrrolidine-2[1]-pyridine):

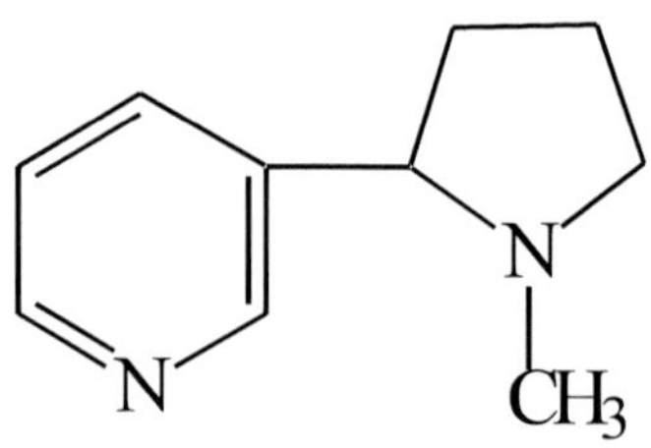

In the sixteenth century, the French envoy to Lisbon, Jean Nicot, an enthusiast and collector of plants, received seeds of an unknown plant from America. It was tobacco (*Nicotiana tabacum*), and its "procession" through the Old World thus began. The active ingredient in tobacco is alkaloid nicotine, belonging to the group of poisons that affect the CNS. It causes fainting that lasts three and more days, spasms, convulsions, heavy breathing and its subsequent arrest. It easily penetrates through the skin and mucous membranes; it is especially dangerous when entering an open wound. LD_{50} (rabbits, intravenously) is equal to 6mg/kg. For people, the lethal dose is 50–100mg. The expression "a drop of nicotine kills a horse" is widely known, although not many know that goats and roe are unaffected by nicotine.

The alkaloids atropine and hyoscyamine, found in *Atropa belladonna* and in other plants of the *Solanaceae* family (henbane, scopolia, mandrake as well as tobacco) influence the CNS, but there are other effects—pathological garrulity, dancing, fits of laughter, fury and rage. In small doses they excite the CNS, and in large doses they paralyze it. Atropine (tropinic ester of tropic acid) has the following formula:

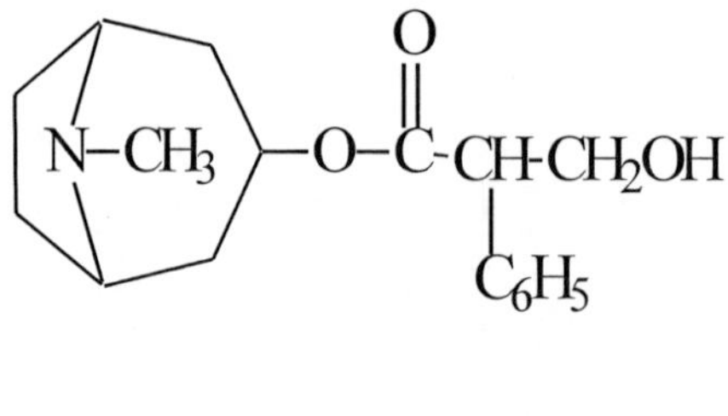

Hyoscyamine contains optically active tropic acid, unlike its isomer—atropine—which is a derivative of tropic acid racemate. Racemate is an optically inactive form, a mix of (+) and (-) tropic acids. For humans, doses of these alkaloids above 100mg lead to respiratory paralysis and death. A characteristic picture of poisoning with these alkaloids is mydriasis (pupil dilation); hot, flushed skin; fever; trembling; and continuous movement of the extremities.

Various methods of synthesis of these three alkaloids have been developed. Atropine is used to suppress muscarine and nicotine action on acetylcholine. Atropine and compounds based on it are antipoisons (antidotes) of organophosphorous chemical warfare agents.

The active ingredient of the one of the strongest plant poisons, aconite ("blue buttercup" or dark blue fighter), is the alkaloid aconitine. For rats, intravenous LD_{50} is 0.11mg/kg; for horses, the lethal dose is 0.004mg/kg; whereas the lethal oral dose for humans is approximately 2–5mg.

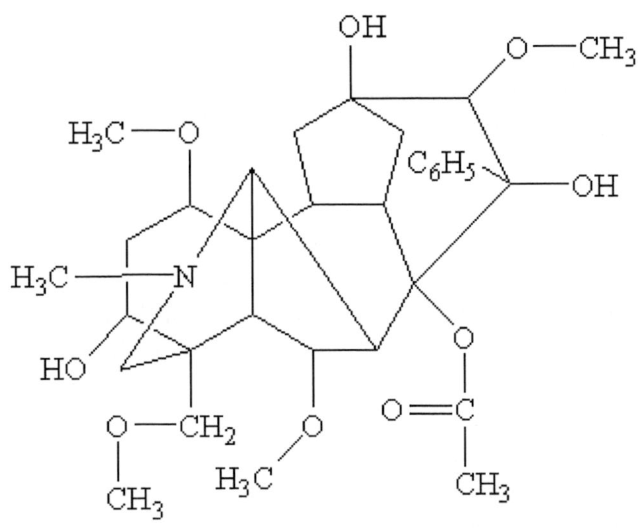

Aconitine

A medical research team at the Buchenwald concentration camp carried out experiments on prisoners to study the action of aconitine nitrate. The prisoners were shot in the hip with projectiles poisoned with aconitine. The first symptoms appeared in 20–25 min (motor excitation and light ptyalism). In 40 min, the ptyalism became stronger and was so intensive that the subjects could no longer swallow their saliva. Other symptoms included nausea and vomiting. A typical symptom was altered sensations of heat and cold. Motor excitation dramatically intensified (jumping up and down, throwing themselves to the ground, rolling their eyes). Then excitation decreased (pupil dilatation). These brutally tortured people died 121–129 min after being wounded. Consciousness remained ante mortem. Death was caused by respiratory paralysis and cardiac arrest. Aconitine is the strongest "nervous" poison. It affects motor, sensory and autonomic nerves, and their initial excitation is replaced by paralysis. It strongly acts on the CNS and leads to respiratory standstill. Aconite is not used in modern scientific medicine. One such poisonous compound is taken from the seeds of

Illicium anisatum L. (Japanese star anise). Doses of 0.04mg/kg (mice, intraperitoneal administration) influence respiration and lead to convulsions. Death by convulsions comes as a result of a respiratory paralysis; LD_{50} is equal to 0.7mg/kg.

In Calabar (Nigeria), the poisonous action of beans of the creeping plant *Phisostigma venenozum* has been known since ancient times. There are two to three seeds in each of its pods (resembling string beans) which contain the alkaloid physostigmine (eserine). These beans were used in passing judgment over people accused of sorcery (hence the term "judgment beans"). The accused were publicly prompted to eat a certain quantity of them. If the person vomited he was deemed innocent; if he died, his conviction considered to be fair. This naive and cruel method of legal proceedings was based on human psychology. In fact, the innocent ate the beans confidently and quickly; therefore, they vomited and the accused survived. The guilty ate the beans cautiously and slowly, which led to intestinal absorption of eserine and subsequent death. Eserine did not find wide use in medicine; however, it played an important role in the development of the science of medicines and poisons. In the 1920s, choline esterase was found in the human body. This enzyme has exclusive importance for the functioning of all nervous systems. It was found that eserine (physostigmine) blocks this enzyme, which leads to abnormalities of the normal course of nervous processes, leading to rapid poisoning. Poisons of such action were named anticholineesterase substances, and their discovery provided the possibility of purposeful synthesis of artificial eserine substitutes. Back-to-back anticholineesterase poisons were produced, including organophosphorous chemical warfare agents, the most toxic of all known synthetic compounds (see chapter 10).

Symptoms include gradual paralysis of muscles. The classical description of eserine poisoning is given in the first scientific guide on toxicology in Russia (E. Pelikan, 1878): "… the victim looks confused, muscles cease to obey him, and he has an unsteady gait, as if drunk. Breathing becomes difficult, pulse decreases, the body cools down and becomes covered with sweat; at last there comes a full relaxation and death, apparently without suffering. If diarrhoeia and vomiting are present, then the life is in most cases rescued. …"

The alkaloid strychnine, along with brucine and other alkaloids, is present in the *Strychnos nux-vomica* tree, native to India, and in many species of glume grass. Brucine is a methoxyderivative of strychnine.

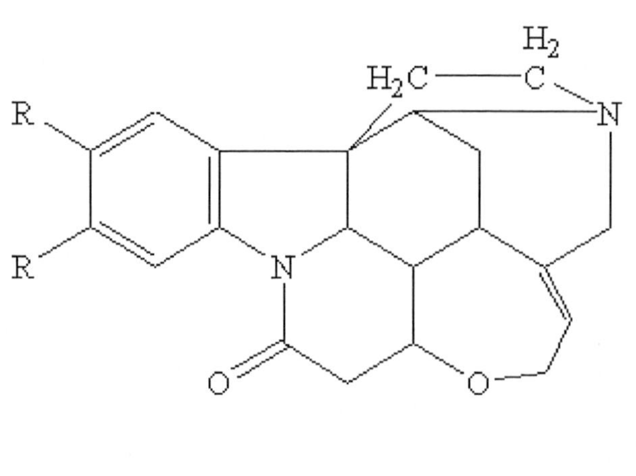

where R=H – strychnine,

R=OCH_3 – brucine.

Synthesis of both alkaloids mentioned above is carried out by several methods. Strychnine is 10–40 times more poisonous than brucine. The toxic action of both alkaloids resembles the action of the tetanus toxin. They raise the sensitivity of sense organs and reflex excitability. With increased doses there is anxiety, trembling extremities, speech abnormality, painful rigidity of the face muscles, facial distortion, and the head is pulled back. With external irritation (light and noise), the first convulsion comes instantly. Convulsions continuously become stronger; they are extremely painful and disturbing. Death comes as a result of emaciation and paralysis of the respiratory centre. For adults, a dose of 15mg can be lethal; for children, 5mg. The use of strychnine and brucine appears in many works of art, as the classical example of the most effective and reliable tool for elimination of the competitor or the enemy. The Indian strychnine tree does not grow in Russia, but poison hemlock or omeg (*Conium maculatum* L.) can be found everywhere. This plant contains the alkaloid coniine (2-n.propyl piperidine), whose action resembles that of curare. *Conium maculatum* L. also exhibits the narcotic effects and toxic features that are peculiar to nicotine. There is some doubt regarding which poison killed the great Ancient Greek philosopher Socrates (see chapter 2), i.e., poison hemlock or cowbane (*Cicuta verosa*). Coniine has a many-sided action: it causes muscular paralysis and drowsiness (curare and narcotic effects), and abnormalities of sensation (numbness and loss of sight and hearing).

It is necessary to note one more specific group of poisons that have a uniquely strong effect on cardiac muscle; their special danger lies in this. What Russian does not remember A.S. Pushkin's poem, "The Upas Tree," with the description of poisoning with its juice? In those days its structure was not known, and its poisonous action was not studied in detail. Now toxicologists know that the active ingredient in the Javanese upas tree is antiarine—the steroid-like substance close in chemical structure to the alkaloids of foxglove (cardiac glycosides including digitalis, digitoxin, and digoxin), strophanthine, and to other strong cardioactive drugs. Upas tree juice, as well as many other plants related to it, has been used since olden times as an arrow poison in Southeast Asia (Malayan peninsula, Indonesia). If a monkey is struck with such arrow, it will fall dead from a tree in two to three minutes. If the heart has stopped and more than three minutes has passed, it is almost impossible to restore its contractility. The discovery of strophanthine's influence on the heart occurred accidentally because of the use of a toothbrush contaminated by African arrow poison during one of the expeditions of Livingstone, the famous British explorer. Foxglove and May lily (lily of the valley), sources of medical cardiac glycosides (compounds of sugars with alcohols, acids and other substances), contains the cardiac poisons digitoxin and convallotoxin, which have a similar action.

Thus, plant poisons, depending on their nature, have a wide variety of toxic effects: one type operates mainly on peripheral parts of the nervous system, others selectively affect brain functions, the third target the heart or liver, and the action of the fourth can cover various organs and systems. Many others are not discussed here; numerous plant poisons are varied in their toxic action, but as a whole they are less poisonous. In comparison with plant-derived poisons, those that developed in the course of evolution of fauna reached higher "perfection" and contain more toxic active ingredients.

8.2. Animal Poisons with Nonprotein Structure

Poisonous substances are produced by animals in special poison-producting organs or in organs that nonpoisonous animals also have (for example, skin, liver, ovaries of different kinds of fish, etc.). Equipped poisonous animals inject poison into an opponent with tools such as special teeth (snakes), jaws (spiders), or stingers (wasps and bees); the non-equipped do not have such special wounding adaptations. Both amphibious and water animals contain highly toxic substances. We will not aspire to examine every poison of animal origin, and we discuss only some nonprotein structures of physiologically active substances of the fauna that are the most interesting in historical, chemical and toxicological aspects.

Among the most numerous and various (regarding the demonstrated effects) of poisonous animals are insects—spiders, scorpions, myriapods, various bloodsuckers (bedbugs and mites), hymenoptera (wasps, bees, hornets), etc. It is speculated that as a result of deadly infestation many historic figures lost their lives, including Roman dictator Lucius Cornelius Sulla (138–78 B.C.), King Herod of Judea (73–74 B.C.), and Spanish King Phillip II (1527–1598). Lice infestation in those days was a frequent phenomenon among privileged classes, especially owing to wearing of wigs. French court ladies during the time of Louis XIV followed a fashion of carrying special sticks, which were used to scratch themselves during balls and other gatherings. People died not directly because of lice bites, but because multiple scratches on the body became infected with pathogenic bacteria, giving rise to abscesses and, eventually, entering the circulation to become a generalized infection of the blood (sepsis).

Abscess-causing bugs are insects with poisonous blood and secretions. There is cantharidin in their body (a typical representative is the Spanish fly, *Lytta vesicatoria*). It is a derivative of cyclohexanedicarbonic acid:

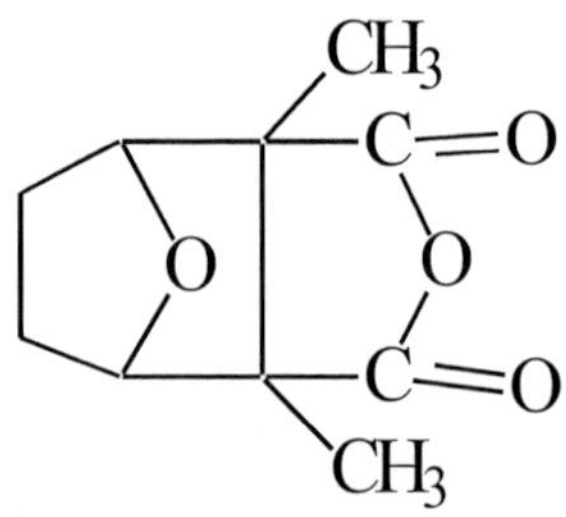

It can be synthesised by reaction of furan with pyroquinine acid. Even on intact skin, cantharidin causes redness, blisters and necrosis. The poison affects different gland organs and serous cavities. Intake causes sialorrhea (drooling or excessive salivation); burning; nausea; vomiting with blood; blood with defecation and urination (hemorrhage); severe pain in the kidneys, urethra and bladder; uterine bleeding; and pathological erection (priapism). Drugs made from cantharidin are related to aphrodiasiacs (*aphrodisiacos*, in translation from the Greek *love*); they are substances stimulating sexual desire and activity. Owing to the latter, the drug "Spanish fly" became popular and, in spite of its side effects, was often used in the Middle Ages by the aristocracy in western and southern Europe. This light golden-green bug is typically 20 mm in size. During the French Revolution, extracts from the

Spanish fly were an integral ingredient of love potions. Side effects of overdose included death. The lethal dose of cantharidin for the human is 40–80mg. Symptoms include uraemic spasms in the kidneys and bladder. Let us notice that, unlike alkaloids containing in their structure one or more nitrogen atoms with the expressed properties of the organic base, the carbon skeleton of cantharidin contains just oxygen as the heteroatom, being an anhydride of dicarbonic acid. If Spanish fly is typical for middle and southern Europe, then for Eastern Europe and especially for the Volga region insect species of the genus *Paederus*, which dwell on the banks and shores, are typical. In spring during floods it seeks refuge in bushes and trees, and accumulates on hillocks, haystacks. Most of all, fishermen and cattle breeders, who spend the greatest part of the year out of doors, suffer from these bugs, which alight on the hands, face, and neck; it is easy to crush them. Affected sites are easy to identify as a trace of the movement of the insect. The areas of skin on which they are crushed have a round form. The skin becomes inflamed, red, and covered with white vessicles. Sometimes the vessicles merge together to become an abscess the approximate size of a coin. Pain and burning of the affected areas are typical. Known Russian parasitologist and expert in animal poisons, F.F. Talyzin, notes a case of a fisherman affected by the poison of *Paederus* whose neck on which he crushed some bugs turned to a solid lesion. The active liquid ingredients of the bug's haemolymph is paederin, and its derivatives contain, along with oxygen-containing heterocycles, a secondary atom nitrogen. Unlike cantharidin, paederin affects the kidneys to a lesser degree, although features of their poisoning are similar.

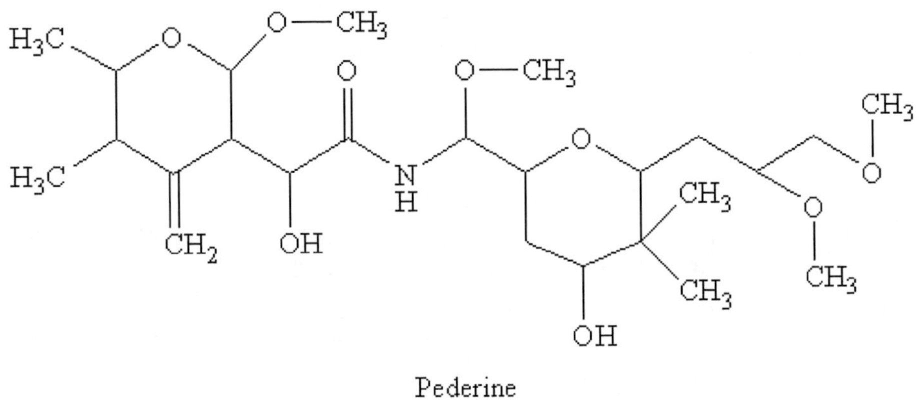

Pederine

Among other poisonous insects, we note only scorpions and spiders, especially karakurt (black widow, *Latrodectus tredecimguttatus*), living in desert regions of Eurasia, Africa, and America. The biology of karakurt interrelations between females and males is interesting. The female is a predator; it eats the insects it catches while the male, smaller in the size, is a vegetarian. Coupling occurs in a female's burrow. After the male quickly tries to escape, the female sprinkles it with a web-like substance, sticking the male's feet together, and then the female eats its partner. Sometimes the male manages to escape to participate in coupling in another burrow. Sexually mature females of the South American karakurt species are the most poisonous. Their poison, according to F.F. Talyzin's, is 15 times stronger than the poison of one of the venomous rattlesnake. The chemical structure of the karakurt's poison, as well as that of the active ingredient of scorpion poison, have not yet been thoroughly examined. The North African species of *Androctonus crassicauda* has a poison that in a quantity of 0.5mg can kill about 200 guinea pigs. The structure of poisons of both the karakurt and the scorpion include albuminous neurotoxins along with numerous enzymes. LD_{50} of *Buthus eupeus* undiluted poison (mice, intraperitoneal) is 3 mg/kg, and for *Orthochirus scrobiculosus* 1mg/kg. The index for undiluted poison of the karakurt is similar at 0.22 mg/kg. Neurotoxins allocated from the poison are more active (by approximately 10 times). For example, the main neurotoxin in the poison of the karakurt is α-latrotoxin, a protein with a molecular weight of ~118,000 and consisting of 1042 amino acid residua. Its LD_{50} (mice, intraperitoneal) is 0.045 mg/kg. In an organism, a complex of neurotoxin-receptor forms a channel for Ca^{+2} which enters the nerve ending and starts a process of neuromediator release. Under the action of the neurotoxin, a boost release of 1000–1500 times is reached; for example, the release of acetylcholine results in its full depletion in 30–50 min in the nerve ending and a full block of neuromuscular transmission. Because of this, neurotoxins are used as "test" substances for studying nerve membrane functioning mechanisms. The active ingredients of karakurt and scorpion poisons have expressed species specificity. One of them selectively paralyzes insects (insectotoxins), others affect mainly mammals. The primary structure of insectotoxins is rather more simple than neurotoxins for mammals; insectotoxins contain, accordingly, 33–36 amino acid residua (versus 65–67) with a molecular weight of approximately 4,000 (versus 7,000), in stabilized intramolecular disulphide bonds. The multicomponent composition and polypeptidic character of poisons of these kinds of insects are similar to the poisons of protein structures that are discussed in chapter 9 in detail. In the examination of the chemical structures of nonprotein poisons, we continue with the example of poisons of amphibians: frogs, toads, tritons and salamanders. These amphibians do not have piercing adaptations, they do not bite, and their only protections are their poison and smell, which repel enemies when under attack. Salamanders and tritons contain poison in the grainy cutaneous gland located behind the eyes and on the back. The principal active incredient of the poison is samandarine; it is a typical alkaloid, somewhat resistant to hydrolysis. Small fish fall asleep in water in which the salamander has let out the poison. The composition of the poison includes steroid alkaloids—samandarine, samamdarone, etc., along with serotonin and hemolytic proteins. The characteristic trait of the active principal structure of salamander poison is the presence of a seven-member azepine heterocycle with an oxazolidine ring.

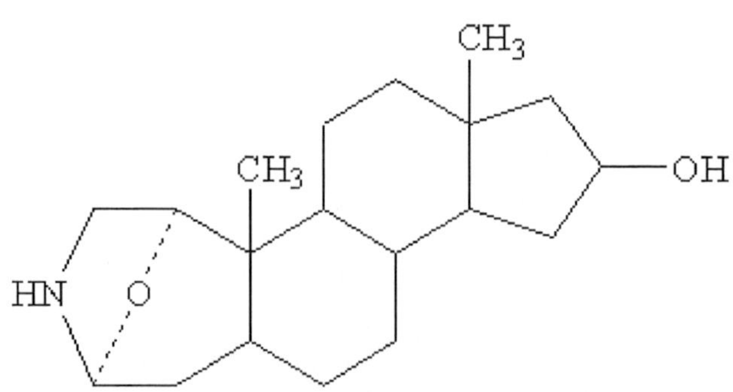

Samandarine

The toxicity of the undiluted poison (LD_{50} mice, intraperitoneally) is 20–30 mg/kg. LD_{50} of samandarine for mice is 3.4 mg/kg; for rabbits, 1 mg/kg; and for dogs, 0.9 mg/kg. Upon contact with the tongue of a dog, the toxin causes a deadly poisoning with symptoms similar to the action of a poison that has entered under the skin. The poison is very actively absorbed through the intact tunica mucosa, causing a convulsive syndrome typical of salamander poison, early signs of which provide an effective warning, whereupon treatment with benzodiazepines (seduxen, etc.) can provide an effective intervention. According to existing data, the poison also has a bacteriostatic action in relation to pathogenic microorganisms, including *Staphylococcus aureus*, *Bacillus anthracis* and *Vibrio cholerae*. Samandarine effects the CNS, originally exciting it, and then paralyzing the centres of the medulla.

Some kinds of frogs and toads belong to a group of poisonous amphibians. In nature, there are up to 250 kinds of toads. Only three of are known in the European part of Russia: ordinary (grey dairy maid), green and cane. It is well known that toxic toads have numerous skin glands—warts or colonies of granules, parotid glands behind the eyes, and "spades" on the hindfeet. Toad skin gland poisons are allocated on the body surface through excretory channels in the form of white foam. The poison is a yellowish liquid, with an intolerably bitter, sickening taste and an unpleasant smell. The poison from glands can be squeezed out with tweezers, but its quantity is insignificant; therefore, for the study of poison, toad skin is removed, dried, pounded and subjected to extraction with the subsequent separating of a mix of toxins. The dried poison of a green toad remains active for an extremely long time (more than 25 years, according to F.F. Talyzin). Toad poison represents an area of great interest in pharmacology and toxicology, first of all, because there is a mix of some independent toxins in it. Skin excretions of toads can be divided into two groups of substances: a) compounds that are derivatives of tryptophan (bufotenine which, along with a generalized poisonous action, causes psychosis; see chapter 10 concerning this group); and b) substances that do not contain nitrogen and affect the heart (bufogenines and their derivatives with suberic acid and 2-amino-5-guanidinovaleric acid [arginine]), so-called bufotoxins of the structures mentioned below, and others. According to some sources, the acetoxy group of the bufotoxin molecule is not at the 5th carbon atom of the steroid skeleton; it is at the 16th carbon atom of the cyclopentanoic cycle. Alternative positions of the acetoxy group are noted with asterisks.

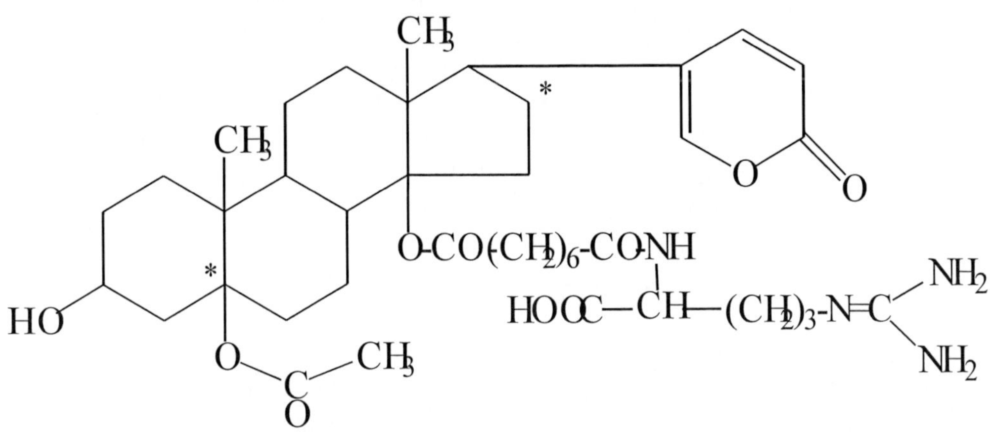

Bufotoxin affects the heart, and in this respect let us compare it with the plant-derived cardiac poisons strophanthin (a glycoside mentioned earlier) and scillaren (a glycoside from sea onions; see chapter 1). The lethal dose of bufotoxin LD_{50} for a cat (intravenously) is 0.3 mg/kg. It has strong resorptive action, and poisoning leads to an increase in blood pressure, pulse, vomiting and spasms. Death is caused by ventricular fibrillation.

Among the many chemical compounds that have been found in toad poison is the hormone adrenaline, in a quantity with a surprisingly high value of 5–7%; in the adrenal glands of the human its quantity is four times smaller.

One of the strongest poisons of animal origin is kokoe, a mix of toxic steroid alkaloids from the skin of Colombian frogs *Phyllobates bicolor* and *Phyllobates aurotaenia*. In one of numerous expeditions (December 1963–January, 1964) in the jungle of western Colombia, 2,400 frogs were caught, and from their skin 30 mg of the active principal ingredient, batrachotoxin, was isolated. The intensive work of research collectives and of noted animal poison researchers, John W. Daly and Bernhard Witkop, established the spatial structure of batrachotoxin with the use of mass spectral analysis, NMR, IR- and UV-spectra, chromatography on silica gel, and mathematical processing of data on diffraction of X-rays with confirmation of analysis, as shown below:

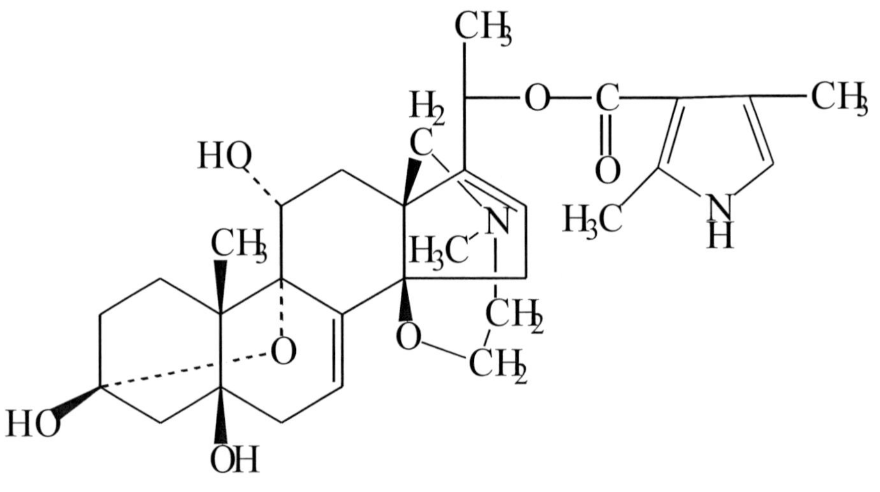

There are four main toxic steroid alkaloids in skin extracts of kokoe: 1) batrachotoxin A $C_{24}H_{35}NO_5$ (LD_{50} 1 mg/kg, mice), whose structure was determined by spouses Isabella L. and Jerome M. Karle with the help of X-ray crystallography of 20α-p-bromobenzoate; 2) pseudo-batrachotoxin, an extremely unstable alkaloid of unknown structure, which in storage spontaneously turns into batrachotoxin A; 3) batrachotoxin $C_{31}H_{42}N_2O_6$, the main toxic active principal component (LD_{50} 0.002 mg/kg, mice), which represents 20α ester of batrachotoxin A with 2,4-dimethylpyrrole-3-carbonic acid, and is the most powerful of presently-known natural cardiotoxins (ED_{50} $\leq$ 0.5 tsg/kg, intravenously to anesthetized dogs); 4) homobatrachotoxin or isobatrachotoxin $C_{32}H_{44}N_2O_6$ (LD_{50} 0.003 mg/kg, mice) represents 20α ester of batrachotoxin A with 2-ethyl-4-methylpyrrole-3-carbonic acid. Homologs of batrachotoxin from batrachotoxin A and various substituted pyrrole-3-carbonic acid have been synthesized. One of them—20α ester of 2,4,5-trimethylpyrrole-3-carbonic acid—

appeared to be more stable and two times more active than batrachotoxin (LD_{50} 0.001 mg/kg, mice); all other homologs are much less active. One of the conclusions of this work states that for physiological activity the presence of 3β-hydroxy-3α,9α-epoxy-groupings is necessary.

The presence of batrachotoxin is typical only for frogs of the species *Phyllobates*; it is not found in other related species *Dendrobates*, *Colostethus* or *Prostherapis*. The poison irreversibly blocks motor layers of elevator muscle, resulting in convulsions. Death comes from respiratory paralysis.

Saxytoxin is a paralytic poison close in strength to batrachotoxin; it is an active principal ingredient of some sea mollusks of the *Saxidomus giganteus* species, *Gonyaulax catenella* oysters, etc. It is found that the toxicity of Californian *Saxidomus* owes to its eating of one species of monocellular flagellar algae (dinoflagellate) and its tissues are capable of storing and accumulating the toxin received from the flagella for a long time. *Saxidomus* poison taken from tissue was named saxytoxin. This poison, having no effect on molluscs, represents a mortal danger to humans. In 1988, Japanese researchers discovered a species of sea bacteria that are producers of saxytoxin. Symptoms of saxytoxin poisoning are similar to symptoms of carare poisoning, but curare antidotes are not effective in this case. The action of saxytoxin as an inhibitor of cholinesterase, appears as tingling and numbness of the lips, tongue and fingertips; relaxation of muscles of the occiput, arms, feet; and in suffocation. Death comes from respiratory paralysis. With oral ingestion of saxytoxin, humans are more sensitive than animals, and the lethal dose is equal to $(4.0–7.0) \cdot 10^{-3}$ mg/kg. The toxicology of saxytoxin has been studied in the Edgewood Arsenal in detail. The poison drew the attention of experts in the area of chemical weaponry because of its rather low molecular weight compared with other toxins, which gave hope for its synthesis or its toxic derivatives. These hopes were not justified, even though the structure of saxytoxin was finally determined in 1975—it is a derivative of guanidine. Saxytoxin and some other low-molecular-weight toxins (tetrodotoxin, mycotoxine T-2, palytoxin) are capable of entering through the skin, although its lethal dose for cutaneous administration has not been established; however, it has been determined that it is at least two orders more than its lethal dose with parenteral administration.

Derivatives of guanidine also include two highly active toxins—tarichatoxin and tetrodotoxin. As it was discovered, these are two names for the same powerful neurotoxin. In 1930, the embryologist Victor S. Tvitti found that the Californian triton of the *Taricha torosa* species is very poisonous, paralyzing even related species of amphibians—for example, the tiger lizard. In the beginning of the 1940s, it was found that the poison is present in the lacrimal glands of the triton and in its eggs. In the beginning of the 1960s, approximately 250,000 Triton eggs (~100 kg) were gathered, from which 330 mg of pure toxin was isolated by multistage clearing.

The same toxin is contained in the eggs of triton species *Taricha rivularis*. The structure of the poison called tarichatoxin appears to be identical to the structure of tetrodotoxin, allocated earlier from the Japanese fugu fish (pufferfish). The toxicity of this fish was described in 2500 B.C. by Egyptian pharaoh Ti. Chinese historian Ivao Tany described the toxic properties of fugu fish more than 200 years B.C. (Han dynasty).

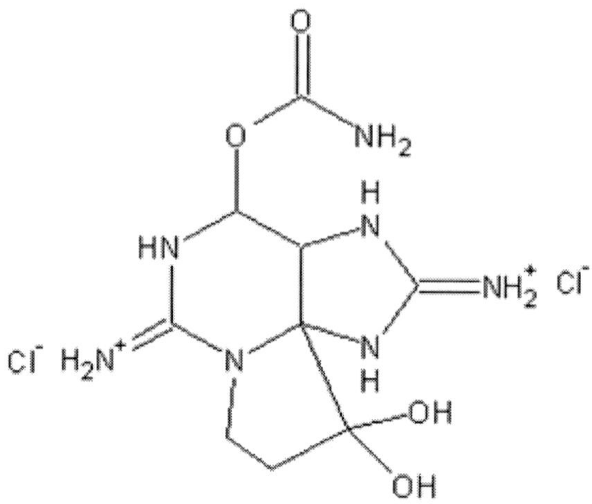

Structure of saxytoxin dihydrocloride

This fish belongs to the tetraodontid family (the best-known representatives are maki-maki, dog fish, fugu, blowfish, etc.), found on the shores of Japan and the Hawaiian Islands, in the Mediterranean Sea, and on the shores of Mexico and Florida. It eats twigs of live coral. Taken out of water or when under attack, fish of this family are capable of inflating, swallowing air or water. According to the Japanese Ministry of Agriculture, Forestry and Fisheries, for the period of 1956–1958 alone, 715 poisonings from the use of this fish in food took place, 420 of which (59%) resulted in death, despite the efforts of skilled medical personnel. This fish is very fragrant and tasty, and after proper cooking it is considered a delicacy in Japan. Cooks are granted a license to prepare this fish only after training and passing an examination. The basic source of poison is the roe and sex glands, but the toxin is also present in the skin, liver and gallbladder in small amounts. During spawning, the toxicity of the sex glands increases, and birds can die from ingesting as few as one to two eggs. Some tribes of the Hawaiian Islands used fugu fish bile as arrow poison. Symptoms of poisoning were described by James Cook during his second expedition: vomiting, extremeties becoming blue and numb, fatigue, sickness, hyperhidrosis and death from respiratory arrest. The identities of tarichatoxin and tetrodotoxin have been confirmed by their similar physical and chemical properties; by NMR, IR and mass spectrum analysis; by optical rotation and chromatography of toxins and their derivatives; and by identifying poisoning symptoms and toxicity levels. For both toxins, LD_{50} is equal to 0.008 mg/kg (mice, intraperitoneally). Both toxins are among the strongest emetics; vomiting takes place only if a dose is less than 0.0003 mg/kg (dogs, intravenously). A sublethal dose (0.001–0.005 mg/kg) to anesthetized cats, dogs or rats in some seconds reduces blood pressure, and skeletal muscles cease to react to irritation of motor nerves. Higher doses lead to respiratory arrest and full block of the neuromuscular system. The paralysis of skeletal and smooth muscle appears to be the direct action of the toxin on the nerve axon, independent ganglion and neuromuscular functions, unlike the site of application of action (for example, curare) (see Figure 2). The specified symptoms are evidence that both tetrodotoxin and saxytoxin interrupt the passage of signals along nerve tissues. This was shown even more than a century ago by noted physiologist Claude Bernard. And, at last, tetrodotoxin-tarichatoxin is many more times effective than another known local anesthetics (for example, the axon is blocked by cocaine at a concentration of 500 micromoles per litre, and the toxin is effective at a concentration of only ~ 0.003 micromoles per litre). Tectine, an anesthesia developed by Canadian pharmaceutical company International Wex Technologies based on tetrodotoxin-tarichatoxin, has passed clinical trials. The structure of this compound as betaine orthoether with a polycyclic structure is in accordance with a number of analytical and toxicological data. The same structure was independently offered by R.B. Woodward:

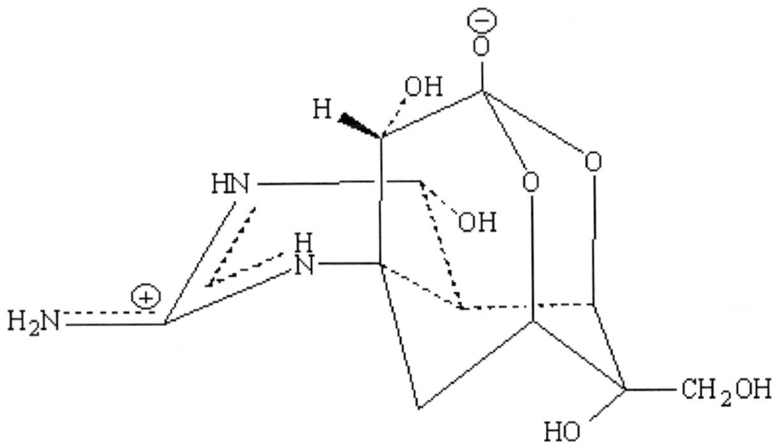

Tetrodotoxin

The toxin contains, unlike the majority of alkaloids, a non-quaternary nitrogen atom in the form of $N^+(CH_3)_3$ groups. It has a positively-charged guanidine fragment and oxygen, both in the form of hydroxyl groups, and in the form of oxygen-containing six-member cycles, derivatives of 1,3-dioxane (see chapter 6). In some cases of various animal tissues (Californian salamanders, Australian octopuses, and some tropical toads), despite the absence of genetic affinity between them, they produce same poison—tetrodotoxin. As in the case of both tetrodotoxin and saxytoxin, a positively-charged guanidine group, simulating a sodium ion, can penetrate into the channel to allow sodium ions to pass into the axon, but the rigid multi-channel structure of the rest of the molecule blocks the channel, halting the distribution of potential along the nerve. It is supposed that the mechanism of toxic action of tetrodotoxin is caused by the influence of the toxin molecule on the properties of the axon's external surface parts, by not entering the channel or, as S.P. Gabuda supposes, by changing the structure of the water solutions structure adjoining the axon. Taking into account the inability to enter the channel, structural parts of tetrodotoxin, saxytoxin and some other poisons (less effective in defining active doses, but also blocking transfer of a nerve signal) have absolutely different chemical and spatial structure, and it is possible to suggest that there are other networks of sodium channels that are ideally apropriate for such kinds of poisons. It is erroneous to assume the existence of special acceptors for them, by analogy with saxytoxin. In connection with it, in our opinion, more probable is S.P. Gabuda's hypothesis based on a change of structure (phase condition) of the water solutions surrounding or adjoining the axon (see also section 12.1).

The structure of tetrodotoxin was offered in 1964, and a year later the first publication about the toxicology of the even more powerful poison, palytoxin, appeared.

Palytoxin is 50 times more toxic than tetrodotoxin and 10 times stronger than batrachotoxin. Palytoxin was found by scientists of the University of Hawaii, and it was examined in detail at the Edgewood Arsenal. The data gathered by a group of scientists led by Dr. James Vick about the toxicity of palytoxin was published in 1970. In the beginning of the 1980s, the chemistry of palytoxin was studied and its formula was identified. American and Japanese experts synthesized palytoxin. Synthesis demonstrated the experimental skill of the technologists, but did not improve the possibility of its industrial production. Hawaiian scientists isolated palytoxin from spineless coral polyps. Another group of scientists found that one of the bacterial cultures isolated from *Palytoa toxica* polyps is a producer of palytoxin. The morphology of this microorganism is similar to that of *Vibrio*, sea species of which are producers of tetrodotoxin, the other highly toxic nonprotein poison. Palytoxin, in comparison with other toxins of nonprotein structure, has a molecular weight of 2680, 19 times greater than the molecular weight of sarin and more than 2,000 times more toxic. Toxicity depends on the route of entry. Extremely low lethal doses are noted with intravenous injection. With endotracheal injection, the lethal dose is four times greater than that of intravenous injection, which testifies to the effectiveness of palytoxin as an aerosol for inhalation. Dr. Vick's published data about the specific sensitivity of animals to intravenous administration of palytoxin allows an accurate forecast of the level of intravenous toxicity for humans in the range of $(1.0–2.0)\times10^{-5}$ mg/kg. Because palytoxin is a solid substance, its level of dermatoresorptive toxicity cannot be as high as that of inhalation toxicity. Transfer of palytoxin as an aerosol is necessary for its effectiveness because in it does not form pairs in a concentration at which affects are possible, and dispersion of a fine powder of palytoxin is complicated because of its high hygroscopicity. Palytoxin is the strongest haemorrhagic poison affecting kidneys, cardiovascular and respiratory systems, and the gastrointestinal tract; its cardiotoxic and haemolytic action is known also. Lethal outcome in experimental animals is caused by renal insufficiency, uraemia and shock; generalized haemorrhagic diathesis with necrotizing vasculitis and ischemia; congestive cardiac arrest; and massive haemorrhagic pneumonia. It is interesting that cantharidin (the poison of the abscess-causing bugs mentioned earlier) also causes haemorrhage and, along with palytoxin, contains in its structure only atoms of oxygen (among heteroatoms) and does not contain any nitrogen atoms, typical for the majority of other alkaloids and PhAS. Palytoxin has an irritative action on the skin and mucous membranes. It causes skin erythema, edema and even necrosis. With eye contact, lacrimation, irritation, conjunctivitis and, 24 hours later, opacity and ulceration of the cornea occur. A case of human palytoxin poisoning in natural conditions is described as accidental contact of bare skin with coral colonies containing producers of the toxin. The victim felt strong muscular pains and spasms in the abdominal cavity.

As noted earlier, the concent that an increase in a poison's toxicity coincides with the growth of their molecular weight is gaining acceptance. Growth in the molecular weight of a substance dramatically raises the number of possible spatial structures most sterically directly (complementarily) able to interact with certain enzymes or parts of the surface of vital receptors. The more precisely the system "key-lock" coincides, the more effective the physiologically active substance. Let us also notice that the growth of toxicity of natural nonpeptide compounds is observed in the transition from flora to fauna and in the transition from land through amphibious to water or sea inhabitants. Searches for the natural origin of PhAS are ongoing, and the world's inexhaustible nature will present us, as it has happened more than once before, with many more discoveries among natural toxins.

Chapter 9

Toxins of Protein and Similar Structures

Poisons with a polypeptide structure are the most toxic among all known chemical compounds of natural origin. The toxicity of polypeptide poisons, along with nonprotein poisons of plant and animal origin, increases correspondingly with molecular weight. The botulinum toxin (king of all poisons) is a mix of globular proteins with a mean molecular weight of 150,000 (from 70,000 to 900,000, according to different data). The multicomponent structure of poison (i.e., the existence of low toxic or nontoxic compounds in addition to highly toxic structures within it) secures a high level of complex toxic properties. This effect is similar to the preparation of chemical weapons mentioned previously: the introduction of one or more compounds improves the toxic or tactical properties of concrete chemical weapons. Such features of natural poisons have been known since ancient times. Nature itself took care of the preparation, providing optimum conditions for formation, storing and high efficiency. But only poisons with a polypeptide structure have a strongly expressed property-structure interrelation. This feature is especially marked among snake poisons, which have no constant structure and include various enzymes (hydrolase and desmolase), other proteins, albumins, glycosides, peptones, salts of various metals, fats, etc. Various structures of poisons are typical not only for snakes of diverse species but also for snakes of one species living in different territories. This causes a change in the main action of the poison; for example, snakes of the species *Crotalus s. scutulatus* living in California and Arizona do not differ in morphological character. The poison of California snakes has an LD_{50} of 0.25 mg/kg with a dominance of neurologic symptoms. But the poison of Arizona snakes has an LD_{50} of 3.3 mg/kg with mainly local symptoms (edema, necrosis, etc.). These differences are caused not only by a change of proportion of components of the poison, but also by the presence of new substances shown by high proteolytic activity of poison in the case of Arizona snakes and by almost a full lack of proteolytic activity in the case of California snakes. The reason for various toxic effects of snakes of the same species is evidently the conditions of their habitation and distinctions in the nutritive base. As a consequence of the variety of composition, polypeptide poisons have no uniform poisoning characteristics. Sometimes they act as neurotoxins and sometimes as inhibitors of enzymes; they can cause disintegration of blood or affect blood vessels. But it is possible to single out one or several main targets of action in an organism from all spectrums as a rule.

Polypeptide poisons can be divided for convenience into three groups depending on their origin or formation source: toxins of mushrooms, poisons of animals and plants, and bacterial toxins. Comparative data (according to B.N. Orlov) on the toxicity of some natural poisons are given in Table 3.

Table 3. Toxicity of poisons of a different nature

Poison (toxin) and its sourse	**LD_{50} for mouse, mg/kg**
Potassium cyanide (synthesis)	10,000
Muscarine (mushroom *Amanita muscaria* or synthesis)	1,000
Soman (synthesis)	100
Neurotoxin of cobra (Naja oxiana)	75
Neurotoxin of scorpion (*Androctonus australis*)	9
Tetrodotoxin (fish *Sphoeroidas rubripes*)	8
Saxytoxin (from *Gonyaulax* sp. [dinoflagellates])	8
Batrachotoxin (skin poison of *Phyllobates* sp. [amphibia])	2
Typoxin (from poison of *Oxyuranus scutellatus* [snake])	2
Palytoxin (from *Palythoa* sp. [Coelenterata])	0.15

9.1. Toxins of Mushrooms

There are also carriers of toxic origins among two basic subclasses of mushrooms: basidiulic and microscopic (mould) fungi. Toxic components of basidium mushrooms are basically alkaloids. One of them (muscarine) was discussed previously. Fly agaric *Amanita muscaria* also contains a number of other poisons (including polypeptide poisons) along with muscarine. In addition, more than 240 strains of microscopic fungi (basically mould) are known to be producers of almost 100 highly toxic compounds mainly polypeptide in nature. Poisons of mushrooms as well as mycotoxins enter the human organism by the food chain as a rule. The active principal ingredient of death cap (*Amanita phalloides, A. virosa* and *A. verna*) is one of the most well-known protein poisons. This mushroom contains a number of toxins; some of them have been identified. Phalloine (one of the toxic origins of death cap) contains in its structure an indole fragment surrounded by a number of amino acids held with peptide bonds:

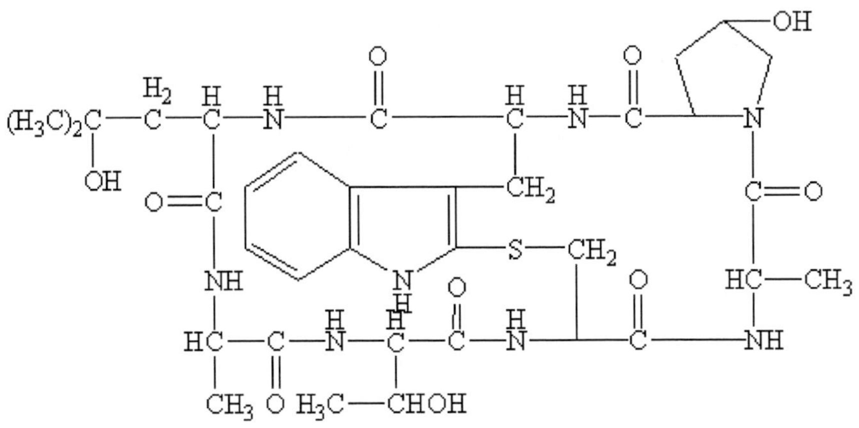

Phalloine

In addition to phalloine, phalloidine ($C_{40}H_{47}O_{10}N_9S$) and amanitine ($C_{33}H_{45}O_{12}N_7S$) have been isolated. Wieland and collaborators isolated amanitine, possibly the main poison of death cap, in the 1940s. Death cap contains amanitine in two forms (α- and β-amanitine). Alhough both toxins contain identical amino acids, the spatial arrangement of amino acids in the molecule differs. As a result, the α-form is four times more toxic than the β-form. Phalloine and phalloidine are 10 times less toxic than amanitine, with LD_{50} for mice intraperitonealy at 0.097 mg/kg. The lethal dose of phalloidine for humans is 20–30 mg. These mushroom toxins as well as other toxins with polypeptide structures are stable enough to withstand hydrolysis and heating, do not decay in the bowels and practically maintain their toxicity during drying and boiling. They are active in organism in the form of either the whole molecule or its fragments with a special spatial-structural arrangement of polypeptide arms. The second important feature of polypeptide poisons contained in fungi and bacterial toxins (as opposed to snake poisons) is a relatively long latent period (from one hour to one day). The first symptoms of intoxication (usually beginning with nausea and vomiting, diarrhea, abdominal pains, tachypnea and loss of consciousness) begin after the latent period. Humans die as a result of the toxic effects on the liver, heart and vascular centre, clearly expressed with oral intake of the poison into an organism. Every summer and autumn, during mushroom season, hundreds of victims of toxic mushroom poisoning arrive at hospitals.

Mycotoxins are more accessible in contrast to death cap poison. There are preconditions for developing the technology of their microbiological synthesis. Toxin T-2 is the most toxic among them, and any attempts to change their structure for the purpose of producing more toxic derivative always leads to a decrease in toxicity.

All mycotoxins including T-2 are 100 times less toxic than chemical warfare agents with a neuroparalytic effect by parenteral administration (intravenously and intraperitonealy). Interest in mycotoxins as potential agents of chemical warfare was raised by the publication of Sterling Seagrave's book, *Yellow Rain: A Journey through the Terror of Chemical Warfare*, timed with the beginning of the campaign connected with the application of mycotoxins during the Vietnam War.

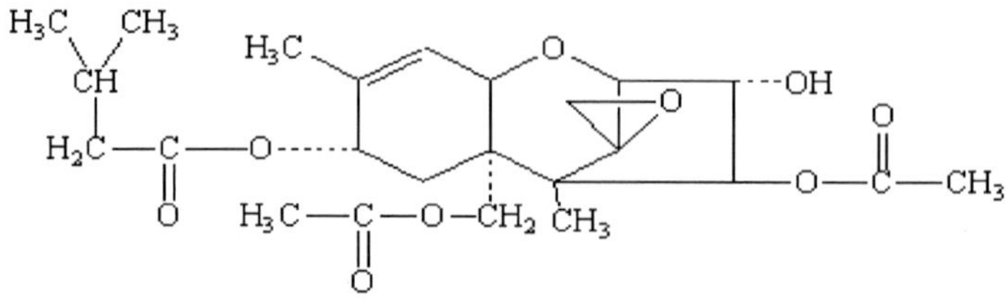

T-2 toxin

The United States government is reproached in this book for missing the birth of third-generation chemical weapons on the basis of toxins in the Soviet Union. Data about the toxicity and other properties of mycotoxins mentioned in the monograph of N.S. Antonov convincingly testify that mycotoxins in all main indexes are worse than modern chemical warfare agents and earlier known toxins. A United Nations report stated that there was no confirmation of the application of mycotoxins as a result of an on-site investigation, and "victims" and their medical reports appeared to be false. Mycotoxins are similar to yperite in toxic effects. Capacity to damage structure, interfere with the functions of cell membranes and to inhibit the synthesis of proteins by penetration into cells underlies the effect of mycotoxins. For this reason, mycotoxins as well as yperite can be categorized as incapacitants with a crippling effect. But mycotoxins were no threat to the English army "in consideration of the existing level of antigas protection of the army," according to R.M. Black and D.G. Upshall (*Chemistry in Britain*, 1988). This means that there is no necessity to create special protection from mycotoxins and, consequently, there is no third-generation chemical weapon.

9.2. Toxins of Animals and Plants

It is necessary to distinguish an order of reptiles—particularly, snakes—characterised by the greatest quantitative and qualitative diversity of individuals among all varieties of poisonous animals of the Earth that possess poisons with a polypeptide structure. There are about 2,200 species of snakes all over the world; from 270 to 400 are venomous. Snakes populate not only land but also the sea. Water snakes live in tropical oceans and seas feeding on fish destroyed by poison. Small animals, especially rodents, are a food source for land snakes. They succumb rapidly from the bite of venomous teeth connected with glands that produce the active principal ingredient. As already mentioned, snake venoms have no constant composition. They differ not only in the proportion of components in the venom but also in individual components and, first of all, in the toxic active principal ingredient. The concept of the "venomous snake" is inexact. It is correctly used not in all cases but only in connection with the effect of snake venom on humans. There are adders whose bite is practically innocuous for humans. A snake might be harmless for people (for example, grass snakes) even though the salivary glands of any snake, including grass snakes, possess poisonous properties that are dangerous for small reptiles, birds and small mammals. The cobra and carpet viper are the most venomous snakes. The lethal dose of cobra venom for humans is 30 mg. In the case of the carpet viper, the lethal dose is 12.3–15 mg (of liquid) or

5mg of dry venom. The quantity of venom in the venom glands of the snake differs depending on the species, climatic conditions, period of time from the previous bite, physiological state of the snake itself, etc. The rattlesnake has maximal content of venom, on the basis of serpentarium practice, of 3.9 ml. When dried—e.g., in a sample weighing 1145 mg after drying—it contains many times the lethal dose of poison for humans. Crude snake venoms are a viscous transparent liquid ranging from colourless to pale yellow or bright green. They coagulate after standing for a long period, and are well dissolved in water. Snake venoms in dried form are powders whose principal active ingredient remains active over a period of ten years. Venom contains many various proteins including toxic ones (cobra venom contains 85% toxic proteins), enzymes (extracted the cobra in a laboratory), fats, pigments, calcium salts (phosphate and chloride), ammonium, magnesium, etc., in addition to water. A venomous snake can kill neither itself nor other snakes of the same species and in many cases even snakes of other species of the same genus. However, it can kill venomous and nonvenomous snakes of another genus. The potency of action of a snake's venom depends on its species, quantity and quality of the venom in the wound, the site of the bite and depth of penetration of the teeth and even on the physical and mental state of the human at the moment of the bite. Venoms of various snakes affect humans and animal organisms differently. The venom of vipers, for example, contains a special compound (hemorrhagin) that destroys the walls of thin blood vessels. Blood leaks through capillaries into surrounding tissues and causes hemorrhages visible even to the naked eye. Other compounds of viper venom (cytolysin) dissolves proteins and red blood corpuscles. An enzyme called fibrin increases the coagulability of blood and leads to the formation of numerous clots in blood vessels. These clots block the lumen of pulmonary and heart vessels and cause death from respiratory arrest or heart attack. Ophiotoxin (a glycoside with the structure $C_{17}H_{26}O_{10}$) can be separated from cobra venom. The LD_{50} of cobra venom for mice (intraperitonealy) is 0.1–0.5 mg/kg. The minimum lethal dose of cobra neurotoxin for mice (intraperitonealy) is from 0.084 to 0.0003 mg/kg (according to different sources) and apparently depends on the separation efficiency of the neurotoxin. The minimum lethal dose of crotalotoxin ($C_{17}H_{26}O_{10} \cdot 0.5H_2O$) separated from the venom of a rattlesnake for mice intraperitonealy is 0.002 mg/kg. E.N. Pavlovskiy showed by calculation that 1.0 g of cobra venom killed a different quantity of animals (in live weight): 1250 kg of dogs, 1430 kg of rats, 2000 kg of rabbits, 2500 kg of guinea pigs, and 8333 kg of mice. One gram of dry cobra venom can kill 20,000 kg of horses or 167 humans weighing 60 kg each. The venom of snakes living in terrotiroes of Russia causes general poisoning of an organism as a rule. Local edema often appears together with a large liquid-filled vessicle after the bite of a viper, blunt-nosed viper, phoorsa or copperhead snake. The vessicle is present for a long time at the site of the bite. The wound does not close up for a long time (a year or more) even if the organism has survived. The same typical picture of poisoning was observed during experimental injecting (subcutaneously into mice) of lethal doses of poison: hyperactivity and anxiety occured after five minutes; shortness of breath, 10–15 minutes later; and flaccidity after 20–30 minutes. The mice became motionless, their head dropped, eyes closed and respiratory rate increased. All mice died 24–48 hours later. Intoxication occurs faster when injecting increased doses of poison; marked dyspnea is accompanied by constrained motion. The subjects fell onto one side 5–10 minutes after injection, and symptoms of paralysis of back limbs and spasms occured. Respiratory paralysis caused death 20–40 minutes later, although the heart continued to contract within three to five minutes after respiratory arrest.

The venom of rattlesnakes is compatible with phytogenic poisons. That fact is used by Indians of South America when manufacturing poison for arrows derived from curare.

Relatively large quantities of snake venom display a poisoning effect on animal organisms and humans, but small doses can be used as medications. Medications used for treatment of pain from rheumatism and nerve diseases, sciatica and intercostal neuralgia; antiplatelet drugs; and other medicines derived from snake venoms have found wide application in medical and everyday practice. In consideration of fact that identification of the chemical structure of the active principal ingredient of snake venoms and their synthesis are rather difficult today even for modern chemical laboratories, snake nurseries (serpentariums), where snakes are kept for extraction of their poison for its subsequent research or application, were created. Along with medical applications, a lot of poison is used for injection of serum (the most effective medicine against snake bite). The study of serum has its own history. In 1887, Henry Sewall was the first to ascertain that it was possible to make pigeons resistant to even sixfold lethal doses by repeated injection of rattlesnake venom. Two years later, M. Kaufman attained immunity of experimental animals to triple lethal dose of viper venom. Three years later, Albert Calmette (a Frenchman) proved that injection of increasing doses of cobra venom preliminarily weakened by heating leads to immunity of animals to poison. Later, this remarkable discovery was tested on horses and then on humans. It was found that the serum of poison of spiders, scorpions and some poisonous insects possess this remarkable feature along with the serum of snake venom. The structure of these poisons has not been sufficnelty determined, even less so than snake venoms. However, the commonality of some properties (including the possibility of prevention of fatal outcome by the instrumentality of serum) speaks about the similarity of the structures of the toxic components of these poisons to the structures of snake venoms. Nowadays, antidotic sera are produced all over the world, especially in those countries in which the bites of snakes, scorpions, spiders and other “exotics” of South and Tropics are prevalent. According to the evidence of medical personnel in India, 10,000 people in this country alone die annually from bites of Russell’s vipers and cobras (98% of them had bites to the shin, below the knee or forearm). In 2003, more than 23,000 people were bitten by snakes, according to the Brazilian Ministry of Health. Human life can be saved only by timely administration of serum (anticobra, antilevantine, etc.). If such help is not given (even in spite of administration of other medicines), victims of poisoning can die two to seven hours later. Anti-ophidic (antivenom) preparations are extracted from the blood serum of horses immunized by certain doses of poison. The disadvantages of produced sera are the necessity to store them in cooled temperatures and some limitation of use for people with an allergy to horse protein. New, more effective preparations against snake venom without such defects are now being comprehensively researched at the Federal University of Rio de Janeiro. Substances extracted from oils of local aromatic plants are the basis for these drugs. Advantages of these antidotes are that they neutralise the poison of all species and come in a powdered form that is dissolved directly before injection. The bites of vipers or Orsini’s vipers rarely cause death, not because the venom of these vipers is less toxic, but because these snakes are rather small. However, a bite of the viper to the neck, head or into a large blood vessel leads to death very quickly. Egyptian queen Cleopatra probably died in this way. According to some legends, she commited suicide by enabling a snake (mamba) to bite her neck.

There are more than 50 species of sea snakes, which differ in degree of toxicity. The bonito, the blue-banded sea snake (this genus numbers 24 species of sea snakes), amphibious sea snakes, etc. are best known among them. The opinion that sea serpents attack humans and often bite them is not true, and has been disproven by Indonesian doctors most often encountering cases of sea serpent bites. As a rule, such snake bites are only an act of defense by direct liberation from fishing nets, and it is difficult to notice snakes among caught fish. Canvas gloves protect only the hands, but snakes bite other unprotected areas, usually the forearm. A. Brem cites the following history in his book, *Life of Animals*: "...in 1837... seamen caught a sea serpent two meters in length, and one of the sailors had been viewing and touching it until it bit him in the forefinger of the right hand. He did not pay attention to the small wound because he was sure that he had already been bitten by a sea serpent in the Mallaksky channel and had not noticed any bad consequences of it. Half an hour after the bite he had breakfast, got dressed and two hours later went to the deck. Here, he suddenly began to throw up; soon his pulse began to weaken and from time to time disappeared completely; his pupils were dilated, but there were iris-contraction reflexes under the influence of light. Cold sweat stood out on his skin. His face became appreciably pale and he more and more evidenced heavy systemic disease. Soon paralysis of the throat considerably complicated breathing. The edges of the wound and part of his hand swelled up a little. A tumour then spread to the entire right side of his body, and his neck together with his face became spotty with dark-purple and grey staining. The doctor prescribed various medicines, but the patient could not take them. About 20 minutes after a bath, attacks of spasms which the patient suffered at the very beginning intensified and his entire body became dark; breathing became much more difficult. ... Further, the sailor lost consciousness and died less than four hours later...." This case is mentioned by us to show that sea serpents are as dangerous as land snakes. The poisonous glands of sea serpents are located behind the eyes, like the poisonous glands of land snakes. In contrast to land snakes, they smell of blubber when captured. This smell does not disappear even after being stored in alcohol or formalin for some months.

As we can see in the short sketch about snake venoms, chemists have somewhat laborious problems in the search and identification of the structures of these poisons. Moreover, the synthesis of venoms is an almost untouched field of science.

Phytogenic toxins-polypeptides, along with albuminous poisons of animal origination, arouse particular interest. Ricin was researched above all among phytogenic toxins. Thanks to military chemists, we have the greatest knowledge in the chemistry and toxicology of ricin. They regarded ricin as a potential chemical weapon since World War I because of its high toxicity and availability (low cost). Ricin is extracted from castor beans. About one million tons of castor beans are produced annually in the world. Oilcake containing from 0.5 to 1.5% of ricin is generated after extracting castor oil from beans. The main manufacturers of castor beans are China, India, Bangladesh and the United States. The technology of extracting ricin from oilcake is simple. Therefore, ricin can be manufactured in various countries, including underdeveloped nations. The latest developments show that terrorists try to arm themselves with ricin because it is accessibile and at the same time a highly toxic poisonous agent. Ricin was intensively researched as a potential chemical warfare agent in England and especially in the United States (where an experimental batch of 1.7 tons was produced) during World War II. The chemical structure, physicochemical and toxicological characteristics of ricin have been determined. Purified ricin is a white odorless powder, easily dissolved in water. The molecular weight of ricin is 440 times greater than the molecular weight of sarin. A molecule of ricin consists of two protein chains which in turn consist of fragments of amino acids and sugars. The two protein chains (A and B) are connected by a disulfide bond which is somewhat weak and labile, especially in conditions of an organism. These features of the disulfide bond were used by Russian scientists when synthesizing medications of with a controllable action (chapter 7). Each of the chains is not toxic in itself, but develops a toxic action only under the condition of the combined action of both subunits as a part of the ricin molecule. The A and B chains, separately injected into an organism, combine spontaneously to form ricin and develope the full spectrum of its native toxic action. It is shown that each of the two ricin chains can form a chemical bond with subunits of molecules of other toxins or even with synthesized polypeptides experimental conditions. As a result, hybrid molecules of toxins that are not found in nature are generated. Relying on this basis, a number of authors consider that the possibility of constructing toxin-like substances with an unlimited wide spectrum of action through generation of so-called "chimeric" molecules has been opened.

The toxic effect of ricin on humans has been well examined because of frequent occurrences of intoxication by castor beans. The minimum lethal dose of ricin for humans is 0.004 mg/kg. The first symptoms of poisoning (hemorrhage of retinas) occur not later than 15 hours after ingestion. Intoxication is accompanied by nausea, vomiting, intense pain in the area of the stomach, spasms, prostration and collapse. Death occurs six to eight days later as a rule. Serious damage to the liver and spleen; hemorrhagic effects in the gastrointestinal tract and lymph nodes of the abdominal cavity; and great changes in the ultrastructure of the kidneys are characteristic for intoxication by lethal doses. The effects of ricin are connected with the inhibition of protein synthesis in the ribosomes of target cells. Lethal doses of ricin by intake are greater than by parenteral administration, and a dermal-resorptive effect is not at all characteristic of it because of its solid state. Data on ricin toxicity from the literature differs for various animals across a wide range (from one hundred to thousandths of mg/kg), owing to the varied detoxication abilities of fermental systems of laboratory animals. That fact is characteristic for any toxin, mainly because of the use of preparations of ricin in experiments with varying degrees of purity. According to experts of the World Health Organization, a lethal dose of an aerosol of impure ricin is similar to a lethal dose of inhaled vapors of sarin, and a lethal dose of pure ricin is smaller than a lethal dose of a compound called "VX." Lethal doses (LD_{100}) of ricin for Cavy, the family of animals most sensitive to ricin, is 0.00005 mg/kg (intraperitoneally), 0.0008÷0.003 mg/kg (intramuscularly), and 0.2 mg/kg (subcutaneously). The lethal dose for cat, rabbit or dog (intramuscularly) is 0.0002÷0.0006 mg/kg. The lethal dose (LD_{100}) for a mouse (intraperitoneally) is 0.006 mg/kg.

Ricin as a potential chemical warfare agent (CWA) has many disadvantages. Because of this, no military has been armed with this highly toxic poison. It is effective only in an aerosol state, and its application in the form of a powder or drops of solution does not cause protection problems, in contrast to protection from liquid chemical warfare agents of neuroparalytic effect. Ricin, being a glycoprotein, dissolves in water with further decomposition. Dispersion of pure ricin or ricin in the form of a solution (up to an aerosol state) by the instrumentality of bursting charges is not effective because of a loss of activity. Effective action of ricin through respiratory apparatus is possible by its dispersion in the form of a fine dust with a particle size of less than 5–10 microns. Producing and preserving such a powder present a number of other problems (clogging and clumping). In the form of a powder or solution, it undergoes deactivation by means of ultraviolet radiation (half an hour of exposure reduces its activity by 1,000 times). For these reasons, the application of ricin for military and terrorist purposes cannot be effective. Known Russian expert in the field of chemical warfare agents, General N.S. Antonov, holds the same opinion. He has pointed out that "...effective application of ricin is extremely unlikely in modern conditions."

9.3. Bacterial Toxins

Some toxins used as weapons occupy an area between bacteriological and chemical weapons and are products of metabolism of microorganisms. As a rule, they are researched in microbiological laboratories along with bacteria, viruses and other biologic matter. But toxins, unlike live causative organisms, are chemical substances with a certain structure and composition, and they can be synthesized in principle. Recent successes in the field of molecular biology and genetic engineering in particular have made the future production of supertoxic toxin-like compounds possible. In 1986, the World Federation of Scientists distributed brochure called "Chemical Weapons and Consequences of Their Application." It was pointed out that the United States allegedly began work on producing military synthetic toxin-like compounds with a toxicity level exceeding VX gases by hundreds to thousands of times and capable of causing human poisoning in concentrations as low as 0.1–0.001 mg/m^3. These predictions did not come true, and we hope that they will never come true. However, new threats connected with the possibility of terrorism have emerged. Therefore, according to the information presented, consideration of the properties of typical representatives of this group of toxins is important. The latest review on natural toxins was written by Eugene Grishin (director of the Institute of Bioorganic Chemistry of the Russian Academy of Sciences) in a collection of works of some well-known international scientists (*Defense against Bioterror*, 2005) devoted to various aspects of the chemistry of toxins.

A number of species of microorganisms producing toxins dangerous for humans are known. Bacilli of *botulinum*, *tetani*, diphtheria, plague and scarlet fever, and some species of *Staphylococcus* and *Salmonella* (microbes causing affects in the bowels), etc. are among them. Comparative data about the toxicity of this group of poisons for various animals and by various methods of injection were systematised by D.M. Gill in 1982.

The tetanus toxin is high-molecular-weight protein produced by *tetani* bacilli called *Clostridium tetani.* This toxin, as well as *botulinum* toxin, is generated by bacteria in appropriate nutrient media. The toxin is extracted and crystallized from filtrates of these media. The crystal tetanus toxin is labile when heated. A lethal one-time dose of concentrated toxin for humans is 0.2–0.3 mg. The effect of tetanus toxin is similar to the effect of strychnine. However, the tetanus toxin, unlike strychnine, apparently does not enter major organs through the blood, but it affects the transforming centers of the motor nervous system through nerve tracts. Intoxication begins with initial non-characteristic symptoms in the form of spasms of chewing muscles and then of all skeletal muscles. Spasms of respiratory muscles cause death from respiratory insufficiency as a result. The tetanus toxin relates to a group of the most toxic substances. It is 3,000 times more toxic than diphtheritic toxin and 300,000 more toxic than VX gases. Toxins of microorganisms as well as other poisons, including those of albuminous structure, maintain a tendency to increase toxicity in conjunction with an increase in molecular weight. For example, toxicity increases among scarlet fever toxin (molecular mass 29,000) → diphtheria toxin (MM 72,000) → tetanus toxin (MM 100,000) → botulinic toxin (MM 150,000). Toxins of *Clostridium botulinum* bacteria are the most highly-toxic substances. Seven antigen types of these toxins have been identified (A, B, C, D, E, F, G), although many researchers consider, not without cause, that there are some other types existing in nature. The toxin of type A is the most examined one. The United States categorized it under code number "X." Botulinic toxins were manufactured on an industrial scale on the basis of biotechnology using bacteria producers of toxins. One-and-one-half million lethal doses of toxin type A, two million doses of toxin type B, and up to 142 million doses of toxin type C can be obtained from 1 ml of culture medium in optimum conditions. Several molecular forms are known for every toxigenic type. Each of them contains a neurotoxin with an approximate molecular weight of 150,000, but there are only nontoxic proteins in associated form. The structure of associated proteins has not been examined. Thus, their role in these as well as in other natural formulations (for example, snake venoms) is apparently related to the stabilization and protection of the neurotoxin and probably in the provision of favorable conditions of delivery of the neurotoxin to target centres. The amino acid order of neurotoxins was determined in the 1980s. The molecule of toxin of type A is (as well as many other toxins of polypeptide type) a two-chain globule containing about 1,500 amino acid residua with a total molecular weight of about 150,000. Two chains are linear polypeptides with a molecular weight of 51,000 and 99,000, respectively. The toxin is partially hydrolyzed in water solutions. As a result, the toxicity of solution increases approximately by 80% after two days. Botulinic toxin can be stored for a long time in dry crystal form without loss of activity and can also be applied by dispersion. Botulinic toxin is the strongest of all known poisons. The mechanism of its effect consists of malfunction of neuromuscular transmission as a consequence of the blockade of the release of acetylcholine in synapses, which leads to the paralysis of muscles. At the same time, the fermentation activity of these toxins and their ability to cause the hydrolysis of synaptobrevine (a protein that is part of the synapse membrane) play a definite role. The development of intoxication by botulinic toxin is well known owing to the somewhat frequent food poisonings of people eating albuminous products of poor quality. Poisoning occurs especially frequently when eating spoiled canned food—for example, mushrooms, kidney beans, peas, cheese or badly-smoked and corned meat and sausage products (the term "sausage poison" came from this phenomenon). The first mass poisonings treated by medical professionals at the end of the eighteenth to the beginning of nineteenth century had been caused by blood pudding and liver sausage. Botulinic microorganisms are resistant to boiling and they evolve without air (anaerobically). Microorganisms require tryptophan (one of the main amino acids in the structure of albuminous molecules) for producing and generating the toxin.

Early symptoms of poisoning occur after a latent period which varies widely and depends on the method of administration and the dose of the toxin. The latent period is 10–72 hours (for oral administration). The duration of the latent period by inhalation can be reduced by increasing the dose of the poison. Botulinic toxin of type A is most toxic among all seven types: LD_{50} is $4.25 \bullet 10^{-7}$ mg/kg; type B ($4.4 \bullet 10^{-7}$ mg/kg) and type D ($6.0 \bullet 10^{-7}$ mg/kg) are less toxic. Toxins of type C ($2.0 \bullet 10^{-6}$ mg/kg), F ($1.25 \bullet 10^{-6}$ mg/kg) and G ($1.0 \bullet 10^{-6}$ mg/kg) are approximately 10 times weaker; type E toxin ($1.04 \bullet 10^{-5}$ mg/kg) is the weakest one. All data on the toxicity of types are given for mice by intraperitoneal injection. The cavy is most sensitive to botulinic toxins among all laboratory animals. The documented fixed lethal dose of botulinic toxin for humans with oral intake is within the range of $1.433 \bullet 10^{-6} \div 1.433 \bullet 10^{-5}$ mg/kg. The following values of predicted lethal doses of toxin for humans are obtained by method of modelling of transfering toxidoses from laboratory animals to humans: parenteral administration, $3 \bullet 10^{-9}$ mg/kg; inhalation injection, $33 \bullet 10^{-8}$ mg/kg; and oral intake, $33 \bullet 10^{-6}$ mg/kg. The first symptoms of poisoning are nausea, headache, fatigability and weakness and, sometimes, vomiting, diarrhea, and vertigo. The effect on the CNS is expressed in disturbance of vision (double vision), and dryness in the mouth with subsequent paralysis of the muscles of nasopharynx and throat, esophagus and other muscles. Speech becomes compromised and sometimes impossible. Salivary and perspiratory glands stop functioning, the muscles of the entire body weaken, and breathing is interrupted. Death comes usually after 10 days (sometimes three weeks later) as a result of paralysis of respiratory and cardiac muscles. Botulinic toxin is 750 times more toxic than sarin and 100 times more toxic than VX gases in inhaled doses. In spite of such high toxicity, in field tests conducted in the United States by dispersion of botulinic toxin over a group of tethered animals, the toxin did not outperform many neuroparalytic CWAs applied in the same conditions, according to the number of deaths. This disagreement between levels of toxicity and results of conditional comparative application of botulinic toxin and, for example, VX is explained by advisers of the WHO. Differences in areas of affect and in properties of compared agents at their conversion into aerosol state are discussed in the report *Public Health Aspects of Chemical and Biological Weapons*. The main reasons for the inefficiency of botulinic toxin are the following: dispersion of aerosol particles of toxin of the most effective sizes in the upper atmosphere; detoxication of the toxin at the expense of environmental factors; and the absence of the possibility of effect through cutaneous membranes. Nevertheless, botulinic toxin was considered until recently the most dangerous in military application, especially effective for poisoning provisions, water, etc. Poisoned water can be disinfected only by boiling for not less than one hour. Approximately one-third of people poisoned seriously by spoiled products die, and the number of fatal outcomes would be much greater (not less than 90%) if there were no antibotulinic serum. It, per se, is toxoid (the neutralised toxin). With its timely application, as well as that of snake serum, it is possible to save the lives of many victims.

Chapter 10

Chemical Warfare Agents

Chemical warfare agents (CWA) comprise a wide, specific group of physiologically active substances intended for destruction on the battlefield and at the rear of live enemy forces. Almost all substances upon injection into an organism cause a physiological effect. Substances that in small doses cause a strong physiological effect are related to poisons. The strongest poisons were chosen for battle. Approximately one-third of more than 15 million currently known substances are toxic, with the potential to disable or kill. Not all poisons can be a chemical warfare agent: for example, alkaloid tetrodotoxin is the strongest poisonous substance; its lethal dose for humans is fractions of a milligram (see Table 1), but technically it is rather difficult to create a great enough concentration in the atmosphere for destruction, and there is not sufficient raw material for its manufacture. Consequently, a poisonous substance can be considered for warfare if it meets the following requirements:

- In small concentration, it causes an appropriate physiological effect.
- It has certain physicochemical properties, low capacity of reaction (especially in relation to water and oxygen in air); during long storage it does not have a corrosive action on the container material.
- It is stable at the elevated temperature necessary for use in artillery, aviation and rockets for delivery to the target and provides the possibility of its transfer as an aerosol by crumbling with explosion or by heating.
- The technology of a chemical warfare agent should be simple and, when necessary, be producible in peace time with use of domestic raw-material.

There are some more additional requirements: difficulty to detect, absence of colour and odor, high ability of penetration through skin and mucous membranes (not just through respiratory organs), difficulty to counteract by means of known methods of protection, etc. There is not one known CWA that satisfies these requirements.

During World War I, more than 50 various CWAs were used; they belong to diverse classes of compounds having a wide variety of physical, chemical and toxic properties. CWAs are classified according to different principles. Throughout the twentieth century, preference was given to one or another group of properties of substances as a basis for classification. Nowadays, for example, physiological classification according to Cornuber or classification offered by Edere and Isten represent historical interest only, and are based on the type of effects caused by CWAs, according to three groups: a) irritants, b) cauterants and c) general poisons. A dramatic widening in the range of potential, and the number of agents produced by the CWA industry in the second half of the twentieth century showed that this classification has a number of essential disadvantages. At present, the number of groups has increased to seven: 1) neuroparalytic, 2) blistering, 3) generally poisonous, 4) incapacitating, 5) lachrimatory, 6) irritating, and 7) psychochemical; however, this classification does not take into account multiple side effects of CWAs because a number of substances can be related to several groups. A more accurate systematization on the basis of the pathological reactions caused by CWAs is possible. The present classification system also does not take into account all factors. Toxicologists have attenpted to classify poisons according to their aciton on organs or enzymes. Generally, classification according to toxic action is broad enough, because it is guided by character of action, warfare properties and neutralizers, which are extremely important for civilians, military personnel and doctors.

Classification according to physical properties—in particular, aggregate state (under normal conditions), method of air infiltration, reaction to steam pressure, stability and behaviour of CWAs on location—can be applied to direct tactical evaluation of CWAs. For that purpose, CWAs classified according to physiological principles were distinguished in battle by marking ammunition with colored stripes or crosses. Such classification is convenient for application.

Because the classifications identified above are not helpful in the study of the chemistry of poison gases, Chugaev suggested grouping CWAs according to their chemical structure and composition. Nekrasov and Yanovskiy, in trying to connect the structure and composition of a substance with its physiological action, offered a chemical (a so-called "toxophore") classification of CWAs. This is based on Ehrlich's representations about the analogy between the action of a medicinal substance or poison on animal organism with the action of a dye that colors tissues. The authors tried to allocate in a molecule of a CWA toxophore a grouping of atoms defining the properties and character of toxicity of a CWA. The groundlessness of this theory was shown with numerous examples, and this approach to connect the action and structure of subsance is now rejected by chemists. Classification based on the systematization of substances according to their typical groups and classes of compounds accepted in organic chemistry is more convenient, and for a number of reasons. Using data from organic chemistry, it is possible to make certain conclusions or even predictions regarding chemical stability, typical reactions and transformations of a specific substance and, as far as the ratio between structure and toxicity that exists within narrow groups of compounds, it is also possible to make a conclusion about the toxicity of compounds in a group. Of course, assigning a CWA or poison to a certain group of organic compounds does not demonstrate confidence in pharmacological laws. Classification that considers biochemical processes in the poisoning of an organism is necessary. At the present time, these processes are studied insufficiently and cannot be a reliable basis for construction of a theory about the interaction between structure and physiological effect of any compound.

There is a classification of CWAs based on the problems addressed by them and their methods of application, i.e., offensive action, defense, diversion, ambush, gound and basin contamination, removal of foliage and destruction of crops (phytopoisons), destruction of materials, etc. However, for military-tactical estimation of conditions on land after use of a CWA, it is necessary to take into account three circumstances: a) character of action; b) damaging action and c) duration of damaging action.

According to character of action, CWAs are divided into two groups: 1) deadly-active and 2) incapacitants. The most typical representatives of both groups are listed above in Table 1, and more in detail will be shown further. The first group includes substances intended for destruction of live forces—organophosphorous compounds of sarin, soman, V gases, hydrocyanic acid, etc.

Among the deadly-active CWAs of the first group, let us examine, first of all, hydrocyanic acid, which was known long before World War I and was already offered as a chemical weapon at that time. Hydrocyanic acid was discovered by Swedish pharmaceutical chemist Carl Wilhelm Scheele in 1872 and he, apparently, became the first victim of it. Serious attempts to use this substance at the battle front were undertaken by Frenchmen in 1916 in response to the use of chemical weapons by Germany. Using hydrocyanic acid on the battlefield did not confirm its high toxicity. During all World War I, France applied ~4000 tons of hydrocyanic acid without appreciable military success because of the low density of its steam and high volatility. After 1939, more advanced methods and tools of application were developed with which it was possible to create at ground surface a high enough concentration of hydrocyanic acid for a long enough time. The exceptional toxicity of this compound was demonstrated for the first time by French pharmacologist Mazhendie. One drop of hydrocyanic acid put on the tongue or conjunctiva of a dog led to its death after two to three deep breaths. Later it was established that this CWA is effective not only upon inhalation but also by applying it to the skin. It is considered absolutely confirmed that the mechanism of action of hydrocyanic acid consists of irreversible inhibition of iron-containing respiratory enzymes. The consequence of their blockage is lack of oxygen in the cells. Delivery of oxygen to the cells by blood is not perceived by enzymes, which leads to the heightened content of oxyhemoglobin in venous blood, accompanied by reddening of the organs and cutaneous membranes in the victim. Death is caused by paralysis of the respiratory centre and, depending on concentration, comes in 15–30 minutes. An absolutely lethal concentration for the human is 0.4 mg/l. At high concentrations, death comes three to five minutes after a brief period of agony. The colour of the victim's skin varies from red to violet. The same signs of poisoning are typical in peroral poisoning with cyanides of alkaline metals. Doses of 110 mg sodium cyanide or 115 mg potassium cyanide are usually lethal for people. With significant amounts of cyanides, death comes in five minutes. In fiction and in special literature on toxicology there are many cases of poisoning, both planned and accidental. Let us show just one historical case that has entered the annals of the science of poisons, as an example underlining the necessity of taking into account the chemical properties and conditions of application of a poison for the achievement of a desired result.

During the reign of Tsar Nikolas II, Grigori Rasputin was given great authority at the imperial court. He was a mystic, monk, visionary and commoner, and a member of the *Khlysty* sect. His promotion by means of favouritism caused envy and anger among the nobility, who tried to eliminate him with the classical methods employed in antiquity and during the Middle Ages—giving him poisoned food. Cream pies and cakes, which Rasputin liked very much, were prepared with many times the lethal dose of potassium cyanide.

However, Rasputin, according to plotters, ingested several lethal doses of this substance with sweets, and the result of the poisoning was merely short-term stomach upset the next morning. The main reason for this fiasco was the plotters' ignorance of the fact that an organism is capable of neutralizing some quantities of cyanides with the formation of almost benign thiocyanates or cyanohydrin. Formation of the latter proceeds easily and quickly with quantitative yields during interaction of hydrocyanic acid or water solutions of cyanides of alkaline metals with ketones and aldehydes:

$$HCN + RCHO \longrightarrow RCH(OH)CN$$

The poisoned cakes eaten by Rasputin contained considerable quantities of sugars, having in their structure an aldehyde group which was actually an antidote; that, along with Rasputin's hearty constitution, prevented not only his death, but also other desired essential consequences.

It is interesting that myriapods of the *Apheloria corrugata* species, using hydrocyanic acid for protection, store it as cyanohydrin of benzaldehyde in one of two chambers of their poisonous gland. The second chamber contains a special enzyme that displaces the balance of the reaction of cyanohydrin formation to the left. Between the chambers there is a musculus sphincter that prevents the accidental mixing of the chambers' contents. Upon excitation, their contents are mixed, and the mixture leaks out through the pores. The process of formation of hydrocyanic acid fumes lasts some minutes with a gradual decrease in the chambers' contents. The fumes of hydrocyanic acid act as protection as the myriapod rolls itself into a ball. The maximum duration of such chemical protection is about 20 minutes, long enough to allow the millipede to creep away from danger.

When examining hydrocyanic acid and its derivatives from the point of view of chemical warfare, it is necessary to underline one essential feature—the presence of constantly operating large facilities in all industrially developed countries used in the manufacture of plastic, artificial fibres, weapons against plant pests, amino acids, etc. This feature, along with performance, explains its limited use by all industrially developed countries up to the signing of the Chemical Weapons Convention on chemical disarmament. Industrial methods of hydrocyanic acid production are widely elucidated in the educational chemical literature, which is why it is not discussed in this text.

The greatest successes in the chemistry and toxicology of CWAs are connected with research in the field of esters of phosphoric and alkylphosphonic acid. The first syntheses of dialkyl esters of fluorophosphoric acid were described in the literature in 1932, and in 1938, in the insecticide laboratory of I.G. Farben, Dr. Gerhard Schrader discovered diisopropyl ester of fluorophosphoric acid. The same ester was synthesised by Bernard Charles Saunders (Great Britain), which he reported at a conference in December of 1941 in London. This product met the CWA requirements of that time and was produced in large volume under the code name "DFP".

Gerhard Schrader, during a search for chemical weed and pest killers (CWPK), also synthesized other highly toxic organophosporus substances: tabun (cyanamide of ethyl ester of phosphoric acid) was identified in 1936. From 1943 to April of 1945, fascist Germany had stock of that CWA in a quantity of 8,770 tons.

In 1939, Schrader synthesized sarin (isopropyl ester of methylfluorophosphonic acid) with an inhalation toxicity approximately five times greater than tabun. At the end of the war, German stocks of sarin totalled 1,260 tons. At the end of 1944, an analogue of sarin was produced in Germany. It was named soman (pinacoline ester of methylfluorophosphonic acid), which is approximately three times more toxic than sarin. Until the end of the war, soman was in the development stage in laboratory and technological research, and about 20 tons of it were allocated for this purpose.

With this newly-created generation of chemical weapons and its organized industrial production, fascist Germany achieved obvious superiority against the anti-Hitler coalition in the area of chemical weapons. Even now, the reasons for Germany's defeat in a war it fought with conventional weapons without trying gain advantage with the help of the newest chemical weapons are unknown.

The United States and the Soviet Union seized as trophies stocks of tabun, sarin, ammunition equipped with them, documentation, and production equipment, and experts quickly organized their own manufacturing of these CWAs. The successes of the German synthetists who discovered tabun, sarin and soman initiated a dramatical growth in the scale of work conducted in the search for new CWAs carried out during the post-war period in the United States, the USSR and other countries. In 1952, Dr. Ranajit Ghosh, a chemist working at the Plant Protection Laboratories of the English company, Imperial Chemical Industries, synthesized an even more toxic substance of the phosphorylthiocholine class with the following general formula:

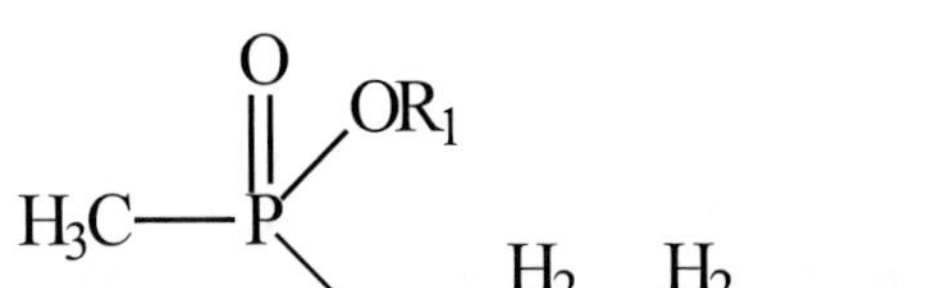

The information on it was transferred to the United States and Canada where, in defense laboratories for a short time, hundreds of structural analogues were produced and studied. The majority of them were highly toxic compounds and, taking into account a complex of physical and chemical properties, in the United States the choice of manufacture was made in favor of O-ethyl-S-2-(N, N-diisopropylamino) ethyl ester of methylphosphonic acid, which was given the code number VX. In the beginning of the 1960s, almost simultaneously in the United States and in the USSR, type VX substances were synthesized. These structures were synthesized independently of each other by Dr. Schrader and Dr. Lars-Eric Tammelin from the Swedish Institute of Defense Research. He was the first who published the information on phosphorylthiocholines that subsequently led to the introduction in the scientific lexicon of the concept "Tammelin's esters." The earliest literary review in the USSR on the properties of these compounds was published by V.V. Smirnov in the appendix to the Russian edition of Bernard Charles Saunders' book, *Some Aspects of the Chemistry and Toxic Action of Organic Compounds Containing Phosphorus and Fluorine*.

Substance VX is approximately 10 times more toxic than sarin with intravenous injection and inhalation. But its main difference from sarin and soman lies in its especially high level of toxicity with cutaneous administration: the lethal dose of sarin and soman with cutaneous application in the form of drip-liquid is equal to 24 and 1.4 mg/kg, respectively; an analogous dose of substance VX does not exceed 0.1 mg/kg. The influence of vaporous substances through the skin also differs by a factor of ten in favor of substance VX. The noted distinctions of toxicological characteristics of these compounds give rise to various approaches to their combat use. Although the magnitude of the lethal dose of substance VX with cutaneous administration is approximately 100 times higher than with inhalation, the significantly greater volume of aerosol cloud affecting cutaneous membranes in comparison with inhaled volumes make up for this difference in values of lethal doses. There is an especially important hidden motive (as the well-known domestic expert in this area, N.S. Antonov, has noted) in the conclusion that CWAs of the VX type are more advantageous to use based on dermato-resorptive application than by inhalation. For the same reason, solid CWAs, which are not capable of producing an effect through the skin, are less efficient than liquid VX-type CWAs, which are equal or even higher in toxicity when given by parenteral (not passing through the gastroenteric tract) injection.

The mechanism of action of biologically active organophosphorus compounds was clarified during World War II in Germany and in England. They show toxic action by blocking choline esterase—the enzyme providing decomposition of acetylcholine, a transmitter (mediator) of nerve impulses. Subsequent research found that result of action of organophosphorus CWA is not only the inhibition of choline esterase (though this is its main defining action), but also suppression and inhibition of other enzymes, such as phosphatase of the kidneys, esterase of the liver, lipase of breast milk, amylase, etc. Inhibition of choline esterase leads to an abundant accumulation of acetylcholine in synapses (the spaces between two nerve cells) of the central and peripheral nervous systems which, in turn, leads to their overexcitement. Overexcitement of the parasympathetic nervous system and smooth muscles and glands connected with it causes a muscarine-like action and overexcitation of sympathetic ganglia and myoneural synapses of transverse striated muscle fibers, causing a nicotine-like effect. Against the background of these effects, the general central action of CWAs has been demonstrated. Let us notice that, along with acute toxicity of OPC (organophosphorus compounds) caused by inhibition of a key enzyme of the nervous system, acetylcholinesterase, it is necessary to define the so-called put-off (postponement) of neurotoxicity of OPCs (PNOPC) that is caused in humans and other receptive kinds of live organisms by a variety of OPCs. Clinical symptoms become apparent seven to eight days after poisoning and consist in disorders of sensitivity and numbness of the extremities which, in 20–21 days, can be develop into partial paralysis. This disease is not connected with inhibition of acetylcholinesterase; OPCs with lower toxicity can have similar toxic effects.

The clinical picture of poisoning with organophosphorus CWAs depending on dose is characterized by the following: 1) in mild cases, miosis (iris contraction), discharge from the nose, increased salivation, headache, shortness of breath, loss of appetite, diaphoresis, sleeplessness, depression and fear; 2) in moderate cases, strong miosis, short-term convulsions, abundant salivation and phlegm, larynx spasms, irregular breathing, strong cough, etc.; 3) in severe cases, the same symptoms described above but in faster sequence, fixed pupils, painful pressure in the eyes, headaches, asphyxia, strong spasms and, in the process of exhaustion, development of spasms and paralysis, and death by paralysis of the respiratory centre and cardiac and circulatory arrest. Clinical signs and symptoms of acute poisoning of all neuroparalytic CWAs are identical. Some differences in symptoms and the sequence of their development depend on the dose and route of injection.

According to G. Schrader, organophosphorus compounds are biologically active if their structure satisfies following conditions: a) the central atom of phosphorus is five-valent; b) the central atom of phosphorus has a double-bonded atom of oxygen or sulphur and, in addition, two alkyl, aryl, etc. groups, either mono- or dialkylamino groups; c) the fifth valency of phosphorus is sated by acyl residue. The general formula below satisfies these requirements:

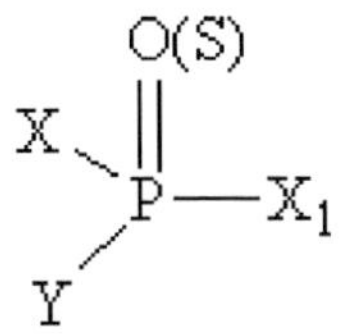

Where X, X^1 = R, RO(S), RNH, R_2N;
Y= halogen, CN, SCN, OCN, residues of phenol, enol, choline, thiocholine etc.

Although for chemists engaged in synthesis of OPCs G. Schrader's key formula is important in the search for biologically active compounds, for all complexes of organophosphorus compounds there are no general laws of toxicity depending on changes in structure. Of course, as well as in other classes of organic chemistry, it is possible to formulate some ratio between change of toxicity and structure within one group or to apply them to other groups. A connection between the toxicity and chemical structure of dialkyl- and di(aryl)fluorophosphates, alkyl-dialkylamidofluorophosphates, esters and monoamido- and diamidoalkylcyanophosphates has been studied in detail. Just as in the case of phosphates, there are similar interconnections between toxicity and structure among O-alkyl-alkylfluorophosphates, phosphorylcholine and their thioanalogs. These dependencies are discussed in appropriate educational and original literature in detail and they are not examined in this text.

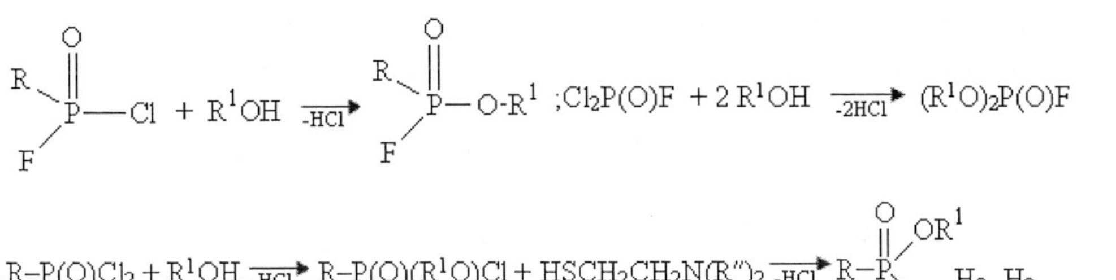

In the literature, there are many methods for obtaining CWAs with neuroparalytic action. We will present the results of only the most rational, based on industrially produced raw materials and characterized by relative simplicity and high yields of desired product. The general method of deriving esters of fluorophosphoric and alkylfluorophosphonic acid and phosphorylthiocholine is described by the following schemes:

Processes of esterification, studied in detail, proceed with high yields and in mild conditions. The basic problem consists of obtaining the initial products—appropriate chloranhydrides. Direct hydrofluoridation of phosphorous-oxychloride is somewhat difficult and also proceeds with low yield (up to 20%) of the desired product. Therefore, in the case of obtaining dialkylfluorophosphate, it is more preferable to first obtain dialkylchlorophosphate, which further should be fluoridized. However, also in this case, the first stage (obtaining chlorophosphate) proceeds with low yields and is complicated with some side processes. Therefore, during interaction with appropriate alcohol, trichlorophosphorus is injected instead of phosphorous-oxychloride, and obtained along with this (with high yield) dialkylphosphite is subjected over chlorination to dialkylchlorophosphate:

$$2ROH + PCl_3 \longrightarrow (RO)_2POH \xrightarrow{Cl_2} (RO)_2P(O)Cl \xrightarrow{NaF} (RO)_2P(O)F$$

In the case of obtaining DFP (where R is isopropyl), the general yield of desired product is ~75%. For obtaining sarin, soman and V gases, it is necessary to create a phosphorus-carbon bond, for which methods of formation were studied in detail at the beginning of the twentieth century (reactions of Arbuzov, Michaelis-Bekker, etc.). One of the most convenient methods is pyrolysis of dimethyl phosphite at a temperature > 100°C; owing to that, it undergoes Arbuzov regrouping. As a result, a mix of methyl ester of methylphosphonic acid and dimethylpyrophosphonic acid is formed. The obtained mix is chlorinated in hard conditions—for example, by five-chloride phosphorus. The yield of dichloroanhydride of methylphosphonic acid (DCA) is about 70%. It is possible to derive sarin and soman from DCA in various ways; the most rational is conversion of DCA into difluoroanhydride or fluorochloroanhydride and its subsequent interaction with corresponding alcohol. Product yields are more than 80%. Phosphorylthiocholines with acceptable yields can also be obtained with various methods, but it is most rational to start with DCA.

Adding to the armory of organophosphorus poison gases with neuroparalytic effect signified an apogee in the development of chemical weapons. The further increase of its fighting strength did not take place for half a century, although during this period extraordinary sums were spent for the search, synthesis and study of many tens of thousands of new structures in laboratories of different countries. This allows the conclusion that discovery of new CWAs surpassing the level of toxicity and lethal action of modern CWAs and having at the same time optimum physical and chemical properties (liquid form, moderate volatility, ability to effectively penetrate the skin, ability to be absorbed by porous materials and by lacquer coating, etc.) is doubtful, and even dismissed by a number of experts. In the well-founded opinion of the Soviet expert in this area, N.S. Antonov—who, in his monograph based on original techniques, generalized and determined the range of the minimum lethal dose for each substance with similar characteristics of toxic action—this boundary in logarithmic coordinates, "LD_{50} (mol/kg) - molecular weight," represents a parabolic curve, and in the most toxic substances of a set there are certain corresponding values of molecular weight. With the growth of molecular weight, the aggregative state of a substance changes. Data file processing of more than 60,000 volatile and liquid organic compounds led to the conclusion that volatile compounds should have a minimum lethal dose not below 0.04–0.06 mg/kg, and calculated that the value of the minimum lethal dose for a liquid CWA was only 0.002–0.004 mg/kg, or just 24 times less than the lethal dose of a VX substance delivered by intravenous injection. Any attempt to create new, more toxic substances than VX (10 times or greater) for chemical warfare is connected, according to the diagram, with the necessity for transition to the synthesis of compounds with much greater molecular weight, which is limited to only solid substances. It follows from this that it is impossible to obtain a supertoxic substance that could be a liquid and, moreover, be a volatile liquid. According to N.S. Antonov's forecast, a significant increase in the potency of a CWA with lethal action is not expected in the near future.

At the same time, for last 50 years, the list of temporarily disabling CWAs was essentially increased in a quantitative and in a qualitative sense. This group includes substances intended for weakening or temporary suppression of an army's fighting efficiency, through their exhaustion and disorganization. The significance of taking into account all factors for achievement of the necessary result and especially taking into account the level of fighting capacity can be illustrated in a known historical example—the result of the Battle of Poltava (1709). It is known for sure that in the Swedish army there was a mass outbreak of gastric diseases, and King Charles XII on the eve of fight had diarrhea. There was hot weather that summer in Moldova and the Ukraine, and water sources quickly bloomed with microorganisms and became dangerous. In contrast to the Swedes, the Russian armies, by order of Peter I, drank water only after having placed a piece of a "flaky" stone in the water's storage container. According to many contemporaries, the emperor was aware of the unique properties, including antiseptic, of a "flaky" stone of Kareliya (nowadays it is known as the mineral schungite), and he was familiar with the only deposit of this mineral in the world in the Russian resort's "Marcialic waters," which was already older than 300 years. In addition to Peter's leadership and organizing talents, he wisely used the factors of exhaustion and weakening of the fighting capacity of the Swedish army, which, along with the tactic of destroying the opponent's provisions along its supply route, helped to save the lives of many Russian soldiers and to win the Battle of Poltava. And although all of the circumstances above mentioned were helped to a certain extent by climatic features, the result—the temporary weakening of the opponent's fighting capacity—can be purposefully attained nowadays with the use of incapacitants. Incapacitants comprise a large group of physiologically active substances with various toxic actions. Unlike substances with lethal action, doses of incapacitants are hundreds of times lower than their lethal doses. A number of products, depending on concentration or infection density (phosgene, yperite, nitrogenous yperite and lewisite), can belong to any group. Incapacitants include irritants, dysregulators and substances with crippling actions which, in turn, can be divided into subgroups (see Figure 17).

Vapors and aerosols of irritants cause irritation of the eyes (lachrimators) and upper air passages (sternites), and their action is maintained only until unprotected people in the area containing irritants will be affected. When targeted subjects are no longer in contact with the infected atmosphere, the toxic effects disappear in a short time. Until recently, adamsite and chloroacetophenone, which were used in World War I, maintained their value as CWAs.

After the end of World War I, intensive research led to the addition of three new, more effective irritants. The first, o-chlorobenzylidenemalonodinitril (CS), along with chloroacetophenone, found wide application during the operations of the U.S. Army in Vietnam.

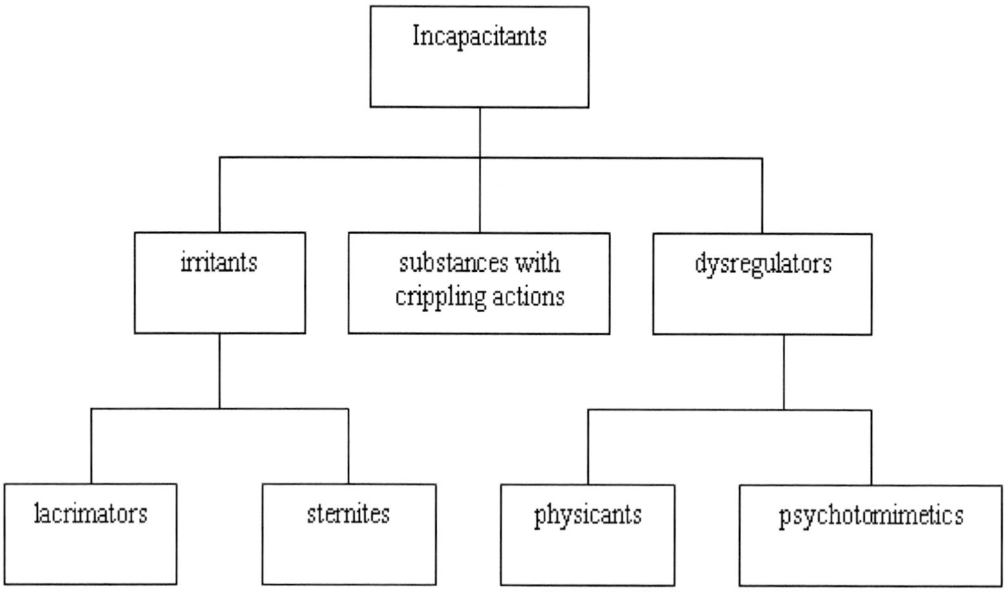

Figure 17. Classification of incapacitants according to character of influence.

It was applied for the purpose of removing the Vietnamese armies and population from areas. It was important in operations and tactics, and for smoking out unprotected personnel from underground refuges. Excessive lachrymation, burning in the nasopharynx and retrosternal pains arrive after 20–60 seconds of exposure to a cloud of vapors or aerosol. Although CS is a solid substance with a melting point of 95°C, it is volatile enough. A concentration of its vapor at 20°C is equal to 0.12 mg/m^3 (at a threshold concentration of 0.05mg/m^3), which leads to vision impairment in people without eye and respiratory protective apparatus in the areas in which a powder of CS is distributed. The concentration leading to loss of fighting capacity is 0.001–0.005 mg/l. The substance affects the skin and mucous membranes, causing strong burning that is aggravated by moisture (sweat, tears, etc.). With prolonged exposure and at high concentration, erythema and blisters form.

In a number of industrially developed countries, CS is used for dispersal, dispersion, etc. Experience with its application, including that gained in Vietnam, showed that CS is not only highly efficiency as an irritant but is also a teratogenic substance. In this connection, in 1973, it was discontinued as a police weapon. Another irritant, chloroacetophenone, is used nowadays as a "police" CWA. In Russia, there is similar substance called "bird cherry." It was widely applied for the first time during mass demonstrations in Georgia and the Baltic Respublic at the end of the 1980s and the beginning of the 1990s in connection with instability in the USSR.

CS is obtained from *ortho*-chlorbenzaldehyde and malonodinitrile:

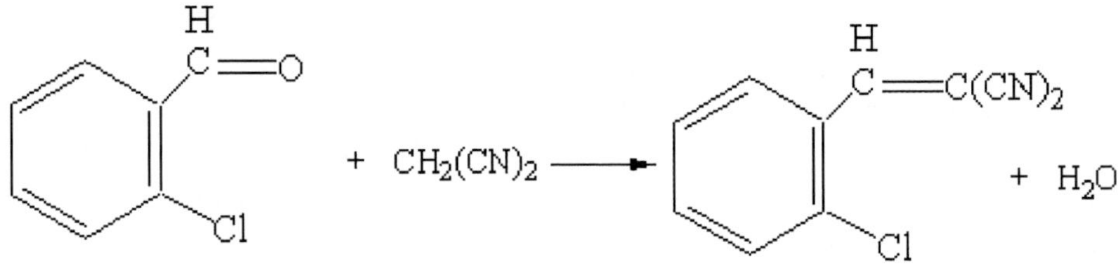

The substance is stable enough in terms of hydrolysis. The speed of hydrolysis decreases in acidic medium, and anions of OH^- accelerate it.

In 1973, a new irritant was added to armoury of the USA and England - dibenzoxazepin (CR). Concentration of its saturated vapor at 20°C is $1 mg/m^3$ or nearly 400 times above its threshold concentration, i.e., though it is also a solid like CS, it is even more effective. In a vaporized or aerosol state, CR has a powerful lachrymation effect in combination with a stinging and burning action and, in comparison with other synthetic irritants, CR creates more expressed discomfort with an extensive complex of painful effects.

In the mid-1970s in the United States, the technology of a new irritant, 1-methoxy-1,3,5-cycloheptatriene (CH), was mastered. Unlike those mentioned above, this substance is a liquid; its irritating action is inferior to both CS and CR, but in a liquid state it can be used in a liquid stream for direct influence on cutaneous membranes.

The group of dysregulators consists of two groups of substances, psychotomimetic and physicants, causing reversible mental or physiological (physical) disorder, respectively. The toxic action of dysregulators can be preserved from several hours to several days with injection of appropriate effective doses in an organism.

The group of psychotomimetics consists of sympathomimetics, glycolates, cannabinols and a number of other compounds. Wide interest in psychotomimetics appeared after Dr. Albert Hofmann, in 1943, synthesized lysergic diethylamide acid (LSD, LSD-25) and accidentally discovered its hallucinogenic properties. A new page in the study of psychotomimetics began with LSD because an insignificantly small dose (0.001mg/kg) leads to psychotomimetic effects. It is necessary to note two more circumstances: since the discovery of the psychotomimetic properties of LSD more than 50 years ago, and despite an intensive and comprehensive search for effective analogues, no other preparation with such high activity has been found. The intensification in research during the final 50–70 years of the last century was brought on by, on one hand, the great interest of industrially developed countries in incapacitating CWAs, and, on the other hand, LSD's psychotic effects resembling schizophrenia. The latter was connected with the possibility of the use of LSD and its derivatives for treatment of schizophrenia or, at least, some types of it, and also for its study by modeling psychopathological conditions. The importance of psychotomimetics as a means for research was not limited by psychiatry. They are no less important for research of the physiology of the CNS, the pathology of higher nervous activity, and psychology. In the most comprehensive review about psychotomimetics in Russia, G.I. Milshtein and L.I. Spivak in 1971 systematized pharmacological, biochemical, physiological and other data (more than 600 references); they compared them with the clinical picture, examined existing representations about the psychotomimetic action mechanism and, especially important, they made some conclusions about the connection of chemical structure with activity. The authors of the review, based on material in the work of Yarovenko, Downing, Yacobsen and Kohen, marked out six basic groups of psychotomimetics, although from the point of view of their estimation, N.S. Antonov allocates only four groups as potential CWAs. The first group of sympathomimetics consists of LSD and its derivatives. From four possible spatial isomers of LSD, only one, corresponding to natural lysergic acid, has high psychotomimetic activity.

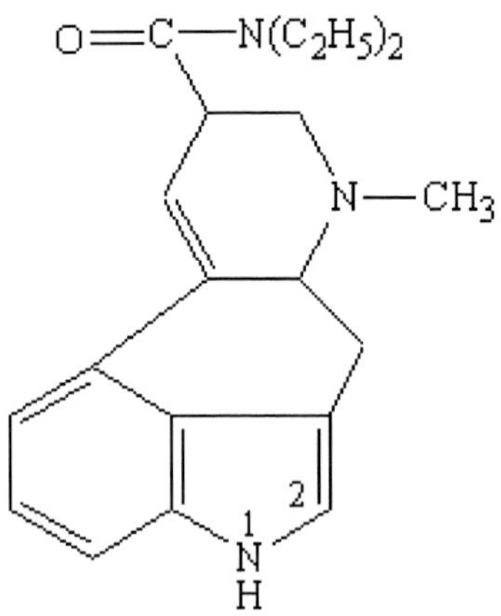

Diethylamide of lysergic acid at dose of 0,001 mg/kg causes psychotic condition of healthy human in 5-10 hours

1-acetyl- and 1-methyl- and 2-brom-diethylamides of lysergic acid also have psychotomimetic effects, but at doses two to ten times greater than that of LSD, and the duration of effect decreases to one to six hours. There are more than 100 presently known amides of lysergic acid that cause psychotic disorders; their effects are weaker and shorter in duration in comparison with LSD. Only in accordance with a clinical picture of an experimental psychosis is it possible to define what test substance was injected. The first monitoring of the action of LSD on a human belongs to its pioneer, chemist Hofmann, who described his sensations as follows: "… in the afternoon I was obliged to stop work in the laboratory and to go home because I felt wonderful anxiety and light dizziness. At home I lay down and I was surprised by the occurrence of a pleasant sensation of intoxication with excitation of the imagination. Light seemed to me too bright; with closed eyes I observed fantastic, exclusively soft pictures with an intensive kaleidoscopical play of colors. This condition continued for two hours."

It is necessary to especially underline the insignificant general-toxic action of LSD. Intravenously, LD_{50} for mice is 45–60 mg/kg, for rats 15–16 mg/kg, for rabbits 0.3 mg/kg, for elephants 0.1 mg/kg, and a monkey died in a neurotic state after injection of the usual dose for this species of 0.02 mg/kg. The majority of researchers in tests on volunteers and during self observation used doses of 0.1–0.25 mg (0.0012–0.003 mg/kg), and, more rarely, 0.25–0.75 mg (up to 0.009 mg/kg). The maximum dose taken by a healthy human was 1.7 mg. The psychotic phenomena with administration of average doses (0.1–0.15 mg) are observed in 30–40 min, reach their peak in 1.5–2 hours, and end between 8–12 hours. The high specificity of LSD regarding its influence on nervous structures allows consideration that this substance affects the synapse. Acetylcholine promotes the transfer of nervous impulse, and adrenaline and serotonin inhibit it. Tranquilizers block the action of adrenaline or release serotonin. Serotonin (5-hydroxytriptamine) has essential importance for CNS activity. Both formation and splitting of serotonin occurs in brain tissues. Hallucinogens, especially LSD, have a similar effect with serotonin and adrenaline, and also can promote adrenaline release. Any malfunction of this difficult balance can cause psychotic symptoms.

Analysis of most data shows that hypotheses regarding the binding psychotomimetic effect of LSD with intervention in serotonin exchange have sufficient proof. At the same time, it is necessary to state the absence of convincing data testifying to the connection of the psychotomimetic effect of LSD with suppression of choline esterase activity; by the same token, the clinical picture of psychosis cannot be explained only by the superfluous accumulation of acetylcholine. Also, the question regarding therapy of lysergic psychosis is not solved, although there are preparations (nicotinic acid, mescaline, and, to a lesser degree, aminazine [(α-dimethylaminopropyl)-2-chlorophenothiazine hydrochloride]) whose application is recommended by G.I. Milshtein, R.A. Ivanova, etc.

The somewhat small amount of synthesized derivatives of lysergic acid is explained by the limitation of raw material. Acid is allocated by multistage extraction of a methanolic solution of alkali from spore formation—the result of cereal culture disease with ergot. The insufficient range of the researched compounds does not allow some essential conclusions about the interconnection between structure and effect. A purely synthetic method for LSD production has been developed; however, it is multistage, and the yield of final product is extremely low.

A completely different picture is observed with examination of the second group of psychotomimetics—glycolates, synthetic preparations with the following structure:

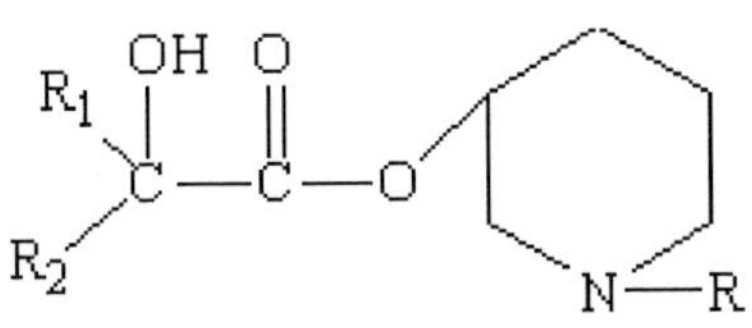

If $R=CH_3, C_2H_5$; $R_1=R_2=C_6H_5$,
than such compounds are psychoactive.

N-methyl-3-piperidile-benzylate in a dose of 0.1–0.2 mg/kg leads to a malfunction of mental capacity for a duration of 10 hours. Replacement of one or both phenyl groups with other aryl cycles, cyclohexyl or cyclopentyl radicals leads to an increase in psychoactivity. G.I. Milshtein et al., on the basis of the analysis of a number of works, including the publications of Abood and Gabel, came to the conclusion that phenylic, tiophenic, cycloalkyl or 1-hydroxycycloalkyl groupings are optimum for R_1 (at R_2 = phenyl). In diphenylglycolates, the replacement of hydrogen in the phenylic ring with chloro-, methyl-, methoxy- and 3,4-dioxymethyl groups completely removes both psychotomimetical and cholinolitic activity. Gabel and Abood consider that the most active substances are those with an undivided pair of electrons in the nitrogen atom of the alcohol part of the molecule which, apparently, for achievement of pharmacological effect, should be connected with any electrophylic site of appropriate receptor surface. Derivatives of 3-quinuclidinol have the highest psychotomimetic activity among examined substances. A decrease in the psychoactivity of compounds depending on the structure of aminoalcohol are in the following range:

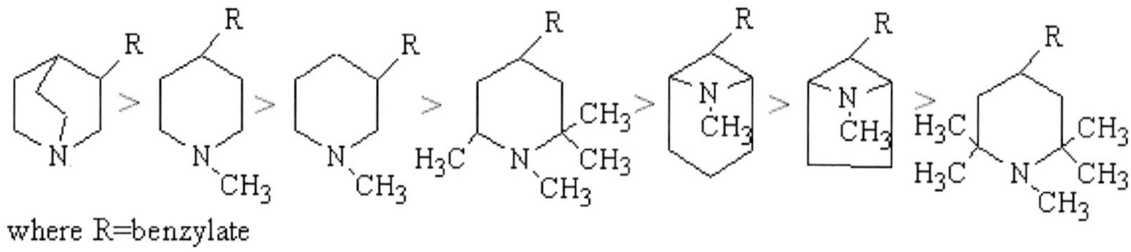

Regarding the mechanism of psychotomimetic action, a direct connection between psychotomimetic and central M-cholinolitic properties has been found, and the high cholinomimetic activity of psychotomimetics of this group and the possible reduction of these effects with preparations that act as inhibitors of choline esterase shows definitively that the cholinolitic mechanism is central in the progression of psychotomimetic effects. If the intensity of malfunctions of higher nervous activity and the central M-cholinolityc activity of psychotomimetics is in direct dependence, then there is no correlation between these properties in the case of peripheral M-cholinolitic activity, in spite of the fact that there are hypotheses concerning the similarity in structure of M-cholinergic receptors in the centre and at the periphery. The metabolic malfunctions accompanying the progress of experimental psychosis, obviously, are not limited by the cholinergic system. A number of hypotheses about the mechanisms action of psychotomimetics have been presented; each of them casts doubt for various reasons, and the creation of a definitive theory explaining the mechanisms of psychotomimetic activity of central cholinolitics, in particular glycolates, is future work. At the same time, the facts known at present allowed G.I. Milshtein to draw the conclusion that the leading link in the system of malfunctions that appear in an organism under the influence of a psychotomimetic of a given type is the selective blockade of M-cholinergic receptors in structures of the central nervous system.

The most psychoactive compounds in this range are N-ethyl-3-piperidile-phenylcyclo-pentyl glycolate and 3-quinuclidinile-diphenyl glycolate (BZ). The first compound and its analogues were obtained and examined in the Likeside laboratory, and subsequently they were studied in detail in the Edgewood arsenal, also on male military volunteers. The psychoses caused by these substances proceeds approximately over a period of 20–24 hours and almost do not differ from authentic mental diseases. The threshold dose for humans (per os) is 5–15 mg to 70 kg of weight. The first signs of poisoning are iris dilatation (mydriasis), muscular weakness, dry mouth and palpitations. In approximately one hour, intensive hallucinations, speech infringements, loss of ability to concentrate, and disorientation appear. Hallucinations (visual, acoustical and tactile) disconnect the subject from his environment, and his movements and behavior are defined by these hallucinations (raising of nonexistent objects, dancing with no existing partner and without music, etc.).

Piperidile benzylates are being developed with a high yield by reesterification of methyl ester of benzyl acid with appropriate aminoalcohols in boiling solvent and in the presence of sodium methylate:

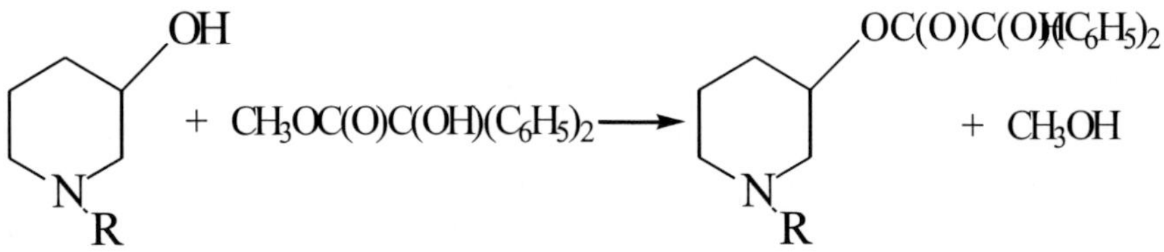

In 1961, 3-quinuclidinile-diphenyl glycolate (3-quinuclidinile benzylate, BZ) was added to the U.S. armory because of its high psychotomimetic activity (threshold dose is 2 mg for humans) and because of its rather simple synthesis. Manufacture of 3-quinuclidinole is mastered by pharmplants, as this aminoalcohol is a component and semiproduct for a number of medicines (acyclidine, etc.). The method for obtaining benzyl acid from accessible benzyl has been known to synthesists for a long time by a classical regrouping according to Gatterman-Wieland:

$$C_6H_5COCOC_6H_5 \longrightarrow (C_6H_5)_2C(OH)\text{-}COOH$$

Synthesis of 3-quinuclidinile benzylate is similar to that of glycolates of piperidine-ole derivatives. By toxicity level, BZ is several times inferior to LSD. The intoxication of a human with BZ is characterized by the expressed inhibition of mental capacity and orientation malfunction in surrounding conditions. The only effective route of administration is inhalation. BZ is a solid that does not penetrate cutaneous membranes, and it is converted to aerosol form by pyrotechnic means. The usual volatility of the substance is not sufficient for achievement of an effective concentration (volatility is $2.6 \cdot 10^{-6}$ mg/m^3 at 25°C). An insufficiently high level of toxicity, absence of dermatoresorptive affect, unpredictability of behaviour of the affected, and the high cost of the substance were the reasons for its discontinuation as a weapon. And though no fewer than 800 incapacitating glycolates were synthesized and examined within the United States CWA development program, not one of them surpassed BZ in number of properties, and the only success was obtaining glycolates with an unctuous consistency capable of penetrating through skin.

The third group of psychotomimetics includes cannabinols, the active principal ingredient of cannabis; 1-hydroxy-6,6,9-trimethyl-3-pentyldibenzopyran (cannabinol) is the parent of some synthetic analogues and, in particular, tetrahydrocannabinol (U.S. classification EA 1476).

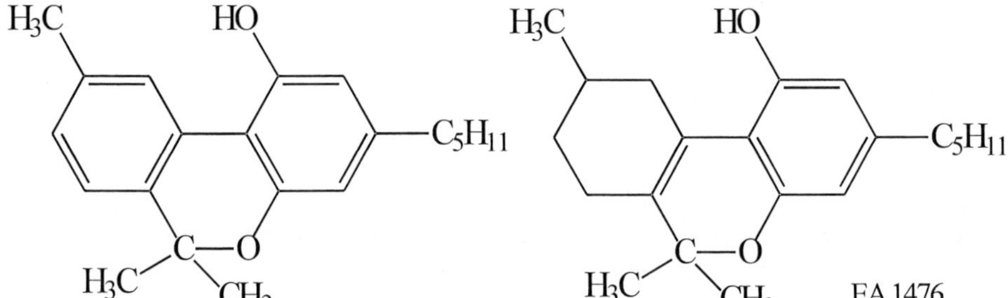

EA 1476

This substance is 10 times less active than cannabinol. In doses of 0.02–0.055 mg/kg it causes hypotension, hypothermia and analgesia, and at doses more than 0.06 mg/kg there are hallucinations. With inhalation, both natural and synthetic analogues of cannabinol are more active than with oral administration. Substance EA 1476 with intravenous injection at doses of 0.001–0.002 mg/kg lowers blood pressure at a value of 20–40 millimeters of mercury, and at a dose of 0.005 mg/kg the human loses fighting capacity at a value of 80%. The intensity and character of influence of EA 1476 isomers on the CNS depends on the arrangement of the double bond in the cyclohexane cycle, and on the type of joint with the ring of pirane and on optical activity. Laevorotatory EA 1476 is two times more active than dextrorotatory. Regarding speed, cannabinols are inferior to glycolates and psychotomimetics of other ranges; their synthesis is multi-staged and difficult, they do not produce effects with cutaneous application and they are hardly interesting as CWAs. However, in recent years, cannabisol was synthesized (derivative of hexahydrocannabinol) with a very high hypotensive activity—the minimum effective dose causing a drop in blood pressure is 0.00001 mg/kg, and an oral dose of 1 mg causes an expressed frustration of mentality.

The fourth group of psychotomimetics concerns known alkaloids and their derivatives, psilocin (4-hydroxy-N, N-dimethyltriptamin):

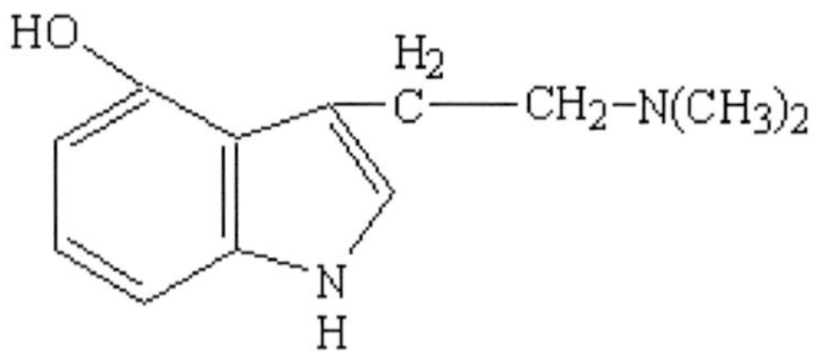

Substance causes psychotomimetic action at dose of 0,1-0,2 mg/kg in course of 2-4 hours

The synthesized analogues of psilocin, triptamine derivatives, have the same or weaker psychotomimetic activity. The same tendency is typical for derivatives of phenylethylamine. The parent of this psychotomimetic group, alkaloid mescaline (the active principal ingredient of some the Mexican mushrooms), causes modeling psychosis with a duration of 10–12 hours at a dose of 5–10 mg/kg. The most active of phenylethylamine derivatives is 2,5-dimethoxy-4-methylamphetamine:

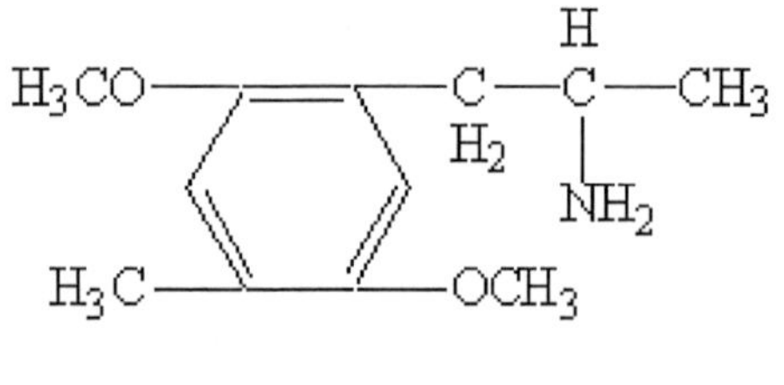

Subsance causes malfunction of mentality at dose of 0,05mg/kg in course up to 10 hours

Other alkaloids—garmine, iohimbine, ibogaine, cocaine, bufotenine, atropine and scopolamine—show weaker psychotomimetic activity than the psychotomimetics mentioned above. This short examination of psychotomimetics must be supplemented with two more synthetic preparations. The first, phencyclidine, or 1-(1-phenylcyclohexyl)-piperidine, was discovered in 1956 and has the following formula:

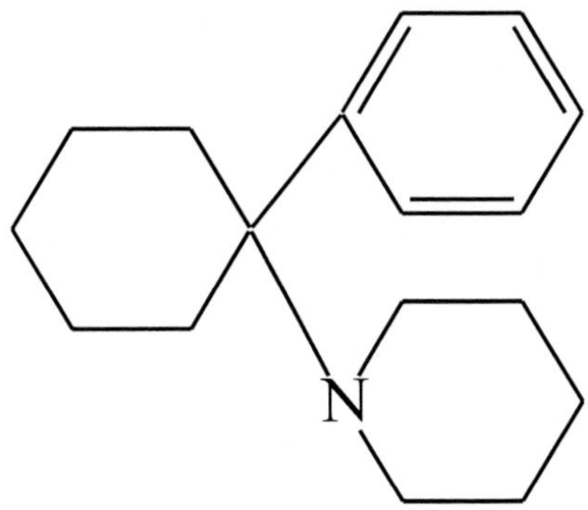

Depending on dose, this substance causes a wide spectrum of toxic effects to humans, from light psychomotor excitation to deep coma. In a dose of 5 mg per human, phencyclidine causes logopathy and decomposition of movement over a course of two to four hours. At a dose of more than 20 mg, convulsions and coma are typical, and with psychosis anesthetization appears, leading to full immobilization. It is inferior to glycolates in accordance with the level of psychotomimetic activity.

One more synthetic preparation was synthesized in China in 1972: 3-methylfentanyl, which is the most powerful narcotic and analgesic (see further). It is 500–2,000 times more active than heroin, and in accordance with level of activity level it surpasses many psychotomimetics.

These successes allow the hope that, among synthetic organic substances, extremely highly active psychotomimetics will be found, the study of which will bring us closer to understanding the mechanism of their interaction with the biological systems of an organism and, finally, it will provide the possibility for effective treatment of mental disorders.

Unlike psychotomimetics, which cause mental disorders, from the end of the 1970s great attention was given to dysregulators—*physicants*, or substances causing somewhat short-term physical or physiological malfunctions: immobilization, catalepsy, imbalance of blood pressure, tremor, long-term exhaustion and regularly repeating desire to vomit, defecate or urinate, etc. Physicants include narcotic analgesics, neuroleptics, tremorgens and emetics.

The group of narcotic analgesics includes derivatives of morphine and fentanyl, which have an immobilization effect. Derivatives of morphine are products of the processing of natural raw material (opium); they have a high cost and are not accessible. Their advantage is high activity (for example, an effective dose [ED_{50}] of 14-methoxymetapone for a mouse, with subcutaneous administration, is 0.000019 mg/kg), safety of use, rapid action and stable effect of immobilization. In the 1980s in Canada, the synthesis of a stronger narcotic analgesic with an unusual structure (ED_{50}, mouse, subcutaneous administration, is equal to 0.0000037 mg/kg) was carried out.

Narcotic analgesics of the fentanyl group 1-(2-phenylethyl)-4-(N-propionyl phenylamino)-piperidine causing analgesia and anaesthesia at doses of 0.01–0.001 mg/kg are toxic enough (for fentanyl, LD_{50} = 3.5 mg/kg). Modification of fentanyl into tens and hundreds of its derivatives were synthesized, among which were found highly effective analgesics.

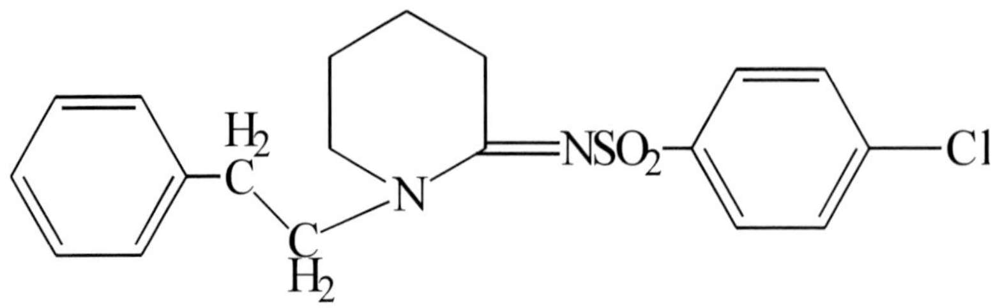

The immobilization dose ED_{50} for various animals for one of them (carfentanyl) is equal to 0.0008–0.02 mg/kg, and with it activity is shown in various routes of administration to an organism, including inhalation of vapors and aerosols. Tret.butyl analogue of carfentanyl has the highest level of analgesic activity (in rats, intravenously, ED_{50} is 0.000021 mg/kg). Another derivative of fentanyl, sufentanyl, causes deep analgesia in humans in a dose of 0.0129 mg/kg, and three minutes after injection of 0.0189 mg/kg causes full loss of consciousness. The analogue of sufentanyl, substance A-3080, is not inferior according to activity level, but is safer with intramuscular administration and able of causing immobilization; for example, for elk, intramuscular administration ED_{50} is 0.00088 mg/kg. This substance represents indubitable interest for workers employed in breeding and migration of large and predatory animals, and for zoologists and researchers of wild animals.

Neuroleptics cause various movement disorders, mainly are akathisia (the urge to move continuously) and acute dystonia (spasms, involuntary clonuses, gait and speech disorders). Among physicants, neuroleptics are the least toxic substances, causing movement disorders in healthy humans 0.5–4.0 hours after injection lasting 6–12 hours and not affecting the level of mental capacity. These include are butyrophenons, phenothiazines and certain tioxantans and benzamides. Neuroleptics are inferior to the dysregulators mentioned above according to activity, and they now represent no special interest.

Tremorgens comprise the third group of physicants; they were actively examined in the 1960s. Hundreds of tremorin analogues were synthesized. The most active was 1-(2-oxopyrrolidine)-4-pyrrolidine-2-butene (oxotremorin). With different applications for different kinds of animals, ED_{50} is equal to 0.05–0.15 mg/kg, wherein a tremor is observed with a duration of one to two hours. At higher doses, ataxia, analgesia, hypothermia and drop in blood pressure, accompanied by peripheral effects (salivation, lachrymation and diarrhea) are noted.

Emetics, comprising the fourth group of physicants, are the substances with strong emetic action. They include two subgroups: a) alkaloids and synthetic substances with non-protein structure, and b) toxins (polypeptides). In the subgroup "a," interest can be represented by derivatives of apomorphine, of aminotetralin, polycyclic nitrogen-containing compounds, and alkaloid ricin. The best known polypeptide emetic is staphylococcal enterotoxin B. It should be underlined that natural emetics have a greater level of emetic activity, longer latency time (hours) and longer duration of poisoning (days). One author of this book, at the age of 10, along with a group of more than 10 peers, ate from one to eight castor beans, thinking that it was edible fruit. In six to eight hours, everybody had strong vomiting with attacks every three to five minutes. Cleansing was ineffective because of the latency period, during which part of the beans' alkaloids were soaked up by mucous membranes. And though part of the beans were vomited up, vomiting attacks nevertheless continued for one to one-and-one-half days and then less frequently for another one-and-one-half days. As a whole, only after approximately three days was it possible to speak about amelioration. The boys were so weakened by constant emetic attacks that they could not eat any food and only forced themselves to drink, at the insistence of the doctor, a solution of potassium permanganate that was given at once at the next urge to vomit. All survived, but the condition of everyone was directly connected with the overall condition of his own health before the incident: three from the group with weakened health (hunger and constant malnutrition in post-war 1946) were in almost critical condition. This case appreciably influenced the choice of the future speciality of one of the authors.

Contrary to natural emetics, synthetic versions differ in speed and short-term period of disability inflicted in humans. However, both synthetic and natural emetics produce effects with various routes of administration, including inhalation. Apomorphine causes vomiting in humans at a dose of 0.08 mg/kg, intramuscularly. The limited availability of apomorphine and its derivatives owes to its natural raw material base (opium). Derivatives of aminotetralin do not have this disadvantage, and they are approximately identical according to activity with the most active derivatives of apomorphine. Recently, an emetic 10 times more active than other synthetic emetics was synthesized:

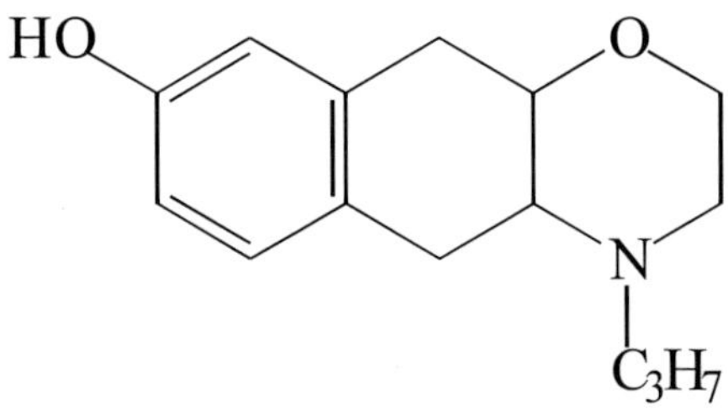

In the United States during the post-war period, staphylococcal enterotoxin (SEB) was examined. Its disabling dose is 2,000 times more active than apomorphine, and an ED_{50} equal to 0.0001–0.001 mg/kg with different routes of administration causes strong vomiting. According to the Biological Weapons Convention of 1972, SEB is forbidden, and we mention it just as an example of an incapacitant with a polypeptide structure.

Along with the irritants, psychotomimetics and physicants considered above, whose effects in moderate doses usually completely disappear, there are substances also having at moderate doses an incapacitating action, but their effects are irreversible and they remain to some extent for the rest of the victim's life, by analogy to the consequences of mechanical or thermal damage. They are called *substances with mutilating effect*, and sulphurous and nitrogenous yperit and lewisite are among them.

In July of 1917, near Ypres, English troops were attacked by German land mines containing yperite. So began a new stage of conducting chemical war—military application of long-term, stable CWAs. Yperite was examined and recommended as a CWA by German chemists Lommel and Steinkopf. This CWA in any aggregative state is able to cause, depending on dose, different effects, beginning with conjunctivitis and erythema, and ending with a possible lethal outcome. Its influence appeared not only in an attack with a "primary" cloud of vapors and drops, but also as victims remained at the site of defeat after hours and days of chemical attack. Unprotected humans remaining in the affected are inevitably subjected to so-called "secondary" defeats. It affects the eyes, the respiratory and gastrointestinal tract and cutaneous membranes. Ordinary clothing does not protect from yperite vapors and drops. And though the first cases of its application in World War I were stunningly effective, in the subsequent process of studying its chemical and toxic properties and development of protection against it, the results of its influence were minimized. According to expert calculations, in the days of World War I, approximately 1.5 tons of yperite were needed to cause one fatality. According to the United States, among 272,000 losses of the American expeditionary corps, 26.8% were affected with CWA, and only 2% of them died. On this basis, the former commanding general of the U.S. Army Chemical Corps Research and Development Command, Brigadier General J.H. Rothschild, referred to yperite as falling within the category of incapacitants in his book, *Tomorrow's Weapons.*

In order to affect the skin, the lethal dose of yperite in steam is equal to 10,000 mg•min/m^3; in liquid it is 70mg/kg. The eyes are somewhat sensitive to yperite steam; at a concentration of 150mg•min/m^3 military personnel are incapacitated because of conjunctivitis and erythema. At small doses, these effects disappear in a few days, and at higher doses there are blisters filled with a colorless or yellowish liquid on the skin which, in a few days, burst and form slow-healing ulcers that ultimately leave scars on the skin that are similar to those left by burns. With higher doses of yperite, conjunctivitis and photophobia lead to the closing of the eyelids and keratoleukoma. Inflammation and bronchitis last for three to four days. At a higher concentration, incessant cough, obmutescence, retrosternal pain, urge to vomit, and hypostasis of lungs are typical for upper airway passages. Lung and eye disorders lead to loss of health and working capacity, people are afflicted with shortness of breath, and they partially or completely lose vision and become vulnerable to infectious diseases. Similar effects are observed in exposure to nitrogenous yperite and lewisite. These incapacitants are comprehensively described in any textbook covering the chemistry and technology of CWAs, as these are the most accessible in industrial production owing to their low cost and high level of effectiveness.

As a whole, the most active incapacitants according to disabling effect reach the level of nerve gases and are exceded only by staphylococcal enterotoxin SEB. Mycotoxins do not represent interest as disabling substances. Even the most toxic among them, toxin T-2, according to the level of disabling dose, is ten or more times inferior to active incapacitants. The activity of yperite is also low, although based on this indicator in the days of World War I it was accepted as "the king of gases." As less active psychotomimetics, tremorgens and other neuroleptics lost their importance. Table 4 there lists the levels of disabling doses of incapacitants in comparison with nerve gases. We can see that the most active among narcotic analgesics, synthetic emetics and irritants reach the level of doses of organophosphorus CWAs.

The quantity of potential incapacitants continuously grows, first of all, because of analgesics, emetics and other substances with similar toxic effect, whereas the prohibition of the Chemical Weapons Convention of 1993 does not extend to their research and application. At the same time, synthetics—the focus of the search for new pharmacological preparations for medicine and veterinary applications—result in many "wastes," which include substances with high incapacitant activity.

Table 4. Doses of toxic agents with disabling effect

Substance	Dose	
	ICt_{50}, mg·min/m^3	LD_{50}, mg/kg
Irritants	0.7–1.0(eyes) 0.15 (respiratory organs) 5.0 (skin)	—
Psychotomimetics LSD Synthetic	 30 125–400	 0.002 (per oral) 0.14–0.3
Narcotic analgesics	0.07–0.35	0.00002–0.02
Neuroleptics	—	0.26
Tremorgens	700	0.15–0.05
Emetics Staphylococcic enterotoxin B (SEB) Synthetic	 0.6 5.0	 0.0004 —
Vizicants (yperit)	150–200 (eyes) 2000 (skin)	—
Mycotoxins (T-2)	—	0.1
Nerve paralytic CWA (organo-phosphour compounds)	5–15 0.09–0.1 (miosis) 1.6 (tremor)	—

In the beginning of the chapter, a number of requirements for toxic agents were outlined, and it was underlined that no one substance met all of them. However, in some cases, it is possible to correct and improve certain properties by creation of mixed forms, which is analogous to the age-old practice of deriving prescription forms of medicinal substances. There were successful and unsuccessful attempts to use prescriptions to increase toxic agents' efficiency in World War I. Highly toxic cyanhydric acid, discussed previously, did not bring appreciable military success to the French because it was difficult to create a high enough concentration. Unsatisfactory physical and chemical properties, especially low density of vapor, compelled the Frenchto add heavier and high-boiling substances to cyanhydric acid. Thus, a mix was formulated that contained 50% HCN, 30% $AsCl_3$, 15% $SnCl_4$ and 5% $CHCl_3$ (*vinsenit*). Also, different mixes of cyanhydric acid with trichloro arsenic (*mantanit*) or a mix of cyanhydric acid with chlorocyanogen (*mangvinit*) were formulated. The Soviet Army was armed with a compound called RK-7, a mix of yperite and lewisite. This compound combines the level of yperite toxicity with the rapid action of lewisite, and hardens at lower temperatures in comparison with yperite. In the United States, a compound was developed on the basis of incapacitants, a solution of psychotomimetic BZ in liquid irritant CH. For the purpose of prolonged action, the U.S. Army used CS in Vietnam in the form of compounds CS-1 and CS-2 with silica gel as the sorbent carrier. With the same success, it is possible to use microencapsulation and other methods of modification of certain physical, chemical, toxic (for example, increase of level of cutaneous activity, etc.), tactical and other properties of any toxic agent. In some cases, these modifications result in the creation of toxic agents not only with optimum volatility, but also in liquid form, which provides good penetration through the skin and other barriers and allows realization of its application in explosive ammunition rather than the usual pyromixtures for solid CWAs. Certain interests represent the insertion of polar solvents into the structure of compounds (for example, dimethyl sulfoxide, capable of penetrating easily through intact skin, or "azone" [1-dodecylaza-cycloheptane-2-on]), accelerating the penetration of toxic agents through the skin. It is no coincidence that the U.S. Army had a program to develop liquid incapacitants which, unlike solid, can be applied in binary ammunition and transformed into vapor or aerosol by means of explosion. Until the 1980s, all chemical ammunition was equipped with CWAs, produced in special factories. Then, in the United States, so-called binary chemical ammunition was created. It is necessary to suppose that binary ammunition can also be developed in other countries. The principle of action of the binary weapon is simple: the ammunition body is used as a chemical reactor, in which the final stage of synthesis of the CWA from two precursors (initial semiproducts) is realized. The mixing of precursors, for example, in artillery shells occurs as a result of the destruction of the partition between them at the moment of discharge, to preserve the integrity of the ammunition's body. After destruction of the partition, the contents of the container located in the head part of the shell mixes with the contents of the rear container, at first because of the hydraulic blow, and later because of shell rotation in the channel of the barrel and further during flight. In binary aerial bombs, battle parts of rockets and jet shells, various devices are used for mixing, and mixing is carryied out, as a rule, at the moment of a rocket's launch or bombardment. Transition to binary chemical ammunition has a number of advantages at the manufacturing stage, in transportation and storage and even in the subsequent destruction. Precursors are produced in the usual chemical manufacturing facilities, which do not require difficult and expensive systems of safety maintenance, which are obligatory and necessary in the manufacture of CWAs. Binary ammunition has a number of advantages over unitary ammunition, as it allows changing the structure of CWAs even in battle positions by replacement of containers or even a change to binary ammunition for other purposes (smoke, incendiary, agitation, etc.). However, binary ammunition has an uncorrected disadvantage, in particular, with the necessity for optimum time from firing a shot to explosion, which is necessary for chemical reaction; construction of such ammunition does not allow application of the central arrangement of explosive charge, which is the most favorable, and a number of other ammunition lacks. Experts consider that, on the basis of battle efficiency, the use of binary ammunition cannot be equaled and, moreover, surpasses similar unitary ammunition equipped with the same CWA, though the manufacture of chemical contents for the latter is approximately two times more expensive. Binary ammunition was created for oganophosphorus CWAs with lethal action. However, it is possible to use in them as incapacitants, a number of which were not prohibited by the Chemical Weapons Convention. It is possible to believe that the current level of incapacitants' activity can be surpassed in the near future, and there will be a temptation for certain organizations and states to create new kinds of chemical weapons bypassing the Convention. The necessity to create an effective mechanism to control such activity that bypasses the Convention is dictated also by other important circumstances. In the second half of the twentieth century, there were qualitative changes in the economy of the majority of the countries of the world in connection with the development and creation of their own petrochemical industry. By the beginning of World War II, no more than 10–15 countries were referred to as industrially developed; at the present time there are already more than 50 of them. The developed chemical and petrochemical industries of these countries is based not only on a comprehensively branched infrastructure, but also on the wide use of modern technologies and, in particular, "double-purpose technologies" in which short-term manufacture can transition from general peace-time economic production to manufacture of chemical weapons, and vice versa. The difficulty to control such infringements of the Convention is obvious. For this reason, it is impossible to stop at the current level of chemical disarmament. Continual, all-around and effective international control of activity of certain chemical organizations and enterprises is necessary, although it is difficult to attain under modern conditions.

10.1. Destruction of Chemical Weapons: History, Problems, and More

The problem of destruction of natural poisons was not present before the development of laboratory synthesis as a source and tool for their study. However, after the appearance of the first samples of new synthetic poisons, their timely and purposeful transformation into nontoxic substances (degasation) became necessary. The process of degasation was connected at first with the destruction of the toxic principle of synthesized products, and subsequently gained wider understanding and began to include all processes that serve the purpose of removal of a CWA or poison from any environment and surface of any object. Chemical and physical means of degasation are being developed for the realization of this process. Nowadays, such means target diversified substances in different aggregative states, and include solvent washing, sorption and other agents capable of removing toxic agents from decontaminated objects and simultaneously transforming them into nontoxic compounds. It is necessary to distinguish degasating substances from antipoisons or antidotes used to counteract poisons directly in a human organism. Development of the chemistry and technology of antidotes began to be included in the sphere of research and manufacture not only of traditional antidotes, but also in the creation of complex, protective and preventive compounds that allow healthy people to resist the effects of toxic substances. The chemistry and technology of degasating tools grew simultaneously with the development and perfection of poisons and became an independent branch of the science dealing with problems of indication (qualitative and quantitative detection of toxic agents in different environments) and degasation of toxic agents, and, for the last 50 years, all aspects of their destruction.

For the first time, the question of destruction of chemical weapons (CWs) arose after the end of World War I in the period of preparation and acceptance of the Chemical Weapons Convention regarding CW prohibition. Beginning with the Brussels Conference of 1874, a great number of declarations and decisions have provided guidelines regarding the prohibition of CWAs and bacteriological weapons of war. However, it was not until the

Geneva protocol of June 17, 1925 that the basis of future international agreements in this area was achieved.

Former adveraries still had large stocks of unused CWAs, both at manufacturing facilities and in army warehouses in the form of equipped ammunition. Moreover, questions regarding the use of already-built and functioning devices of CWAs demanded an urgent solution. Some countries did not sign the Geneva Convention, and a number of those who signed, including the USSR, reserved the right of a reciprocal "chemical" response to an aggressor. There were prerequisites for substitution of a CWA, its destruction and its assimilation (transition or repurposing of a CWA to the category of chemical semiproducts used for production of nontoxic products that had wide application in everyday life and engineering). Objectively, this substitution was stimulated, on one hand, with large financial and industrial investments with no prospect of compensation and, on the other hand, with the presence of effective examples of assimilation of chemical products used as CWAs in World War I. For instance, various valuable and sometimes unique products in industrial volume, such as chlorine, phosgene and cyanhydric acid, found broad use. This circumstance allowed maintaining a necessary inventory of a number of CWAs, which were formally designated as semiproducts of national-economic use.

The circumstances mentioned above stimulated the search in the 1920s for methods to assimilate, first of all, the largest stocks at that time and production capacities of yperite and arsenic-containing toxic agents (Clarke I, diphenylchloroarsine; Clarke II, diphenylcyanogenarsin; lewisite, β-chlorovinyldichloroarsine; and adamsite, 10-chloro-5,10-dehydrophenarsazin). However, in spite of numerous research studies, effective means of assimilation of these substances have not been found. Certain hopes were set on yperite use in the manufacture of thiokol rubber; however, they were not justified, and the same held true for arsenic-containing toxic agents. Because of the high toxicity of an overwhelming number of their derivatives, they were not found at all acceptable in the sphere of economic use. At the same time, in the 1920s and 1930s, some simple, reliable and effective tools and methods of degasation of different objects and protection of army personnel and civilians were developed. These included degasators, gas masks, antidotes and other protection tools for people.

Thus, during this period, despite certain scientific and technical and political movements in the solution to the problem of prohibition and destruction of CWs, industrially-developed countries continued to work on perfecting these agents, and the problem of their destruction, assimilation and degasation became a local issue. The ongoing threat of their application and rise of operating manufacturing facilities was clearly demonstrated by fascist Italy in 1935–1936, which produced and applied its own CWAs, including blistering agents, in the war against Abyssinia.

The next period, from the end of World War II until the 1980s (activization of work on the new agreement project), brought new features in the interpretation of the problem of CW destruction. Along with continuation of work in perfecting a new generation of CWs in the 1950s to the 1970s, community demand regarding chemical disarmament became more and more persistent, which began to gain government attention. International protocols related to prohibiting the development, manufacture and accumulation of stocks of bacteriological (biological) and toxic weapons and their destruction were set in place with the Biological

Weapons Convention, signed on April 10, 1972 in Washington, London and Moscow. Main approaches, principles and concepts of this document were used and developed taking into account specific features of chemical weapons. Successful and effective work on the Convention project was also promoted by a range of other objectives. The essential factor that affecting decisions regarding the destruction of CWs was the USSR's and the United States' enormous stockpiles (40 and 32 thousand tons, respectively). The duration of their storage (30 or more years) made the problem of safe storage of CWs more and more critical because of the possible decomposition of toxic agents and the gradual destruction of containers, shells and bombs. And though Russian chemical ammunition, owing to its construction features and material composition, is more stabile than American ammunication in storage, ammunition especially made during World War II began to draw attention. Another essential factor stimulating the development of the Convention was the appearance of new types of weapons based on efficiency which surpassed toxic agents. In addition to that, substantiation and promulgation by Russian experts regarding the impossibility to add to stockpiles of toxic agents (see above) led to the fading of interest in toxic agents as a type of weapon. These factors promoted the acceptance of political decisions by the governments of the USSR and the United States in coming to an effective and universal agreement about toxic agents. The result of collective efforts was the text of the Chemical Weapons Convention on the prohibition of development, production, accumulation and application of the chemical weapons and their destruction, signed on January 13, 1993 by President George H.W. Bush. The representative of Russia signed it on the same day, and after ratification by the State Duma on November 5, 1997, it went into effect. This Convention opened the closing stage in relation to toxic agents—a stage of prohibition, reduction and real destruction.

The Convention is a multilateral agreement on chemical disarmament in accordance with the international control of numerous complex questions and basic requirements of all aspects of this problem. Its main, necessary and key condition and requirement is observance of safeguards in the broadest sense of this definition. Destruction of CWs on an industrial basis should, along with maintaining the safety of people living in territories adjoining CW facilities, provide guaranteed protection of the environment according to national standards concerning safety and industrial emissions. Each state determines in what way it will destroy CWs but the following methods are excluded as potentially dangerous:

- submersion in any reservoirs
- burial in the ground
- burning in open air

The methods above are unacceptable because of possible environmental contamination, and their exclusion is based on practical experience. Let's return to the battle-scarred Europe of 1945. The winning nations received not only the trophy of the next generation of CW technology, documentation, equipment and experts, but also enormous stockpiles of CWs. According to the Potsdam Agreement, the demilitarization of fascist Germany required an urgent solution to the issue of the destruction of these stockpiles. A military directorate in September 1945 accepted a document, the first point of which was: "Destroy, burn and sink in the sea all tools of chemical war." Some months later, a committee of the Allied Supervisory Commission governing military materials developed and accepted a document (November 1945) determining "a way of chemical weapon liquidation by submergence in the sea, as *just one practically-realized way*" at that time (italicized by us). Submergence of CWs was carried out by the military administration of each zone of occupation independently in a number of areas of the Baltic, Northern and White Seas, the Atlantic and Arctic Oceans. The task ended in December of 1947. The total quantity of submerged CWs by the Soviet occupational armies was no less than 11,000 tons, with a prevalence among them of blistering toxic agents (yperite, lewisite). Among the CWs submerged by the Allies were the first organo-phosphorus nervous-paralytic toxic agents (tabun and sarin). A certain quantity may have been used by the Allies for studying and organizing their own research. Up to 1971, no control over the condition of submerged toxic agents by any of the countries was attempted. However, in connection with the activity of "green" interests of the public and publications in the mass media, some practical attempts were undertaken to identity the presence of toxic agents in the ground and waters near the areas in which the CWs were submerged. Primary investigations were carried out by Germany in 1971–1972, Norway in 1989, and Sweden in 1991 in the Skagerrak strait and Denmark in 1992 in Bornholm hollow. Of course, nothing was found, despite a report about the detection of yperite and "its derivatives" by Danes in one of several hundreds of tests of bottom sediment that can be interpreted as an experimental error. Let us also notice that in one of the many hundreds of tests of bottom water in 2001 on the station built in the Skagerrack strait, sarin was found (apparently, qualitatively [*editor's comment*]). In the period from the late 1990s to the beginning of the twenty-first century, within three years a Russian research ship, *Academician Shtockman*, carried out a complex examination of the influence of toxic agents or products of its half-disintegration on the ecosystem of submersion areas in the Baltic (Bornholm hollow, Danish sea channels) and in the North Sea. In a Russian chemical journal, one of the authoritative scientific editions that has regularly addressed different aspects of toxic agent problems since 1990, the oceanologist V.T. Paka wrote that not one of the many hundreds of tests showed the presence of any submerged toxic agents, and did not even detect products of their disintegration. Hydrolysis of flooded organo-phosphorus toxic agents should lead to allocation of methylphosphonic acid and its acidic isopropyl ether in the case of sarin, and phosphoric acid and its acidic ethyl ester of dimethylamidophosphate and monoethylphosphate in the case of tabun. Taking into account the absence of sensitive techniques for direct detection of these hydrolysis products, the author of research studies gives attention to the possibility of identification of organic phosphorus (C-P bond) and an increase in pH in bottom waters. Simultaneously, it is underlined that these signs "are found only near the operating source, and naturally disappear." Taking into account that the basic accumulating products of disintegration of arsenic-containing submerged toxic agents are hydrolytically stable oxide diphenylarsine (hydrolysis product of Clarke I, Clarke II), oxide of 2-chlorovinylarsine, arsenic oxide (hydrolysis products of lewisite) and adamsite, all of which are capable of being in water for many years without decomposition, numerous samples of arsenic were taken and analyzed. It was found that only one identification stood out for limits of background values; thus, as a whole, arsenic was identified in isolated spots in areas of the Baltic and the White Sea. In spite of the absence of toxic agents based on the results of the analysis, the author affirms that "at the same time, results of microbiological research testify to the presence of yperite, and it is especially indicative in the area of the White Sea." In our opinion, according to results of microbiological research studies, it is possible to make a conclusion only about the influence of yperite or products of its decomposition on studied objects, but not about its presence. Thus, the most important and main ecological question is the dynamics of observable changes, i.e., whether worsening of the environment is proceeding or whether the effects have already passed their peak and there is a renewal of the ecosystem. It can be solved only by a system set and comparative analysis of data over several years. Along with such experimental estimation, it is also impossible to exclude the possibilities of the recent intensive theoretical research, elucidated in a Russian chemical journal, concerning mathematical modeling of the transfer of toxic substances in bodies of water or forecasting the technical condition of chemical ammunition stored long-term, etc. The spectrum of opinions on identification of the degree of ecological threat is extensive—from prediction of accidents to zero effect. Starting with established data on the presence of signs of toxic agents and their influence on the ecosystem of their areas of submersion, let us point out that this influence has appeared in varopis volumes and degrees, as predicted by professional experts in the chemistry and toxicology of CWAs. They have completely dismissed the necessity to preserve and build expensive sarcophagi as unproven and invalid. At the same time, it is necessary to confirm the fact of a certain ecological threat at the microbiological level resulting from the submersion of toxic agents and the validity of including in the text of the Chemical Weapons Convention such means of their destruction.

It is clear even to those who are not experts that burial of CWs in the earth will lead to similar results. And this process of destruction will drag on not just for centuries, as in submersion, but for many hundreds or even thousands of years. Open-air burning is also potentially dangerous because of the threat of industrial accidents, equipment malfunctions and failures, and human error. In connection with the circumstances mentioned above, tens of various technologies that limited personnel contact with CWAs as much as possible and prevent their permeation into production areas and the environment were developed by the 1990s. In 1980, Russia, armed with a mobile complex of small destruction crews, removed chemical ammunition from weapons. Its technology was a double-stage method of destruction of CWs, including detoxication of CWAs and subsequent nontoxic reaction mass burning. According to the results of testing these operations (1980–1987), the completeness of destruction of CWAs was sufficient in all cases and environmental contamination was not registered. The reliability of these operations allowed a presentation of it in the residential community of Shihany (Saratov oblast) in 1987 for the purpose of demonstration to the public and to participating nations in negotiations on the Convention project. At the same time, the operations did not completely meet the requirements for industrial destruction of CWs. They were formalized legislatively subsequently in Russia (decree of President of Russia No. 314 24.03.1995) and in the United States (State Act of U.S. P102-484).

Direct burning is the most universal way of destroying CWAs. However, the complex of extremely tough standard requirements for safety and protection of the environment does not make it possible to realize it in our country. Processes of thermodestruction can be realized by many methods:

- by nuclear explosion
- in blast furnaces
- confined explosion
- by burning of liquid formulations in jet engines
- by destruction directly inside ammunition, etc.

Even from this short list, it is evident that each of these processes of thermodestruction of CWAs includes a phase of vaporous or aerosol state and consequently can cause intoxication of personnel and have a negative effect on the environment. Any reliable, ecologically sound, safe, double-stage technology of destruction of chemical ammunition equipped with organophosphorous CWA (sarin, soman, V-gases) must exclude the negative effects of CWAs mentioned above. Such a technology must include partial neutralization of ammunition, full chemical decontamination of equipped ammunition with its subsequent burning, and transfer of the CWA evacuated from ammunition to the detoxication stage. Detoxication is based on reaction of controllable hydrolysis by mixture of water and monoethanolamine (in the case of sarin and soman) and by solution of potassium butylate (in the case of V gases). As a result of hydrolysis, reaction mass is categorized according to harmfulness, from I (high toxicity) to III (low toxicity). Further reaction mass is mixed with calcium hydroxide and preheated bitumen. Calcium fluoride, calcium salts of methylphosphonic acid and its acidic esters are formed basically as a result. The generated bituminous-saline mixture of nontoxic class IV material is packed in metal drums which are removed to a landfill. Russian technology was successfully tested in a joint bilateral expert check of destruction of CWAs of both American and Russian production. Modern methods of analytical control were used during the work, including choline esterase methods of analysis, gas chromatography methods with the use of various systems of detection, along with methods of biological control. All methods showed that bituminous-saline mixtures did not contain CWAs. An international independent commission of experts accepted the Russian double-stage technology of CWA destruction.

A number of methods of destruction of CWAs with blistering effects (yperite, lewisite and their mixes) are known. The majority of them are good for decontamination of relatively small quantities in field conditions. In consideration of this technology, destruction of these CWAs should be based on the principles and requirements accepted for organophosphorous CWAs. The following methods were chosen for industrial implementation: alkaline hydrolysis of lewisite with subsequent electrolysis of reaction mass; ammonolysis of lewisite, yperite and their mixes; and chemical detoxication of yperite and its mixes with lewisite by mix of monoethanolamine and diethyleneglycol with subsequent bituminization of nontoxic reaction mass.

Destruction of lewisite should be connected with the necessity to isolate compounds of arsenic from products of destruction both for the purpose of excluding environmental contamination and for support of the possibility of their peaceful application. A committee of experts qualified alkaline hydrolysis with subsequent electrolysis of reaction mass with generation of metal arsenic (for which world demand is about 1,500 tons per year) or processing of reaction mass with generation of arsenic oxide (world production is 40,000 tons per year) as the most preferable methods of destruction of lewisite. The advantages of this method are the certain destruction of lewisite, inexpensive explosion-proof and firesafe reagents, formation of marketable products, reception of intermediate low-toxic reaction mass (harmfulness class III), and a variety of uses of products of destruction of lewisite.

The process of destruction of yperite and its double (yperite with lewisite) and threefold (yperite with lewisite in dichloroethane) mixes is based on a method of decontamination by water solution of monoethanolamine with formation of low toxic reaction masses. These reaction masses are directed further on bituminization with the generation of solid water-insoluble nontoxic products suitable for burial. We would like to note that each of the discrete operations of detoxication of any CWA (first stage) by the instrumentality of two-phasic method lasts for no more than 10 hours. The functioning of such industrial production in consideration of the quantity of stocks of CWs prone to destruction should last not more than 10 years and come to end on April 29, 2012 according to corrected international obligations undertaken by Russia (based on the decision of an international organization for control of destruction of CWs of November 2003 in satisfaction of a request of Russia and extension of the date of definitive destruction for five years). Russia's financial difficulties, in spite of the assistance of 14 countries, and an unsuccessful start-up of the first created industrial complex for destruction of CWs in 1989 in Tchapaevsk played a major role in this prolongation of terms. The active protest of the public and the population of the region, which has been supported by neighboring regions (this region had forbidden transportation of CWAs within the entire territory), compelled heads of state to find new ways of communication with the populace and press. The phenomenon of mass chemophobia (fear of living permanently in areas of deployment of potentially harmful industrial chemical objects) assumed real material consequences for the first time. The order of SM USSR No. 1564-r of September 5, 1989 adjudicated a change in the line of business in Tchapaevsk into a training centre of education and development of technologies of inert media. A new federal program on the destruction of stocks of CWs was confirmed by decree of the government of the Russian Federation, No. 305 of 1996. The decree ordered destruction of stocks of CWAs with blistering effect to be stored in vessels of the urban village of Gorny (Saratov oblast) and Kambarsky region of Udmurtia, as well as destruction of stocks of organophosphorous CWAs. Intensive research studies, experimental development and design projects were begun. In addition to the development of technologies, equipment, methods and environmental monitoring, the creation of a new legislation for the security of medical, sanitation and other aspects of safe functioning of this new segment of the chemical industry were needed. The Volgograd Research Institute of Hygiene, Toxicology and Occupational Pathology (VRIHTOP) and the St. Petersburg Research Institute of Hygiene, Occupational Pathology and Ecology of Humans (S-PtRIHOPEH) actively participated in this work. They developed and confirmed many instructive-methodological documents for the realization of state sanitary inspections of the design, creation and operation of manufacturing facilities for the destruction of CWs. The ecological and sanitary aspects of the problem of destruction of CWs are discussed in the monograph of well-known VRIHTOP hygienists P.E. Shkodich, V.V. Klauchek and ecologist V.F. Zheltobrjuhov. Experts of VRIHTOP developed and confirmed hygienic standards for destruction of CWAs in industrial and surrounding environments in terms of maximal permissible concentration (MPC), i.e., $MPC_{\text{of air of working zone}}$, $MPL_{\text{on equipment surfaces}}$, $MPC_{\text{of atmospheric air}}$, $MPC_{\text{in water of water bodies}}$, and $MPC_{\text{in soil}}$. Inspection is carried out and the background state of the environment in locations of objects of destruction is estimated. Agile control over change of the background state is also carried out. Mass diversified inspection of inhabitants living in areas of objects of destruction of CWs in the presence of mass situational phobias (chemophobia; analogous to the radiophobia discussed earlier in connection with the Chernobyl disaster) is carried out for the first time. The monograph, *Chemophobia*, by P.E. Shkodich, V.V. Klauchek and V.V. Delarju, discusses inspection and suggests methodical approaches and a system of measures (including psychohygienic) to help the formation of objective public opinion to prevent and minimize socio-psychological tension and uncertainty in ecologically problematic regions, in an effort to strengthen the mental health of the populace of large industrial centers.

A complex of research, design and construction work provided the start-up of the first industrial-scale plant in the country in the urban village Gorny in December of 2002. According to the opinion of Russian and foreign experts, this manufacturing facility has an ecologically friendly technological process, is completely automated, and the system of technological control has no analogues anywhere in the world. This start-up provided the first control stage—destruction of 1% of CWs (400 tons) until April 29, 2003 by Russia. All stocks of yperite from Gorny (622.5 tons) and 10 tons of phosgene stored in Schuchye city (Kurgan oblast) have also been destroyed. Facilities in Kambarka in the Udmurt republic (for destruction and processing of all stocks of lewisite in Russia) and in the Maradykovsky settlement of Kirov oblast (organophosphorous CWAs; the first phase is destruction of aerial bombs equipped with VX, and the second phase is for aerial ammunition equipped with soman and sarin which are scheduled to be destroyed up to the end of 2009) are built and functioning. Other kinds of ammunition equipped with these CWAs will be destroyed until April 2012. The technology of destruction of organophosphorous CWAs directly in bodies of ammunition is the last objective. The gist of this technology is extraction of ammunition from the filling unit, filling the necessary quantity of reagent into the ammunition, capsulation of the filling unit and transfer of ammunition to an intermediate storehouse (depot). Ammunition is returned in three months to the technological facility for extraction of the reaction mass, which is transferred for destruction, and the body of ammunition is transferred for remelting. By April 29, 2007, 8456 tons (or 20% from all CWA), including 3306 tons of lewisite (Kambarka), 4007 tons of VX ("Maradykovsky") were destroyed (originally scheduled for April 29, 2007). Four more facilities will be constructed and 45% of stocks of CWs will be destroyed by December 2009. One hundred percent of Russian stocks of CWs will be destroyed in the final stage by April 29, 2012. Seven CWA manufacturing facilities out of 24 in Russia have been destroyed, 14 have been restructured for peaceful production and others are in the process of restructuring. A Russian chemical journal has provided a lot of information on the process of chemical disarmament of Russia. Regular publications on diverse aspects of destruction of CWs make it possible not only for experts but also for the public to control this process permanently and to become acquainted with the practice of chemical disarmament, with the technology CW destruction, questions of medical and analytical security and environmental safety. The editorial staff devoted the second issue of the journal (2007) to elucidation of the questions mentiond above.

The 2008 G8 summit in Kananaskis promised Russia an allocation of \$20 billion (~50% of planned costs) in financial help in 10 years. Actually, less than 7% has been allocated so far. Of all sponsor nations, only Germany has fulfilled its commitments. The United States promised to take upon itself the biggest share of financing, but has not followed through. Experts consider complications in the destruction of American chemical arsenals as one of reasons for this. Their technologies of CWA destruction are different but are also based on the same coordinated principles and safety requirements. The United States had previously begun a national program of CW destruction. However, it had managed to liquidate only 5% of CW stockpiiles for a period of 12 years after 1986. By 2005, the United States had destroyed 30% of its stockpiles by burning in special (plasma) furnaces on the Johnston Atoll in the Pacific Ocean. The cost of the national program increased from $2 billion to $25 billion. This is the first accepted technology for burning CWAs in the United States. Destroying CWs is much more difficult and expensive than developing and producing them. Subsequently, it became clear that combustion products were very harmful for the environment and human health because of their content of carcinogenic compounds and dioxins (chapter 11 and section 12.4). It is remarkable that the United Staets continues work in the search for safer methods of destruction of CWs—in particular, catalytic methods based on reactions of hydrolysis and oxidation; i.e., the United States uses the same approaches developed by Russia.

In conclusion, we will notice that in spite of big scientific, technical, organizational, legal and especially financial difficulties and strict terms, Russia meets its full obligations as outlined by the Chemical Weapons Convention, and the state of this work at the present stage does not cause doubts ergarding their successful and timely termination.

The political importance of the Convention currently in force in securing multilateral international cooperation in the confidential chemistry and technology of CWAs is great. The authors sincerely hope that the cooperative atmosphere that has been developed will promote an increase in the level and efficiency of international control over work in this field after the conclusion of all stages of CW destruction.

Chapter 11

Harmful Substances in the Environment

Along with CWAs manufactured in the middle of the last century in industrially-developed countries, the chemical industry manufactured large quantities of highly toxic products belonging to a class other than CWAs. Today, the chemical industry continues to produce them. Some are applied as additives or components of CWAs (for example, dichloroethane mixed with yperite and lewisite). However, the overwhelming majority of them are now widely used as intermediate products in the synthesis of industrial and domestic goods (varnishes, colorants, plastics, solvents, medications, agricultural pesticides, etc). In the mid-1960s, the terms "harmful industrial compound" (in the United States) and "industrial poison" (in the USSR) were introduced to classify them. Classification of the latter was originally based on different characteristics of their toxic effects (Table 5).

Table 5. Classification of industrial poisons

Character of toxic effect	Typical compounds
Nervous (neurotropic) toxins	
with physical toxicity	Hydrocarbons, benzine, fatty spirits.
with chemical toxicity	Methyl spirit, hydrogen sulphide, aniline, tetraethyl lead, dioxane, fluoroacetate, tricresyl phosphate.
Irritative	Caffeine, strychnine, ammonia.
Transmitter action (blocking communication of activation between nervous cells)	Nicotine, atropine, organophosphorous compounds.
Hepatic (hepatotropic) toxins	Chlorinated hydrocarbons (carbon tetrachloride, chloroform, dichloroethane, bromobenzene), phosphorus, selenium.
Blood poisons	
reacting with hemoglobin of blood	Carbon monoxide, nitro, nitroso and amino compounds of aromatic series and their derivatives.
causing erythrocytoschisis	Phenylhydrazine, arsenious hydrogen.
disturbing bone-marrow hemopoiesis	Benzene, toluene, xylene, chloroethyl amines, plumbum and its inorganic compounds.

Table 5. (Continued)

Character of toxic effect	**Typical compounds**
Enzymatic poisons	Cyanhydric acid and its salts, arsenic and its compounds, dissociating salts of bivalent mercury (sublimate), organophosphorous compounds (thiophos, metaphos).
Irritative poisons	
affecting upper airways mainly	Chlorine, chloropicrin, ammonia, dimethylsulphate, fogs of acids, acrolein, sulphurous gas.
affecting deep airways mainly	Nitrogen oxides, phosgene, diphosgene, aromatic hydrocarbons, silicate dust.
Poisons cauterizing and irritating skin and mucous membranes	Mineral acids (sulfuric, hydrochloric, nitric), some organic acids (formic, acetic), caustic alkalis (caustic soda, caustic potash), oxides, anhydrides, chromates, bichromates, phenols.
Allergens	Dichlorobenzene, some compounds of nickel, many derivatives of pyridine, p-phenylenediamine, some alkaloids.
Carcinogens	Coal tar pitch, 3,4-benzpyrene, methylchloroanthrene, benzanthrenes, some aminoazo compounds, benzidine, chlorobenzidine, β-naphthylamine, some acridines, fluorene.

This classification allowed prediction of the character of effects in humans by some industrial products but did not connect these effects with quantitative toxicological indexes and the timing of effects of concrete chemical compounds on facility employees when manufacturing and in possible accidents. In consideration of the deficiencies in the above-stated classification, the term “strongly influential poisonous substance” (SIPS) was introduced in the USSR. This term refers to compounds applied for economic purposes that could lead to air pollution and cause mass effects of people after large-scale emission.

Work on identifying harmful industrial substances and SIPS for the purpose of safeguarding and protecting facility staff and others during accidents began during the same period in both countries. The maximal permissible concentrations (MPC) of products in the air surrounding a working zone were used substantially as basic criteria in rating SIPS. The American list included about 400 chemical products, and the list of the USSR included more than 100 products. The smaller number of substances on the USSR list is explained not only by the limited assortment of manufactured products but also by the fact that substances with $MPC_{w.z.}$ of about several mg/m^3 and more were rated as SIPS. They included chlorine, sulphurous anhydride, ammonia, phosgene and a number of other compounds similar to them in physical and toxic properties. In the middle of the 1980s, a list of Dangerous Chemical Substances (DCS) was developed in the USSR. It included, along with SIPS, substances that are very dangerous when permeating an organism but which could not cause mass affects by means of short-term inhalation. The list was developed because of the growth in the number of accidents connected with the use, first of all, of methanol and dichloroethane in factories.

Thefts of methanol from reservoirs and pipelines and their subsequent use in alcohol-containing production caused not only serious harm to health but also fatalities. In connection with it, new criteria for rating DCS as SIPS were developed. That fact caused a reduction in the number of SIPS.

According to the Provisional List of SIPS (1988), 34 compounds were rated as SIPS. In 1991, the list of SIPS was reduced to 21 compounds because of exclusion of scarce compounds or compounds used in factories in small amounts and not causing danger to people in the event of an accident.

In 1994, the term "dangerous chemical substance" was introduced to replace the term SIPS by State Standard R 22.0.05-94. Dangerous chemical substances refers to chemical compounds that could cause acute or chronic human diseases or death by direct or mediated effect. This term proved to be not absolutely successful, as all harmful compounds used in industry concerned this class of compounds. Most of them are not dangerous during accidents. Accidents that had occurred at the end of the last century at chemical facilities in Russia and abroad showed that extraordinary situations could arise not only as a result of atmospheric emission of DCS but also when they penetrate water supply sources. DCS that are easily soluble in water, and those with high boiling points and low speed of hydrolysis are most dangerous in this case. On the basis of the information stated above, the necessity for separating the group of substances that can cause extraordinary circumstances arising from accidents from the list of DCS became evident. Therefore, State Standard R 22.0.05-94 in consideration of modern international terminology introduced the term "emergency dangerous chemical substances" (EDCS). The standard definition of an EDCS is a dangerous chemical compound applied in industry or agriculture that can cause environmental contamination in concentrations affecting a living organism (toxic doses) in emergency emission (pouring) of it. EDCS are subdivided into substances according to possible method of penetration into a human organism, as follows:

- with inhalation (EDCS IE)—penetration through respiratory apparatus
- with perorals (EDCS PE)—penetration through mouth
- with skin-resorption (EDCS SRE) —penetration through intact skin

Using the full abbreviations indicating the method of penetration into an organism makes pronunciation and illustration in documents. Therefore, abbreviation without the prefix EDCS (i.e., IE, PE and SRE) is used in practice.

It is difficult enough to define the unique list of all EDCS because possible penetration of compounds into an organism depends not only on the physicochemical and toxic properties of these compounds but also on their manufacturing, storage and application technologies. In some chief documents concerning civil defence and security in extraordinary situations, we can see that a number of other widely-available DCS are added to compounds from the list of SIPS mentioned earlier (from Table 5): a number of components of propellants, standard CWAs, methyl isocyanate, dioxin, methyl spirit, phenol, benzene, concentrated sulfuric acid, aniline, toluylene diisocyanate, and metallic mercury. Modern classification of dangerous chemical substances is given in the diagram below:

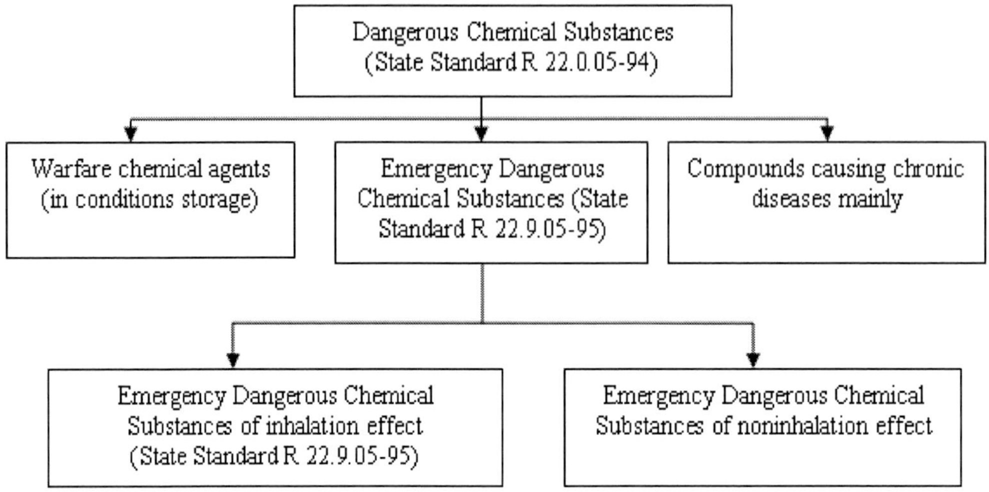

The list of emergency dangerous chemical substances and maximum permissible concentration of the most widespread EDCS in the air (mg/m^3) are given in Table 6. The cited values MPC are ascertained on the basis of results of domestic toxicological research studies and do not differ substantially from similar indexes of industrial dangerous chemical substances approved in international practice.

A number of compounds can cause harmful effects on an organism even at low concentrations with long-term (chronic) contact, along with compounds dangerous in accidents (as it has already been noted above). This is especially characteristic for production work connected with manufacturing, application or storage of harmful compounds. State Standard 12.1.007-76, called “System of Professional Safety: Harmful Substances” (republished in September 1999 with amendments Nos. 1 and 2) is functioning in the Russian Federation today. The given standard is valid for harmful substances contained in raw materials, products, semiproducts and production wastes and determines general safety specifications for their production, application and storage. The standard is not valid for harmful substances containing radioactive and biological substances (strains, microorganisms, etc.).

Harmful substances are subdivided into four classes of danger by degree of effect on an organism: First—extremely dangerous substances; second—highly dangerous substances; third—moderately dangerous substances; fourth—minimally dangerous substances.

A substance is rated according to a certain class of danger as a result of complex consideration based on indexes given in Table 7. This rating is given according to the index value matching the highest class of danger.

This state standard prescribes obligatory inclusion of toxicological characteristics of harmful substances according to specification, standards and production regulations of all industrially made chemical products.

Table 6. List of Emergency Dangerous Chemical Substances

Name of EDCS	MPC in air of working zone	MPC in air of populated locality, single	MPC in air of populated locality, daily
1. Nitric acid (concentrated)	5.0	0.4	0.15
2. Ammonia	20	0.2	0.04
3. Acetonitrile	10.0	—	0.002
4. Acetonecyanhydrin	0.9	0.2	0.001
5. Hydrogen chloride	5.0	0.02	0.01
6. Anhydrous hydrogen	0.5	—	0.005
fluoride	0.3	0.005	0.01
7. Hydrogen cyanide	1.0	—	0.005
8. Dimethylamine	1.0	—	—
9. Methylamine	1.0	—	—
10. Methyl bromide	20.0	—	—
11. Methyl chloride	0.5	—	0.03
12. Acrylic acid nitrile	1.0	0.3	0.3
13. Ethylene oxide	10.0	0.5	0.5
14. Sulphurous anhydride	10.0	0.008	0.008
15. Hydrogen sulphide	1.0	0.03	0.005
16. Carbon disulphide	5.0	0.2	0.2
17. Hydrochloric acid (conc.)	0.5	0.035	0.003
18. Formaldehyde	0.5	—	—
19. Phosgene	1.0	0.1	0.03
20. Chlorine	0.7	0.007	0.007
21. Chloropicrin			

According to state standard, the term "harmful substance" refers to a compound that can cause industrial injuries, professional diseases or deviations in the level of health by contact with a human organism in the case of breach of safety specifications. These industrial injuries, professional diseases or deviations in level of health can be discovered by modern methods both in the working process and in the period of remote terms of life of present and subsequent generations (amendment 2 of March 1989).

Control over the content of harmful substances in the air of a working zone should be conducted in accordance with State Standard 12.1.005-88, "General Sanitary and Hygienic Requirements of Air of Working Zone," with amendment No. 1 accepted in June 2000. A list of harmful substances with designation of size of MPC in the air of working zone, primary aggregative state in conditions of manufacturing, class of danger and specificity of effect is given in obligatory attachment No. 2 of this state standard. The list contains the above-stated indexes for 1,103 chemical compounds and continues to widen. Roughly safe levels of effect (RSLE) are stated for approximately 500 harmful substances.

Table 7. Indexes of classes of dangerous substances

Name of index	Rate for class of danger			
	First	Second	Third	Fourth
Maximum permissible concentration (MPC) of harmful substances in air of working zone, mg/m3	Less than 0.1	0.1–1.0	1.1–10.0	More than 10.0
Medium lethal dose by introduction into stomach, mg/kg	Less than 15	15–150	151–5,000	More than 5,000
Medium lethal dose by contacting with skin, mg/kg	Less than 100	100–500	501–2,500	More than 2,500
Medium lethal concentration in air, mg/m3	Less than 500	500–5,000	5,001–50,000	More than 50,000
Coefficient of possibility of inhalation intoxication (CPII)	More than 300	300–30	29–3	Less than 3
Area of acute effect	Less than 6.0	6.0–18.0	18.1–54.0	More than 54.0
Area of chronic effect	More than 10.0	10.0–5.0	4.9–2.5	Less than 2.5

In consideration of the rather large number of harmful substances in industry, we should separate out other groups of substances (along with EDCS) representing direct or indirect high danger for humans or the environment taking into account criteria other than $MPC_{w.z.}$ There is no doubt that environmental pollution can cause very serious consequences for the health of people. The consequences of the "chemicalization" of the environment for human life has attracted attention recently. The reduction in the numbers or even almost full disappearance of different species of animals situated in high trophic levels as a rule (birds of prey, seals, etc.) has served as a signal. A new interdisciplinary branch of science about environment—chemical ecotoxicology (the science of the spread and effect of anthropogenous chemicals and products of their transformation in the ecosystem)—appeared because of the tendency to better understand the interaction between properties of chemicals and their effect not only on humans but also on natural biota. Recognition of this fact by a number of countries led to the necessity to raise questions about the global escape of pollution. The international report, the Montreal Protocol on Substances that Deplete the Ozone Layer (1987), became the beginning of such an approach to this problem. The necessity to conduct such an international conference was made evident by the recent determination of the destruction and thinning of the ozone layer of the earth's atmosphere by a number of industrially made products (freon 11, freon 12, carbon tetrachloride, etc.). Considering the special importance of the ozone layer for the protection of all life on earth, the conference took unprecedented measures to move forward with a worldwide effort to halt production and use of ozone-damaging chemical substances. Russia signed and complied in corpora with the report of the Montreal conference. The overwhelming majority of countries of the world supported the decision of the conference by ending production and use of freons not only as refrigerants of refrigerators but also as a spraying medium (propellant) of a numerous assortment of aerosol preparations, the basic source of ozone damaging freons in the atmosphere.

The Stockholm convention officially went into effect on May 17 2004. The list of SOCs (stipulated by the Convention) and some of their characteristics are given in Table 8.

Table 8. List of stable organic contaminants

No.	Structural formula	Trivial name, aggregative state	Toxicity of technological product	Comment
1	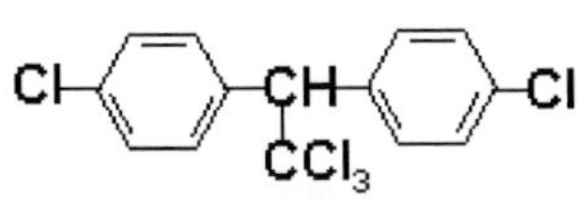	DDT Melting point 109°C	LD_{50} 250–400mg/kg (oral intake, different animals)	Insecticide
2	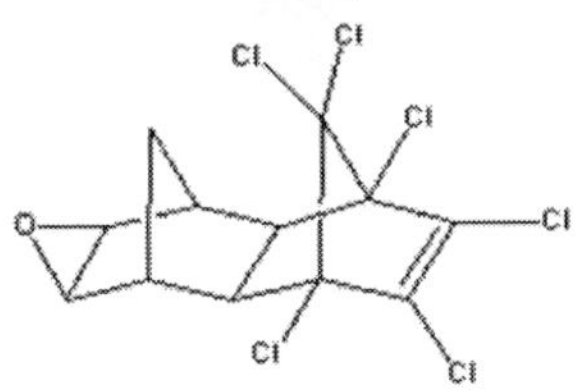	Dieldrin Melting point 176°C	LD_{50} 25–50 mg/kg (different animals)	Insecticide
3	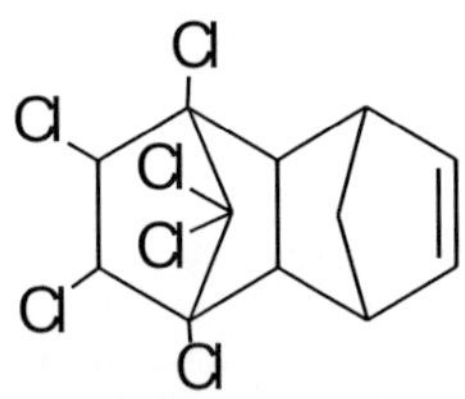	Aldrin Melting point 105°C	LD_{50} 40–50 mg/kg (different animals)	Insecticide
4	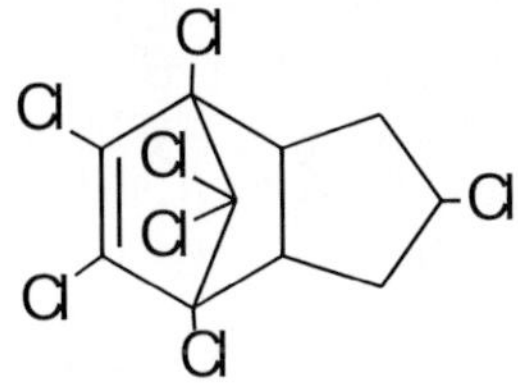	Chlordane oil boiling point 175°C at 267 Pa	LD_{50} 300–500 mg/kg	Insecticide
5	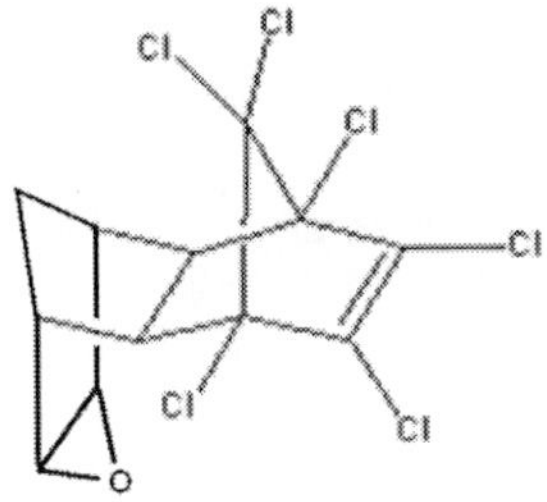	Endrin Melting point 200°C (decomposed)	LD_{50} 7–10 mg/kg (rabbits)	Insecticide

Table 8. (Continued).

6	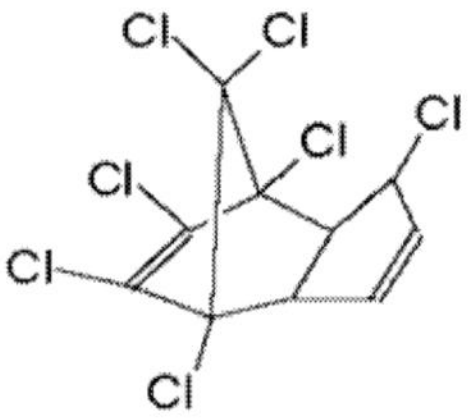	Heptachlor Melting point 96°C	LD_{50} 60–300 mg/kg (different animals)	Insecticide
7	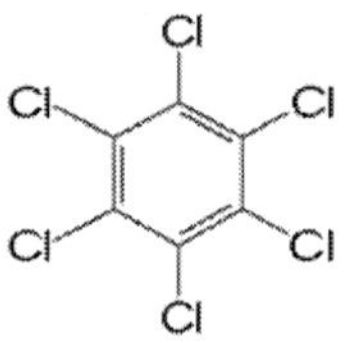	Hexachlorobenzene Melting point 231°C	LD_{50} 1700 mg/kg (different animals)	Fungicide
8	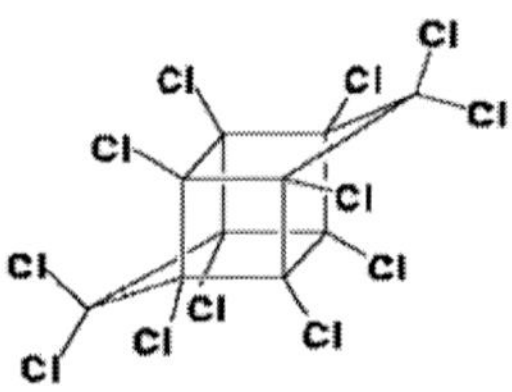	Mirex Melting point 485°C	LD_{50} 300–600 mg/kg (different animals)	Insecticide
9	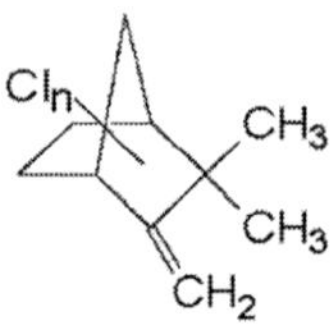	Toxaphene Melting point 65–90°C	LD_{50} 60 mg/kg	Insecticide
10	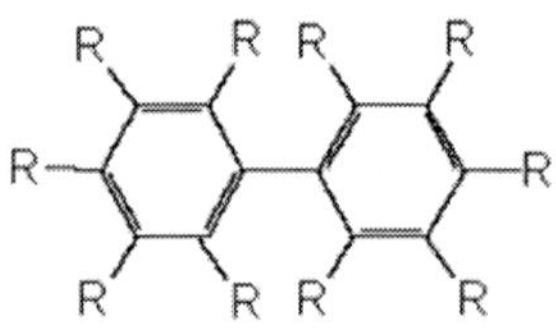	Polychlorinated biphenyls (PCBs) R=Cl, H.	Similar to dioxane in toxicity and mechanism of effect	Dielectric in composition of transformer oil, plasticizer
11	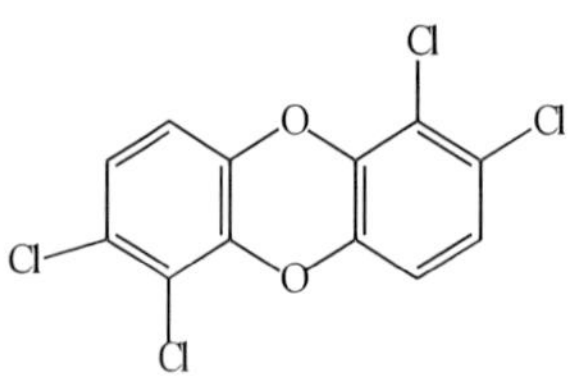	Polychlorinated dibenzo-p-dioxins (PCDDs) Solid	LD_{50} 0,002 mg/kg (guinea pig)	Combustion product of chlorine-containing organic compounds
12	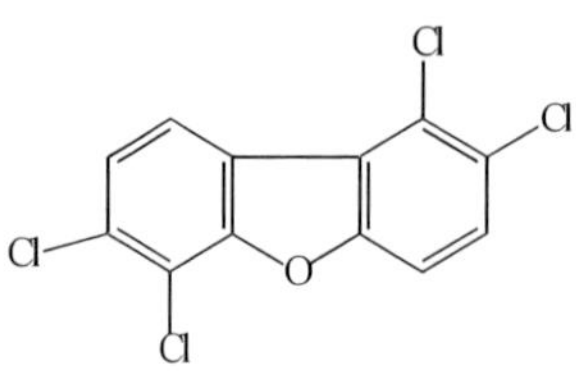	Polychlorinated dibenzofurans (PCDFs) Solid	LD_{50} 5–10 mg/kg (guinea pig)	Combustion product of chlorine-containing organic compounds

These 12 SOCs became a topic of the Stockholm Convention on Persistent Organic Pollutants (May 2001). Representatives of more than 90 countries including Russia signed this document.

This initiative, under the aegis of the U.N., was continued later. Twelve stable organic contaminants (SOCs, called the "dirty dozen") were chosen from numerous highly dangerous chemical substances: polychlorinated biphenyls (PCBs), dichlor-diphenyl-trichloroethane (DDT) and other chlorine-containing highly harmful substances.

A number of general properties are characteristic for SOCs: all of them are toxic compounds, are rated as compounds in the first and second classes of harmfulness in accordance with State Standard 12.1.007-76 (extremely harmful and highly harmful substances). SOCs can accumulate in tissues of living organisms (cumulative effect), can be transferred through food chains and can persist for long time in the environment, decaying extremely slowly in natural conditions. Moreover, SOCs are transferred over long distances under the influence of various natural factors. They are found even in such regions as the Arctic and Antarctic where they've never been produced or applied. The snow cover of Antarctica alone has accumulated more than 3,000 tons of DDT by the present time. Detection of SOCs in human milk has creased a special cause for concern. At the very beginning of the 1950s, it became known that the milk of almost all (94%) of examined women in the United States contained SOCs at an average concentration of 130 mkg/l. In the 1960s and 1970s, similar findings were also reported in examinations of other regions of the world (Ukraine, Finland, Estonia, and Moscow). SOCs affect all protective systems of an organism: nervous, endocrine and immune systems. These compounds cause effects in extremely small doses. Atoms of chlorine both in the side chain and mainly in the cycle are the basis of the toxophore group in these compounds.

The exceptionally low reactivity of atoms of chlorine of the alicyclic and especially the aromatic cycle with respect to nucleophilic reagents (including reactions of hydrolysis) causes the highest stability of such compounds. Production of number of organochlorine pesticides of agriculture was halted by Russia during the Soviet period because of the above-stated negative properties. However, a considerable quantity of unfit, obsolete, forbidden and featureless organochlorine pesticides remained in the territory of many regions of the country. The storage conditions of organochlorine pesticides do not meet elementary nature conservation and sanitary and hygienic requirements in the overwhelming majority of cases. Valid data about the quantity of organochlorine pesticides, unfortunately, are absent. However, according to estimates of independent experts, from 100 to 300 tons of such substances are stored in nearly every agricultural region of Russia. DDT comprises the greatest portion of them.

Problems connected with the recycling of PCB, used as a dielectric in transformers and capacitors of electrical supply networks, are especially complex. The high toxicity of PCB has been known for a long time. Therefore, strict norms of maximum permissible concentration (0.5 mg/m^3 in the United States and 1mg/m^3 in the USSR) of their content in the air of working zones were determined. Detriments caused by these toxicants to natural ecosystems were not realized at once. Therefore, it was not until the 1970s that all countries of the Baltic Sea basin, the United States and many other countries either completely prohibited manufacturing and import or took over strict control of them. Special research studies show that these ecotoxicants were present in humans almost everywhere in the 1970s, and that pollution of the environment by them is global in nature. As well as in the case of organochlorine pesticides, one of the basic methods of migration of PCB is atmospheric transport. According to inventory under the Arctic Monitoring and Assessment Programme (AMAR), there is no less than 14,000 tons of PCB in approximately 840,000 capacitors in the Russian Federation. Thus, no less than 20,000–30,000 tons of SOCs are found in Russian territory. More than half of them are present in electrotechnical equipment (capacitors and transformers).

Article 3 of the Convention stipulates for each country: 1) banning production and use of new pesticides or new industrial chemical compounds that develop characteristics of stable organic contaminants along with prohibition of production, use, export and import of SOCs except for the purpose of *their ecologically safe removal*; and 2) acceptance of measures *for ecologically safe removal* of SOCs located in their territories. Article 6 explains the concept of *ecologically safe removal* of SOCs as follows: "...waste like this, containing stable organic contaminants, must be destroyed or transformed irreversibly (must not develop properties of stable organic contaminants) or must be destroyed by other ecologically safe methods (if destruction or irreversible transformation are not ecologically preferable variants or content of stable organic contaminants is low)...."

The main method of removal of SOCs in Russia is burial in special landfills at present. The problem "About Compliance with the Stockholm Convention on Stable Organic Contaminants (SOC)" was considered at a conference in Omsk on January 24–25, 2007. The meeting stated that work on SOC burial in Arkhangelsk, Kursk, Vologda, Magadan, Tyumen region, Republic of Karelia, Republic of Sakha (Yakutia) is finished. Active work by Republic of Tatarstan was discussed. A total of 1075.9 tons of SOCs was removed from republic limits and taken to a special landfill (financing of works from the budget of Republic of Tatarstan accounted for 52.1 million rbl.) over a period of four years.

It is clear that burial of SOCs in the ground does not lead to their destruction but only pospones the question of how to deal with the problem of their disposal, and the threat of migration of SOCs from burial sites remains. Unlike the bituminous burial of minimally-harmful products (resulting from the technology of CW destruction accepted by Russia), the burial of SOCs of first and second classes of harmfulness (including bituminization) cannot even theoretically secure their safety for the environment. In this connection, we conducted a critical analysis of existing methods of destruction of SOCs for the purpose of finding a method of ecologically safe elimination of SOCs in Russia.

Considering the similarity of the basic toxicological and physicochemical properties of SOCs and CWs, the problem of elimination of SOCs is very similar to the problem of destruction of CWs described above. Without comparison of American and Russian technologies of CWA destruction (section 10.1), we would like to note that the method of combustion used in the United States, in spite of the apparent simplicity, proved to be expensive because of the formation of carcinogenic compounds and dioxins, which required further destruction. In this connection, the United States proceeded with a search for safer methods of destruction of CWs similar to methods developed in Russia.

Compounds 11 and 12 (Table 8) deserve special attention. The high persistence and extremely wide spectrum of biological effects of polychlorinated dibenzodioxins and dibenzofurans (hereafter called dioxins) became the reason for their separation into the category of *superecotoxicants*. Along with other SOCs, they accumulate in fatty tissue, in cells enriched by lipids and some cell proteins. They circulate for a long time with cellular elements of blood, penetrate into milk, pass through the placental barrier and are very slowly metabolized. The toxic effects of dioxins are connected with their ability to form strong complexes with receptors of steroid and thyroid hormones. The multiplicity of target cells for dioxins in various tissues also defines the variety of systemic toxic effects.

Practically any process of combustion leads to the formation of dioxins. The absence of information about the harmfulness of these stable organic contaminants leads to the following: people unintentionally contaminate the environment with dioxins at home, on dachas and in gardens by burning plastic bottles, polymeric products and household dust or when using capacitors soiled by PCB. The lack of system of laboratories for analysis of provisions for the presence of dioxins leads to free penetration of toxic products into food. High-temperature synthesis of these compounds is caused not only by burning of chlorine-containing materials but also by combined burning of non-chlorine-containing organic materials and inorganic chlorides. The total content of dioxins is 2,100 ng/g in flue ash and up to 1,540 ng/m^3 in smoke fumes.

The content of dioxins is slightly lower in emissions of polychlorinated dibenzofurans: 1,300 mg/g and 1,320 ng/m^3 accordingly. The MPC of dioxins in furnaces burning household rubbish is 0.1 ng/m^3 (ng, nanogram, or 10^{-9} g) in the majority of countries. It is known that burning chlorine-containing organic compounds leads to the formation of dioxin content, which in combustion products is much greater. As a result, this leads to secondary environmental contamination. Moreover, the type of high-temperature process used does not matter: flame reactor; flame reactor with additional plasmous heating of reaction mixture; flame reactor with plasmous afterburning of gases of combustion; a plasm-arc reactor, etc. Two factors are very important here: 1) the transition of an SOC into a vaporous or aerosol state and, hence, the additional danger of intoxication of personnel; and 2) the negative effect of secondary waste on environment.

At present, there are three plants for high-temperature utilization of chlorine-containing organic waste in Russia. One of them (stationary plasma-chemical plant) works at NPO "Technolog" (Sterlitamak). The second one is a movable installation of thermal destruction of liquid and suspended solid dangerous waste containing PCB and pesticides created by the Central Scientific Research Institute of Machine Building (TsNIIMash, Korolev of Moscow region) on the basis of the rocket engine of the multi-use spaceship, *Buran*. The third installation was created in OAO Khimprom of Volgograd for thermosterilization of liquid nonutilizable organic waste (including organochlorine waste) and was running until 1997. The manufacturing scheme of the last installation provided for three-stage cleaning of smoke fumes for harmful refuse and aerosols after thermoaggregate: an evaporation-irrigating scrubber, absorber, and antiaerosol filter. Modes providing complete thermosterilization of waste (of seven manufactures, including two of organochlorine manufactures—chloride vinyl and trichloroethylene) are fulfilled.

Unfortunately, we have no data on the efficiency of the first and second installations mentioned. Only the Bashkir Republic ecological research centre in the European part of Russia, aside from organisations in Moscow and St. Petersburg, have experience in identification of dioxins in the environment, a modern technical base and qualified personnel. The centre is accredited by Gosstandart (GOST) of Russia in technical competence and independence for analyses of dioxins by the technique of EPA 1613 (number of registration certificate in public register ROSS. RU. 0001. 510275). Results of analyses of gas emissions and sewage content of dioxins when thermoneutralizing liquid organochlorine waste at OAO Khimprom (Volgograd) carried out by this ecological centre confirmed that emissions of installation conform to sanitary and hygienic requirements in this index. The installation decomposes organochlorine waste into carbon dioxide and chloride hydrogen when working in optimum mode. The content of dioxins in smoke fumes is 0.052–0.054 ng/dm^3, which is two times less than the stated MPC of dioxins for garbage furnaces in Europe. Experience in operating furnaces (including garbage furnaces) in developed countries has shown that high burning temperatures (more than 1100°C) and rapid cooling of smoke fumes (tempering) promoted a decrease in the content of dioxins in smoke fumes but did not prevent their formation. The nature of organochlorine components does not influence formation of dioxins. It is necessary to note that the completeness of destruction of organochlorine waste without secondary environmental contamination is provided in the last mentioned installation only for liquid waste. However, the majority of SOCs are solid substances and they are also found in electrotechnical products.

The plasma arc centrifugal installation RAST 8 by the company Retech Systems LLC in the United States is one of the best installations in the world for destruction of SOCs including PCB-containing equipment and other harmful waste. Its technology is similar to that of chemical weapons destruction used in the United States and does not guarantee against secondary environmental contamination by dioxins. Three regions of Russia make a claim to acquisition of this plasma arc installation: Volgograd, Cherepovets and Yaroslavl. Yaroslavl scientists offered a number of modernizations of installation promoting an increase of its technical and economic indexes. However, the modernizations require a detailed study of the ecological consequences of operation of this installation.

Russia developed a method of destruction of CWs (section 10.1) based on catalytic hydrolysis of corresponding CWAs under somewhat mild conditions. CWAs of different classes of element-organic compounds (including compounds in harnessed form, i.e., packed products of ammunition) must be destroyed according to a common base of technology.

Thus, a certain community of technologies and problems of destruction of CWs and SOCs is noticeable. This makes the reaction of nucleophylic substitution of atoms of chlorine in SOCs a possible method from the point of view of using created substances for destruction of CWs for destruction of SOCs.

The crucial question of realization of this method is fidning the technology for substituting atoms of chlorine in SOCs in conditions close to conditions of destruction of CWs in operating equipment.

First of all, it is necessary to research the conditions for the substitution of a chlorine atom in an SOC containing a minimum number of chlorine atoms in cycles of DDT and PCB. This is logical not only because of the rather large quantity of these compounds (more than 50% of all SOCs in Russia) but also because of the possibility of further use of minimally-harmful products of substitution as raw materials or semiproducts of organic synthesis. Unfortunately, substitution of chlorine atoms in an aromatic ring can usually occur only at high temperature under the effect of strong bases. Milder conditions of reaction of nucleophylic substitution can be secured either by catalyst selection or by activation of aryl chlorides by preliminary introduction of strong electron-seeking substituents into *ortho-*, *para* or into both *ortho-* and *para* positions of a benzene ring.

In consideration of the fact that a rough quantity of SOCs appropriate for destruction is about 30,000 tons (the value must be specific according to region), the operating facilities for CW destruction can be used for liquidation of SOCs after April 2012 (the prescribed date of termination of CW destruction), and their operation can be continued depending on the number of facilities involved for a period stipulated by the Stockholm Convention (until not later than 2028).

Important advantages of the considered approach to the problem of destruction of SOCs are not only reduction of capital expenditure for creation of installations of destruction but also 1) the possibility of using already developed scientific-methodological approaches of CW destruction for creation of laws and regulations regarding ecological and health impacts of destruction of SOCs that are missing today; and 2) using trained and highly skilled staff. The continuation of operation of existing facilities will guarantee continued employment.

Nucleophylic substitution of chlorine in SOCs containing six or more atoms of chlorine in cycles will be connected both with a considerable decrease of completeness of removal of atoms of chlorine and a lower possibility of separation and further use of products of substitution. Methods of burning are preferable, excluding secondary environmental contamination with products of decomposition, including dioxins in this case.

Thus, analysis of existing approaches to the problem of destruction of SOCs makes it possible to draw a conclusion regarding the use of existing facilities for the destruction of CWs for safe, reliable, ecological and less expensive destruction of the majority of SOCs (DDT and PCB, most importantly) in territories of Russia. Residual SOCs can be destroyed by high-temperature neutralization at any installation, taking into account the restrictions noted above and on conditions that secondary waste will meet domestic sanitary and hygienic requirements of dioxin content.

A number of other pollutants (including sulphurous anhydride from the list of EDCS and nitric and carbon oxides) along with groups of ozone-depleting substances and SOCs cause certain dangers to environment. Large amounts of these substances are released into the biosphere and to the earth's atmosphere. According to estimations of experts, about one billion tons of acid gases and aerosols are released annually into the atmosphere by chemical, metallurgy industry and transport alone. The share of pollution remediation costs caused by transport totalled about 8% in 2004.

However, the share of costs for remediation of pollution caused by transport can match industry's contribution owing to a huge annual increase in the quantity of motor transport (including the Russian Federation) in the near future. Acid rain is a consequence of the self-cleaning ability of the atmosphere. The problem of acid rain was discussed for the first time at the 1972 U.N. Stockholm Conference on the Human Environment. Western air streams bring 5–10 million tons of sulphur dioxide (a quantity comparable with that made by the European part of Russia) to the territory of our country. Remediation of acidulation of soils after acid rains in northwest part of Russia alone reached 100 million rbl in 1984. The toxic effects of sulphur dioxide on human are diverse. They begin with irritation of the upper airways, and long-term exposure even in small concentrations leads to bronchitis and other diseases of the respiratory system and to a decrease of the immunobiological reactivity of organism. The detrimental effects of sulphurous anhydride increase in presence of carbon monoxide and nitrogen oxides in the air.

Carbon dioxide has also attracted great attention. Its constant mass dumping, according to the opinion of a number of ecologists worldwide, promotes or is even a main cause of the observable "greenhouse effect." The ubiquitous warming of the earth's climate and its negative consequences (a rise in sea level and drought in some regions leading to their transition to semideserts) has caused alarm and stimulated the activity of scientists to determine the principal causes of such warming. Technogenic consequences of human activity and periodic changes in the geographical coordinates of the magnetic poles of the earth and other factors are noted among such reasons. At the same time, incremental increases in the level of carbon dioxide in the atmosphere over the last 100 years (especially in last 30 years) total ~ 25%, mainly from the burning of fossil fuel. This tendency of constant increase continues today.

Today, almost everybody knows about environmental pollution by harmful substances. Mass media (press, radio and television) have tried to inform the population. It is obvious that it is practically impossible to present a thorough review of what, how and in what quantities contaminants pollute our biosphere. Mankind has thrown away more than 4,000,000 xenobiotics (alien anthropogenous substances) into the biosphere by the present time, and continues to throw away 6,000 substances daily. It is clear that specific weights and proportions of various harmful substances causing environmental contamination are not equal. However, it is necessary to emphasize one more group of contaminants—heavy metals. This group usually includes metals with a density value greater than that of iron: lead, copper, zinc, nickel, cadmium, cobalt, antimony, tin, bismuth and mercury. Their emission into the environment occurs mainly as a result of burning mineral fuel. Almost all metals are found in coal and oil ashes. And considering the modern scale of fossil fuel use, the conclusion comes to mind that coal burning rather than metallurgical manufacture is the main source of emission of many metals into the environment.

For example, the annual burning of 2.4 billion tons of black coal and 0.9 billion tons of brown coal causes dispersion of 200,000 tons of arsenic and 224,000 tons of uranium together with ashes, whereas world industry manufactures 40,000 tons of arsenic and 30,000 tons of uranium. Many of such substances are poisons and health hazards in redundant quantities in an organism. It has been determined that many of these metals cause diseases such as cancer: arsenic, carcinoma of the lungs; lead, cancer of the kidneys, stomach and bowels; nickel, cancer of the oral cavity and large bowels; and cadmium, practically all forms of cancer. According to L.G. Bondarev, the smoking of cigarettes and tobacco pipes all over the world causes the emission of from 5.7 to 11.4 tons of cadmium into the environment. This substance also causes an increase in blood pressure. The somewhat greater incidence of cerebral hemorrhage in Japan in comparison with other countries is connected with the emission of substances including cadmium.

The scale of metal contamination of the biosphere and the possible negative consequences of this process for human health are described in numerous examples in Bondarev's monograph. Toxicological and other aspects of the effect of heavy metals are described in the third volume of the seventh edition of the handbook *Harmful Substances in Industry* and in the last edition of *Harmful Substances in the Environment* (11 volumes).

Nowadays, the problem of pollution of the biosphere by harmful substances is one of the major concerns impacting the destiny of mankind. Therefore, solving the problem of environmental contamination (under the aegis of the U.N.) can and should be continued. Decreasing and preventing emissions of dioxides of sulphur and carbon and addressing the problem of environmental contaminations by heavy metals, especially those most dangerous to human health (arsenic, lead, nickel, cadmium and mercury), must be included in the primary tasks.

Chapter 12

Natural and Synthetic PhAS

In essays on the historical development of the chemistry of poisons, we stopped at the beginning of organic synthesis—the creation in the laboratory of chemical compounds whose structures are identical to those found in nature or are new and not found in the world around us. Along with scientific interests driving the minds of scientists, significant efforts of chemists have been directed toward practical results—the synthesis of chemical structures with certain biological properties. It is quite natural that the primary information communicated by scientists regarding their properties and structure derive from mankind's historical experience.

12.1. Morphine and Its Analogs

Morphine is an organic molecule which, for centuries, held the leading place in an arsenal of means used by doctors for alleviation of the most severe pain. Morphine is the basic component of opium and it was used since ancient times (see Chapter 1). When used as an anesthetizing agent, morphine is 50 times more potent than aspirin (acetylsalicylic acid), the most popular medical anesthetizing preparation.

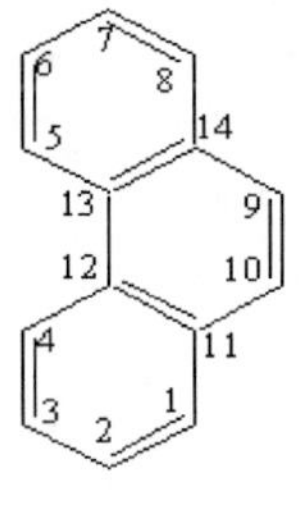

Phenantrene

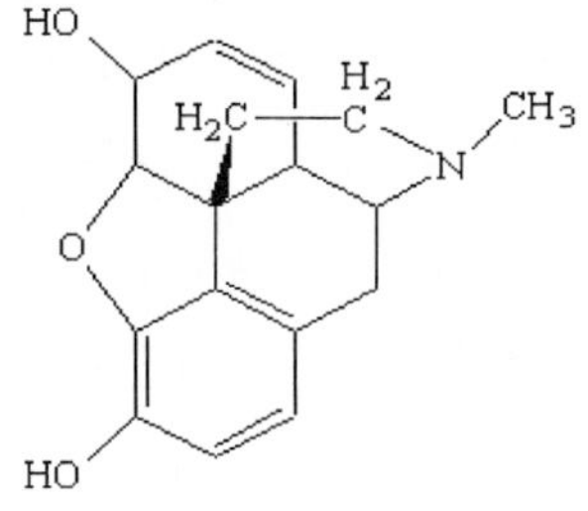

Morphine

The basic disadvantages of morphine are respiratory suppression the tendency among users to cause pathological addiction. In spite of these drawbacks, morphine has been used in medical practice from time immemorial. In the pure state, it was extracted from opium in

1803. In 1925, Englishmen J.M. Gulland and R. Robinson proposed the structure of this mysterious molecule. The molecule, seeming at first sight very complex, appears simple enough if it is consiered a derivative of phenantrene. The skeleton of morphine differs from the skeleton of phenantrene mainly owing to the presence of the bridge –N-C-C– between atoms 9 and 13.

The structure offered by Gulland and Robinson did not precisely establish the connection site of this bridge. Now it is precisely known that it is attached to the 13th atom. The reason for these difficulties was the fact that a molecule of morphine in hot hydrochloric acid decays, and, more significantly, rearranges with displacement of the carbon bridge, forming apomorphine. In the beginning, scientists did not suspect such regrouping and considered that morphine and apomorphine have an identical carbon skeleton:

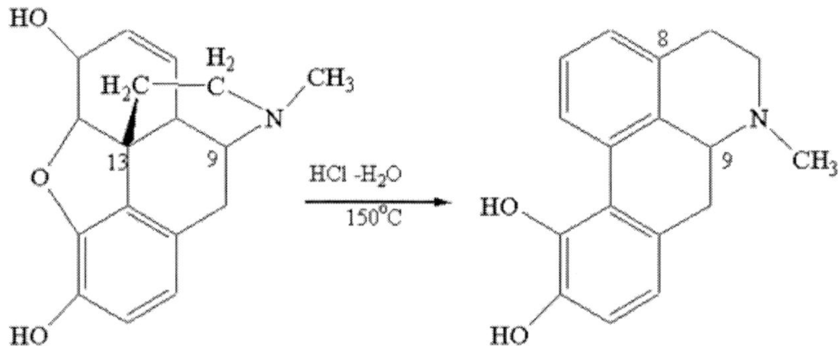

Morphine Apomorphine

The full synthesis of morphine, carried out by Gates and Tschudy in 1952, confirmed its structure. A key stage in this synthesis was the Diels-Alder reaction between butadiene and a derivative of 1,2-naphthoquinone with the formation of a carbon skeleton of phenantrene with the assistant in the corresponding position, which then, as a result of some reactions, is transformed into the -C–C–N– bridge of morphine. Synthesis of morphine in the laboratory is a very slow and labour-intensive process. Nevertheless, the morphine molecule was and remains the center of attention in a huge number of laboratory research studies. The basic purpose of these studies is to alter the structure of the morphine molecule with the synthesis of a substance that would demonstrate only one particular physiological property. In the case anesthesia, such a derivative would exclude respiratory depression and pathological addiction, reveal the most effective narcotic analgesic, possess temporary paralytic properties, or, finally, possess high emetic (ability to cause vomiting) activity. For the latter effect, the structure of apomorphine can be used. This substance causes vomiting with intramuscular administration in a dose of 0.08 mg/kg, and an incapacitating dose is ICt_{50} = 1000 mg•min/m^3. Replacement in the structure of the apomorphine methyl group at the nitrogen atom with ethyl or propyl leads to derivatives surpassing the emetic action of apomorphine by 25–50 times. Successes in the synthesis of emetics are considered in Chapter 8, and here we shall note that the use of apomorphine as a base initial structure for synthesizing various derivatives or use of its structural fragments has led to some success in the search for new emetics. Structures of morphine and its derivatives were also widely used in the search for narcotic analgesics with paralytic effects. Extremely high analgesic activity was demonstrated in a structural adaptation of morphine synthesized by Englishman K.W. Bentley, which possesses 10,000 times stronger action than morphine. One milligram of this substance is capable of making a wild elephant obedient.

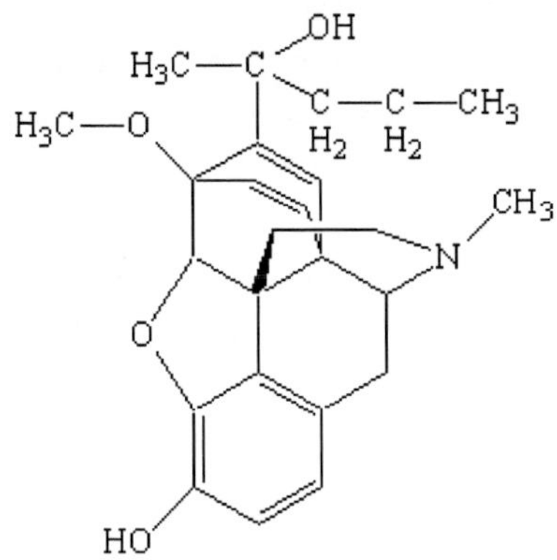

Bentley substance

Even higher analgesic activity among derivatives of morphine is demonstrated by 14-metoxymetapon, for which ED_{50} (mouse, hypodermically) is 0.000019 mg/kg.

Two well-known simple derivatives of morphine are codeine and heroin. Codeine represents methylmorphine (methoxy-group in position 3 instead of hydroxyl) and heroin is diacetylmorphine (acetylation of hydroxyl in both positions 3 and 6, as in acetylation of salicylic acid in the synthesis of aspirin). Codeine is present in opium, but in insignificant quantities, and its methylation of morphine is widespread. Codeine is less habit-forming and is applied as a local anesthetic and as a narcotic in the composition of cough medications. Heroin is not found in nature; it is derived from morphine and is so dangerous from the point of view pathological addiction that in the United States its manufacture and import even for medical purposes are forbidden by law.

Molecules of the majority of morphine derivatives exist in two stereo-isomeric forms, but only L-isomers possess anesthetizing and euphoric activity, whereas rotation to the right (D-isomers) does not produce such properties. This stereospecificity speaks well about the existence in an organism of a special receptor capable of distinguishing the mirror isomers as derivatives of morphine, along with the overwhelming majority of other physiologically active substances both synthetic and natural. It has been established that similar stereospecific receptors exist in all vertebrate animals—from primitive fish up to the monkey and the human. Moreover, it appears that the organism independently synthesizes, in certain cases, substances with action similar to morphine, so-called encephalines. In chemical terms, these are polypeptides, which contain the same fragment of a morphinic "key"—a hydroxyl group and a nitrogen atom a precise distance from it. Encephalines are emitted from special neurons and, after connection with stereospecific receptor, cause relaxation of smooth muscles and euphoria. A molecule of morphine incorporating into the same receptor causes a similar effect even if there is no stimulus for pleasure—for example, in the case of illness.

The successes reached recently in the partial separation of "good from harm" in molecules similar to morphine are connected with the discovery made almost 80 years ago, the value of which was not determined for another 50 years. In 1915, Uber J. Pohl, a chemist from the University of Breslau, replaced the methyl group at the nitrogen atom with an allyl group in a codeine molecule. The resulting N-allylnorcodeine counteracted respiratory suppression in animals that had been given morphine. It was not until 1942 that the same was done with morphine: N-allylnormorphine, known under the name nalorphine, was derived from morphine. Nalorphine not only counteracts respiratory suppression, but also acute poisoning—the effects caused by administration of morphine. Therefore, during overdose, administration of this preparation quickly alleviates symptoms. Unfortunately, nalorphine did not demonstrate anesthetizing action on animals. In 1954, at Massachusetts General Hospital, to surprise of medical researchers and unlike earlier results, nalorphine demonstrated an anesthetizing an effect and did not cause addiction in humans. It was the first example of the synthesis of a powerful anesthetizing medication that did not cause dependence. However, the success was short-lived; further research studies have shown that clinical doses of nalorphine cause hallucinations.

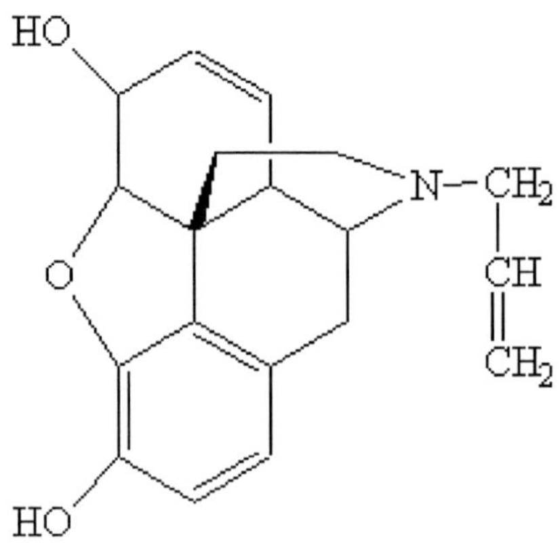

Nalorphine (N-allylnormorphine)

It is assumed that an element identical in structure to a molecule of morphine also binds to a receptor. However, within the limits of the lock and key theory, it is extremely difficult to understand how a chemically inert allyl grouping can change the properties of a substance so considerably. It is established that the property of the antagonist, nalorphine, possesses only one stereo-isomeric form, wherein the allyl-group continues to the top rod of the T-shaped molecule. Another isomer, in which the allyl group is oriented perpendicularly to the top rod, shows properties of a weak narcotic. This connection remains unclear: What kind of interaction between “key” and “lock” (receptor and morphine or its antagonist) should be responsible for a real configuration of an inert, waterproof part of the nalorphine molecule? Possibly, hydration can play a certain role as both “key” (morphine) and “lock” (receptor), as demonstrated in Professor S.P. Gabuda’s analysis of the sizes of sodium channels. Hydration, of course, brings certain “handicaps” in the process of restoration of the true form of a receptor, changing the configuration of cooperating molecules. But, actually there is probably one more major factor connected with the character of hydration and solubility derivatives of morphine and their complexes with receptors in water. The account of this factor has allowed the doctor of physical-mathematic sciences and known expert in the field of nuclear magnetic resonance, S.P. Gabuda, to qualitatively explain at last the variations of narcotic activity of opiates along with the toxic activity of some poisons. The essence of this explanation is based on established facts: For some types of substances, the area of existence of their homogeneous water solutions is limited by temperature and concentration, outside of which the substance drops out in a deposit in solid or liquid form (the phenomenon of stratification). It is extremely essential that the borders of the area of homogeneous solutions are very sensitive to the presence of some substances, even insignificant quantities of which can sharply displace the phase border of divisions of a solution—i.e., the substance, either in emulsion or dissolved, drops out of a solution and is removed from the zone of reaction. Such a substance also should be an inhibitor of an opiate receptor; however, its action will be based not on individual interactions with molecules of the besieged substance, but on displacement of the physical and chemical balance of a solution. The final solubility of amines and substances similar to them is closely connected with the formation of water "cells" around molecules of a dissolved substance. The stability of water "cells" and, hence, a solution depends on the structure of molecules that were subjected to hydration in solutions of substances. Undoubtedly, any changes in the structure of these molecules can displace the borders of stability of a solution. Such changes are also related to changes in the spatial configuration of a nalorphine molecule with a change of position of the allyl group. In this connection, S.P. Gabuda postulates that, as an antagonist of morphine, nalorphine operates as an inhibitor, displacing the border of stability of a water solution both in morphine and its analogues; as a result there is a stratification—the original loss "in a deposit" of a narcotic substance. A direct experimental confirmation of this phenomenon represents an almost insolvable problem, but in an indirect acknowledgment of a hypothetical model of inhibition of morphine by nalorphine, the author explains through the known fact of the potentiation (strengthening) effect of nalorphine in the presence of sodium and lithium ions and its indifference to ions of kalium, rubidium and cesium. A brief analysis of the influence of stratification on the effects of the action of tetrodotoxin and saxitoxin nervous poisons is considered in section 8.2. As a whole, phase transitions in solutions are accompanied by processes of reorganization of a structure in thin layers of water on a surface of biological molecules can be used as the basis of an explanation regarding the important effects of some PhAS, including competitive inhibition and toxic and narcotic actions.

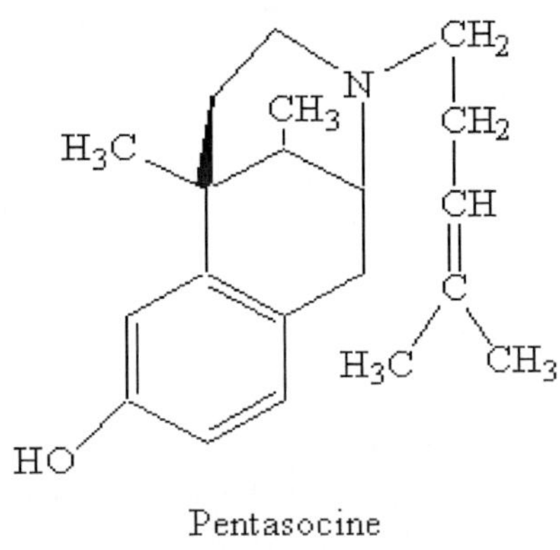

Pentasocine

One of the most effective substances derived on the basis of the structure of morphine is pentasocine:

It is less efficient than morphine in alleviating postoperative, cardiac and other types of pain. It does not cause development of pathological addiction, but this preparation does not qualify as an ideal means of anesthesia, as it causes respiratory suppression. Thus, the search for an ideal anesthesia without side affects will continue.

Along with morphine, it is possible to cite many examples of synthetics that are built on the structure of natural substances. Let us consider only two of the best-known examples. The structure of cocaine, an alkaloid of the coca plant from South America, represents a derivative of tropane (cyclohexane in which the atom of nitrogen forms the bridge between atoms of carbon in positions 1 and 4).

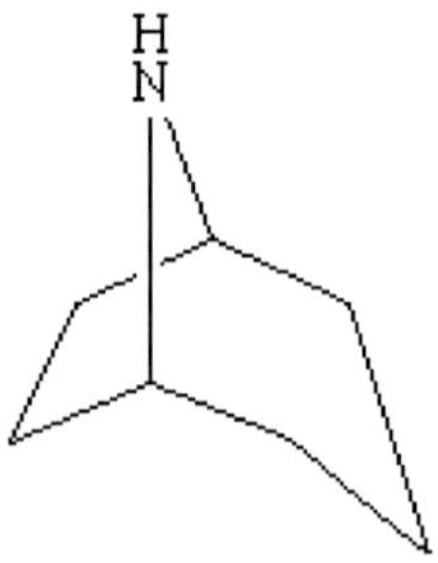

Tropane

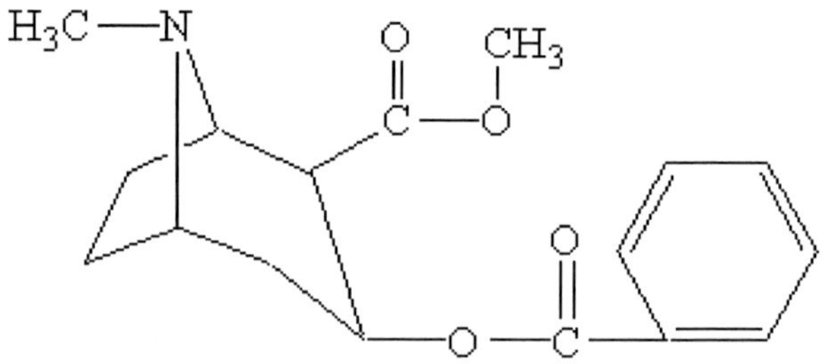

Cocaine

As a result of the successes of organic chemists in the synthesis of structural analogues of this narcotic, novocaine is now widely known and widely used as an anesthetizing preparation that has the anesthetizing properties of cocaine but does not lead to dependence, a detrimental property of cocaine.

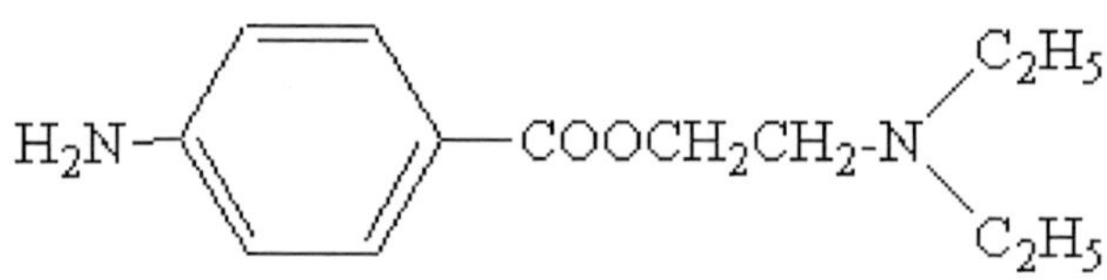

Novocaine

In studying the connection between the structure of a natural cocaine molecule with pharmacological action, it has been established that the anesthetizing effect is shown not with the entire cocaine molecule, but with a separate group within it, representing an ether of benzoic acid and tropanol, an amino alcohol. Research studies have shown that similar ether of benzoin acid renders an anesthetizing effect stronger than the cocaine, but simultaneously causes irritation. This drawback is absent in ethers of p-aminobenzoic acid, which preserve the same physiological action. Thus, a group of synthetic local anesthetizing medical products has been produced—anesthezine, novocaine, dicaine and others. The medical replacement of cocaine with novocaine has resulted in positive social consequences: cocaine has become much more difficult to procure, resulting in a lower rate of abuse.

12.2. Quinine and Its Derivatives

Another example of a marvelous molecule found in nature is quinine. At one time, preceding the discovery of quinine (approximately 300 years ago), malaria was a real scourge even in countries and towns that did not fit the climate profile for circulation of this disease—for example, Rome, London and other cities. Quinine had shown remarkable curative action in the treatment of malaria, whose victims suffered exhausting repeated attacks of the disease and eventually died. It also inflicted a crushing blow to the false medicine of Galen's doctrine, which for 1500 years directed doctors in the use of laxatives and blood release. Quinine in nature is found in the bark of the quinine tree, which comes from Peru. The bark of this tree contains three alkaloids close in structure to quinine—quinidine, cinquinine and cinquinidine, which are also active against activators of malaria. The exceptional popularity of quinine is a consequence of chance—it was picked out first from these four alkaloids. A molecule of quinine composed from parts of quinoline and quinuclidine has a bridge between them of an alcohol-containing atom of carbon (carbinolic bridge).

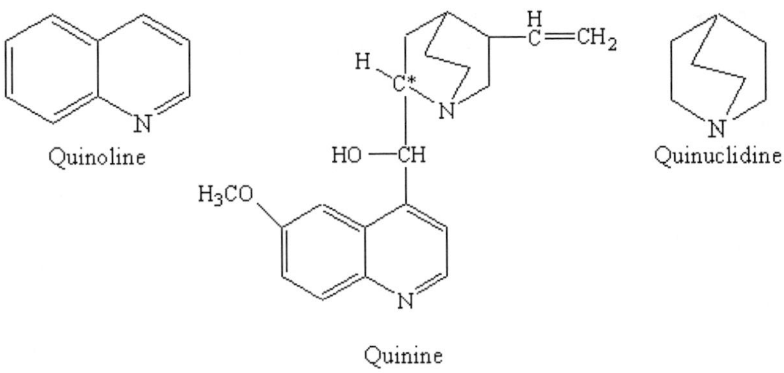

Cinquinine and cinquinidine do not contain a methoxy group in the quinoline part of molecule, but quinine and quinidine differ from the configuration of an asymmetric carbon atom in the quinuclidine part (position marked with an asterisk). Many suppositions exist regarding how the curative anti-malaria properties were discovered in the bark of the quinine tree. Among the more tangled and vague origins of the circumstances surrounding this discovery, some historians have guessed that Indians of South America had known about the anti-malaria properties the quinine tree bark before the discovery of America, but had hidden this fact from Europeans in the hope that the disease would destroy the alien conquistadors. Others have affirmed that the Indians didn't know about the medicinal properties of the bark and did not need it, since malaria was brought to the Americas by the Europeans. The first written information about the remarkable action of this remedy appeared in 1633 in the chronicles of Augustinian monk Antonio de la Calancha in Lima. He wrote that the bark of the quinine tree has the color of cinnamon, and if ground into a powder and prepared as a drink, it cures fever. More than 12 years passed before a Jesuit priest, Father Bartolomé Tafur, brought samples of the bark of the quinine tree to a church meeting in Rome, inhabitants which then without exception suffered from malaria. The rapid success of medical treatment with quinine bark impelled Jesuit priests in South America to begin sending quinine tree bark to Rome, where it was called the "bark of Jesuits." Pilgrims visiting Rome received little packets of powder that alleviated their suffering. In this way, news about the new medicine quickly spread throughout Europe. Doctors, well-indoctrinated by Galen's laws, did not want to hear about the Jesuit tincture. In 1655, for the first time, a conclave in Rome took place with no deaths from malaria among the participants, although at this time in London malaria continued to decimate the population. The continuing spread of the use of the life-saving powder had religious implications. When Oliver Cromwell, an avid adherent of Protestantism, was ill from malaria, he was reluctant to try the Jesuit remedy on religious grounds. He died of malaria in 1658. Still across 12 years a certain Robert Talbor, an unknown but enterprising apothecary's apprentice from London, began to prepare and sell quinine tree bark powder as his own remedy, amid public outcry about the dangers of the "Jesuit powder." Quickly acquiring popularity, he earned enemies among his colleagues, who accused him of antigalenism, and he almost lost his career. However, there was a happy outcome. King Charles II had been ill with malaria and appealed to Talbor, who cured the king with the powder. As a result, Talbor was knighted and given the title of king's doctor. Only after his death was the secret of the preparation revealed, and gradually the bark from Peru gained general acceptance. The next stage in man's struggle with malaria was appear produce on the 1820 year quinine from the bark of quinine tree, when Pierre-Joseph Pelletier and Joseph-Bienaimé Caventou. They did not patent their method, but helped set up manufacturing facilities to extract and sell pure quinine which, for the first time, gave the world an anti-malaria remedy in sufficient amounts. We have not yet thoroughly examined the question about determining the structure of quinine and its synthesis, which is a fascinating story. Let us note that a threatening deficit of quinine in the years during World War II accelerated the realization of its complete synthesis, carried out by Robert Burns Woodward and William von Eggers Doering in 1944 (see Chapter 4). Complete synthesis of quinine is extraordinarily complicated and is probably never used as the source in practice. Simultaneously, a successful intensive program was carried out in search of simpler synthetic anti-malaria medical products, which provided the Western allies a means of combating this illness. During this time, the synthesis of quinine remained a classic example of organic synthesis, based on a series of discoveries and achievements of scientists from different countries within more than 100 years. The search for easily-synthethized derivatives of quinine began in Germany during World War I, mainly because of the inaccessibility of sources from South America. German chemists began with methylene blue, which possesses a small degree anti-malaria activity that became known in 1891. As a result of some updating of various parts of the initial molecule, the first synthetic anti-malaria preparation was produced, and was given the name pamaquine. Pamaquine represents a 6-methoxyquinolinic fragment of quinine, containing in position 8 a dialkylaminoalkylaminic group:

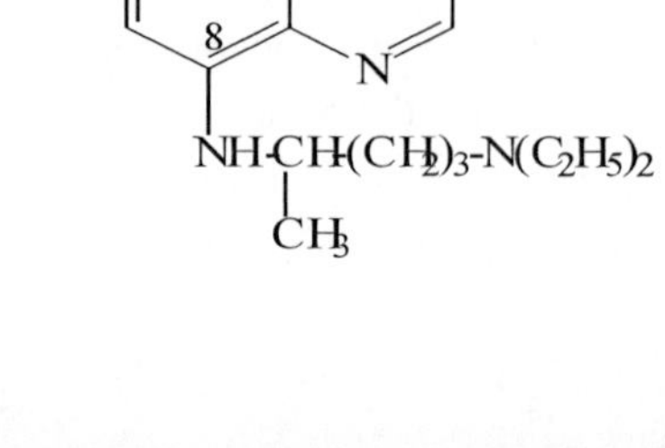

Further research studies have led to the creation of a less toxic and more effective preparation (atebrine) for outbreaks of malaria. The simplified variant of atebrine—chlouroquine—was used in World War II by the British and American armies as an anti-malarial agent. However, neither chlouroquine, atebrine, nor even quinine could prevent outbreaks of malaria type P-vivax, which led to repeated research into the structure of pamaquine. Therefore, pentaquine and then primaquine were created, and these treatments became the safest and strongest representatives of class 8-aminoquinoline.

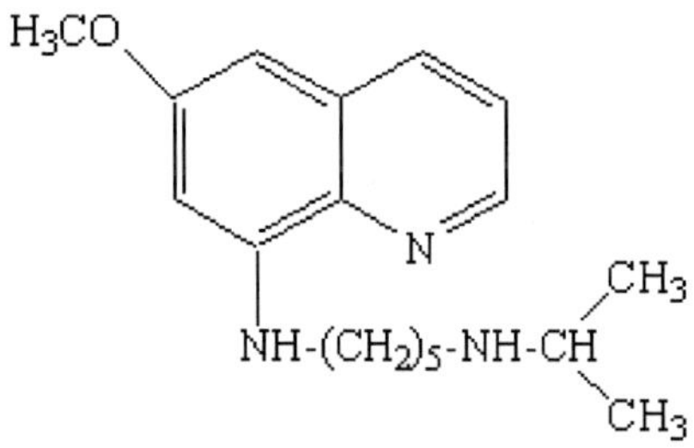

Pentaquine

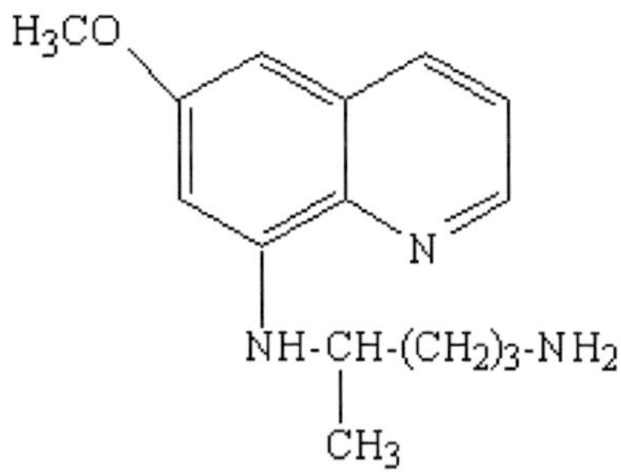

Primaquine

As a result of research studies, England during the same time had been synthesizing substances of a completely different type that also possessed anti-malarial activity—for example, chlourguanide:

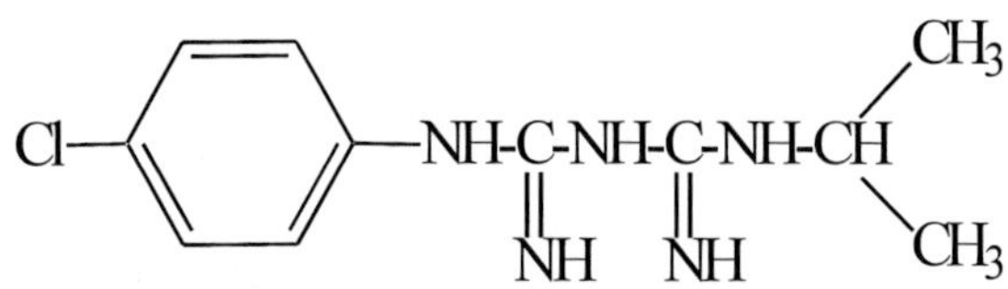

However, treatment with these preparations led to the regular evolution of different kinds of malaria activators, which again compels addressing a natural anti-malaria preparation, i.e., quinine. Therefore, the search for effective synthetic structures continued.

12.3. Synthetic Structure of PhAS

Examining the logic of the creation of new medicinal compounds with the examples of morphine and quinine, it is necessary to underline that an analogical approach was used in the production of synthetics and for other PhAS with various properties, as well as for substances with high toxicity. Synthetic poisons with a nonprotein structure, as shown earlier, were derived by modifying the structure of a natural poison or by adding fragments of its structure to other groups, selected to achieve desired properties. The assorted synthetic poisons gave rise to new structures that absent in nature, i.e., fluorphosphonates and phosphoryltiocholine, examined in Chapter 10. It should be emphasized that it is possible to develop highly toxic compounds by combining established and new chemical substances only a few years after their discovery. In 1992, Czechoslovakian toxicologists were investigating the toxic properties of phosphororganic compounds of hybrid structure by adjoining fluoranhydrides to sarin, but as nitrogen-containing adjoining structures to the VX gases. The most toxic among them appeared to be 2-dimethylaminoethyl-(dimethylamido)-fluorphosphate. With intravenous injection of mice and rats, LD_{50} is equal to 0.0276 and 0.011 mg/kg, respectively.

In order not to arouse suspicion, in the wartime chemical laboratories of leading countries, chemists synthesized and tested toxic properties of all or the overwhelming majority of possible hybrid structures, including the most toxic phosphor-organic compounds, analogs and homologs of sarin and VX substances. No compounds were found that were essentially superior in their level of toxicity.

By the character of toxic action and level of toxicity, phosphor-organic poisons were positioned closer to the take-up position of carbamates. The chemistry and toxicology of these compounds had been studied for more than a century and are now well known. It has been established that the toxicity of carbamates increases according to the diagram below:

A) compounds, having only carbamates group > B) carbamates with one quaternary ammonium group > C) bis-quaternary ammonium carbamates

Among the well-known arylcarbamates, the most toxic is that which has in the composition of the molecule two symmetrically situated groups of arylcarbamates, into each of which is a quaternary ammonium group, the last in combination with the polymethylene chain's characteristic length (see Chapter 7). With intravenous injection of carbamates, the most toxic have an $LD_{50} \leq 0.005$ mg/kg. Interestingly, on the basis of the extremely low level of lethal doses in the bis-quaternary arylcarbamates, N.S. Antonov has not forecast the production of new alkyl- and arylcarbamates, which, based on toxicity, essentially surpass those known at present.

The original approach to the pursuit of highly toxic compounds is the synthesis of substances that have the volumetric, skeletal, and polycyclic character of a molecule. Jointly with morphine-like substances, a group of bicyclical derivatives has the following general formula:

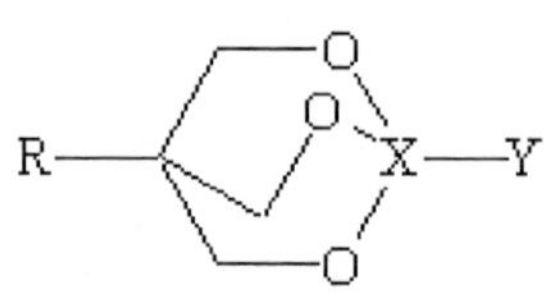

Bicyclophosphates: X=P; Y= (O=), (S=); R= alkyl.

Bicyclocarboxilates: X=C; Y= alkyl, phenyl, alkylphenyl; R= alkyl.

The first communication about the high toxicity of the bicyclophosphates is cited in 1973 by J.E. Casida et al. To distinguish highly toxic organic phosphor poisons, the toxic action of bicyclophosphates is not connected with inhibition of cholinesterase fermentation, but with the influence on other vital systems of an organism, in particular, on the chlorine ionic channels of GABA receptors. However, the blocking mechanism of the ion conducting channels still have not been elucidated. It is supposed that its compounds can connect with structures inside the channels or direct conformable changes accompanying breaches of ionic conduction of channels by the decrease of chlorine crossing neuronal membranes with its successive depolarization. It was found that tret. butylbicyclophosphotionate decreases the conduction time in the chlorine ionic channels of GABA receptors in the open state. Bicyclophosphates are convulsive poisons. Upon entering an organism, they cause suffocation, tremors and tonic spasms, which quickly change to cramps. Death results in 2–20 minutes. The level of toxicity of bicyclophosphates for all species of animals is approximately identical. For that reason, the lethal doses found experimentally in animals are presumed to carry over to humans. As early as 1976, dependence was established between the structure and toxicity of bicyclophosphates. The most toxic among them were discovered (i.e., R=isobutyl, sec.butyl and tret. butyl). The highest level of toxicity is found in bicyclophosphates with a branched out R-group. LD_{50} with intraperitoneal injection of mice and rats for tret. butylbicyclophosphate is 0.053 and 0.036 mg/kg, respectively.

Bicyclophosphites, having a three-valent atom of the phosphor group, determine the toxicity level of bicyclophosphates. Any alterations in the composition and construction of the base cycle structure of bicyclophosphates involve an invariable decrease in the toxicity of such compounds. The introduction of atoms of sulfur or nitrogen instead of oxygen, or substituting an atom of phosphor with arsenic or silicon, lead to a decrease in toxicity. The toxicity of carboxyl analogs of bicyclophosphates were discovered in 1985 and it was proven that their properties are analogical. They, along with bicyclophosphates, are hard substances and also possess convulsive action. The most toxic among bicycloortocaroxylates turn out substances with LD_{50} (mice, intraperitoneal) 0.06 mg/kg.

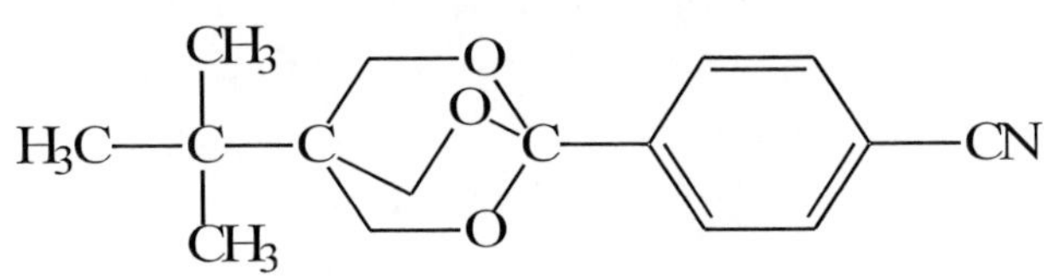

The strongest convulsive poisons, which block chlorine ionic channels of neuronal membranes, concern 2,2-di(threefluormethyl)-3,3-dicyano-5,6-dichlourbornane; the common name is norbornane.

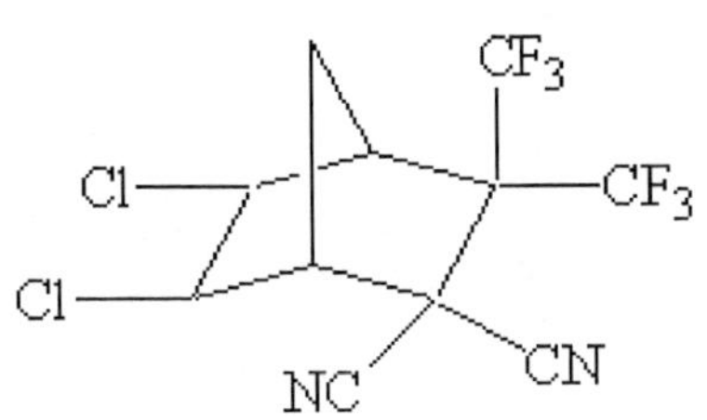

This compound has called clonuses cramps across some hours after introduction.

The toxicity of this substance has no essential species difference, and depends little on route of administration. The toxicity corresponds approximately to that of VX and sarin. LD_{50} (rats, intramuscular) for VX is 0.0096, sarin 0.095, and norbornane 0.1 mg/kg; intravenously in dogs, the values are, respectively, 0.006, 0.012 and 0.045 mg/kg; intramuscularly in cats, the values are 0.0038, 0.014 and 0.069 mg/kg, respectively. The duration for development of convulsive syndrome for norbornane differs from other convulsants—chlorine ion channel blockers are probably specific and noncompetitive and do not reverse connection with protein carriers of ions of the GABA receptor complex.

A sufficiently high level of toxicity is found in geteronorbornane derivatives, which have an oxygen atom or an atom other than carbon in their structure instead of a bridge atom of carbon. Among the representatives of this group that deserve attention are the previously-mentioned cantharidin and 7-oxobicyclo(2,2,1)heptanes. For the latter, LD_{50} (mice, intraperitoneally) ranges from 0.31 to 1.5 mg/kg. The toxicity of substances in this group essentially depends on the spatial configuration of the molecule, so *ekzo*-configurations are more toxic than *endo*-derivatives. The difference in their levels of toxicity is as great as a factor of 400. Reserves for pursuit of highly toxic substances among derivatives of norbornanes so far have not been exhausted. Using the adamantine carcass structure series for production of PhAS by analogy with the carcass structures of tetrodotoxin (see section 8.2) has been considered.

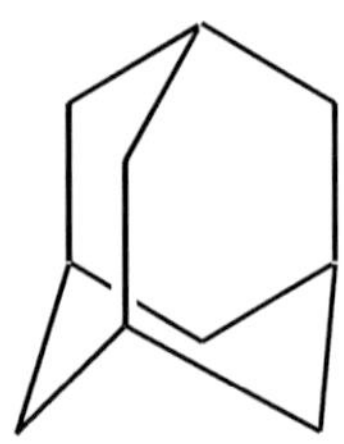

The highly lipophilic properties and the volume structure of radicals of adamantine have allowed modification of the pharmacologic action of a large of series antimicrobial, antiviral, anticancerous, analgesic, neural and other remedies.

12.4. Dioxins

Structures with flat construction have not been fully exhausted; an example may be dioxin or 2, 3, 7, 8-tetrachlourdibenzoparadioxin:

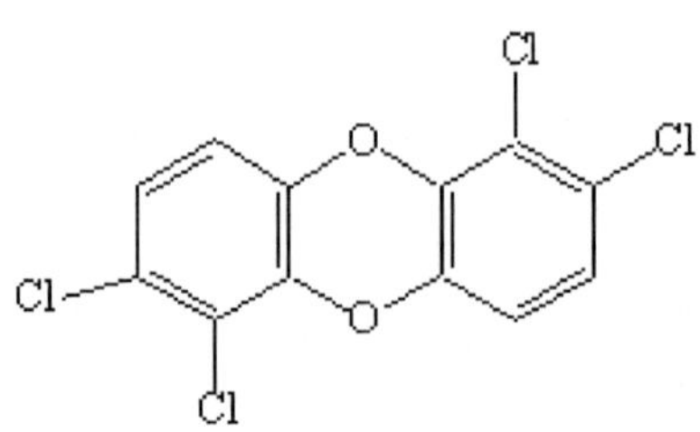

Dioxin

This highly symmetrical and flat structure was determined by X-ray investigations and quantum-chemical calculations, and calls forth manifestation of this compound's extremely complex chemical and physical properties. Chemically extremely inert, it does not decompose acids or alkalis even by warming. It is thermically stable up to 700–750°C, and is nearly insoluble in water (0.008–0.480 mkg/l). It is a hydrophobic compound, which easily forms cation radicals and is capable of donor-accepting interaction; this is why dioxin easily and effectively accumulates in components of soil, which is their basic place in nature. Dioxin has been found in archival samples of soil and plants collected from 1877–1927 in quantities corresponding to contemporary levels of soil pollution in villages and suburbs. Dioxins have never been produced on an industrial scale, but are widespread from Antarctica to the Arctic. Comparatively recently, scientists, inspecting the liver and other inner organs, discovered a disturbingly high level of polychlorinated chemicals (for example, DDT), along with dioxins. Dioxin in an organism is not metabolized and moves extremely slowly. Biodegradation of dioxin in soil microorganisms and bacteria also takes place extremely slowly. The period of semi-disintegration of dioxin in soil ranges from 10–12 years. It is capable of accumulation in the tissues of plants and animals and migrates by the food chain, displaying cumulative properties. Dioxin is one of the most toxic poisons. It is capable of striking any organism, from microbes to humans. With a concentration of a few mkg/kg, dioxin possesses antibactericidic action. Fish perish in water containing 0.1–3.0 mkg/kg of dioxin, but negative affects on birds are observed at a dose of 0.5 mg/kg. Lethal doses of dioxin strongly change depending on the species of animal. The most sensitive are guinea pigs, in which the LD_{50} (per os) is 0.0006–0.002 mg/kg. The LD_{50} for mice is 140–190 times larger than for guinea pigs. So much variation in the lethal doses for animals does not allow reliable extrapolation of this data for humans. It is generally considered that there is no safe dose for humans, and the degree of risk of injury is directly dependent on the dose. In the last 60 years, as a consequence of diverse disasters caused by chemical enterprises and because of the direct influence on people of herbicides based on derivates of dichlour- and threechlourphenols, scientists have received a great amount of data on the toxic effects of dioxin. A typical example occurred in 1976 in Seveso, a town near Milan, Italy. An accident took place at the Hoffman-LaRoche chemical plant, which had been producing herbicide 2,4,5-T. The explosion caused suffering not only among the workers, but also the local inhabitants. Based on calculations, three to four kilograms of dioxin were released into the environment, which contaminated an area of 20 km^2 with a population of 38,000 people. Dioxin was found in soil, atmospheric dust, bottom sediments, tissues of animals and vegetation, cow milk and people. Seven hundred people were evacuated from the region of contamination, and use of agricultural areas was prohibited for a prolonged period. Three mln m^3 of contaminated soil were collected and buried in a specially-built underground repository, an arrangement made in the most contaminated area of the territory. The most common observable signs of dioxin poisoning in animals and humans are the following: loss of appetite, general weakness, weariness, depression and catastrophic loss of weight. Death results after a few days or even weeks depending on the dose. Less than lethal doses cause specific injury to an organism—for example *chloracne*—a reflexive inflammation of the fat glands of the skin. This chronic disease is accompanied by dermatitis and formation of ulcers that do not heal. Often it is accompanied by *porphyria,* a chronic disease with characteristic formation of skin blisters, increased photosensitivity and brittleness of the skin. It is caused by a deficiency in one of the enzymes that converts porphyrin into heme, resulting in a buildup of porphyrin in the liver, urine and excrement. In high levels of poisoning, strong pains in the area of heart and extremities and severe damage to the liver, spleen, and immune and central nervous systems have been observed.

The structure of dioxin provides the possibility of a wide choice for synthesis of its isomers and various derivatives. Products of chlorination of its basic structure (dibenzodioxin) number only 75. Among all isomers of chlorination, 2,3,7,8-tetrachlordibenzo-paradioxin is the most toxic. Among other polychlor- and polycyclic compounds, the closest in properties including toxicity are 2,3,7,8-tetrachlordibenzofuran:

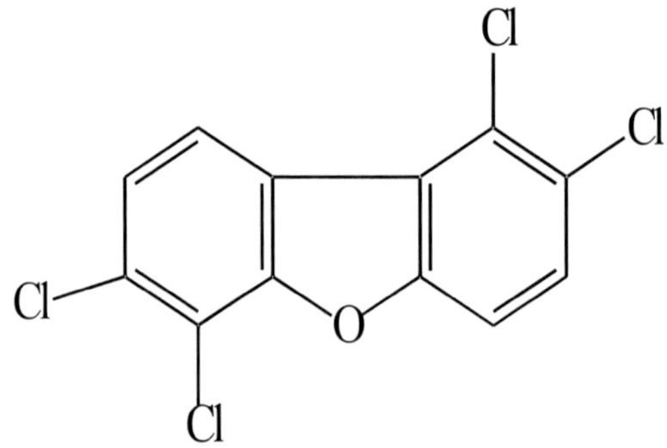

The most toxic among this group of substances observed to cause symptoms have a symmetric structure with atoms of chlorine in lateral positions, as in the case of dioxin. A huge number of other kinds of derivatives of dioxin and dibenzofuran with other atoms of haloids, alkyl-, acyl-, sulpho-, nitro-, amino- and other functional groups lead to less toxic substances. Synthesis of these substancses, one must think, haunts common scientific interests, though one can't dismiss the probability that the search for toxic substances in this group was carried out with the aim to determine the production potential of warfare agents. Dioxins (in this instance and hereafter, this term refers to dioxin and its furan analogs), based on their general characteristics, fill the modern production demands of warfare agents. They possess a high level of toxicity, approximately the same level of warfare agents with nervous paralytic action. The stability of dioxins surpasses all modern warfare agents and they are sufficiently easily adapted for ordinary industrial production, but the creation of antidotes is problematic. In spite of that, dioxins may some day soon be examined as warfare agents and not only because of the Chemical Weapons Convention regulations in force. Their disadvantages include the following: serious defeats are not possible simply due to their effects on the skin; they can be applied only as aerosol; guaranteed reliable protection of troops and civilians requires filter gas masks; effects last for a considerably long period (days and even weeks), precluding use in a moving army or front operation.

Principal sources of dioxin contamination in the environment are 1) the chemical industry, metallurgy and traditional thermal power stations, which employ high-temperature chemical processes with organic and inorganic compounds with one or a few atoms of chlorine (including molecular chlorine), leading to the formation of dioxins; 2) the cellulose-paper industry, which uses chlorine or its derivatives for whitening cellulose; 3) in automobile fuel, to which tetraethyl lead and 1,2-dichlorethane are added; and 4) rubbish-burning plants, which generate dioxins from less dangerous wastes. The recent Stockholm Convention determined principal ways to secure ecologically safe methods to ward off the formation and minimize dispersal of these compounds into the environment (see Chapter 11).

Dioxin and its furan analogs have a striking genetic apparatus; they possess powerful mutagenic, immunodepressant, carcinogenic, teratogenic and embryo-toxic actions. The principal mechanism of action in an organism takes place with the intake of water and food across the gastrointestinal tract (90%) and with air and dust in the lungs (~10%). These compounds circulate in the blood, are taken up by adipose tissue and lipids of all cells without exception, and reach the fetus in utero across the placenta, causing a negative influence on the development of, in particular, the nervous system. When breast-feeding, the child also ingests these compounds, as they accumulate in adipose tissue and milk fat. Nursing mothers lose 20–40% of their previous level of dioxins. Dioxins interfere with the processes of division and specialization of cells; provoke development of oncological diseases; have profound breaches all change processes; result in immune deficits; and interfere in the function of reproduction, often leading to sterility in men and women. It is necessary to classify dioxins as biophysical poisons whose interactions with definite biotargets are not typical, but which are inclined to form associations with different compounds of endogen character.

As a consequence of these specific physiological properties, dioxins presents a serious threat as a possible means of ecological war. The ability of dioxins to influence a large territory over a long period of time with very little expenditure of a compound and simultaneously influence yield, fodder, domestic animals and water springs may turn large regions into uninhabitable space. That is why dioxins, as potentially dangerous compounds, should be placed under the same level of absolute control as dangerous warfare agents, and the 2001 Stockholm Convention is slowly but surely addressing it.

12.5. PhAS and Their Targets

Examining the successful synthesis of any PhAS, one must emphasize that purposeful synthesis of planned structures would not be possible without knowledge of the biotargets of these substances and understanding the mechanism of their interaction with the systems of an organism. But there are exceptions—for example, the mechanism of action of aspirin, one of the most widely-used medicines in the world.

12.5.1. Aspirin and Sulpha Drugs

The synthesis of aspirin by acetylation of salicylic acid was realized by Charles Gerhard in 1853 in Strasbourg, and in the course of the next 40 years this did not attract attention.

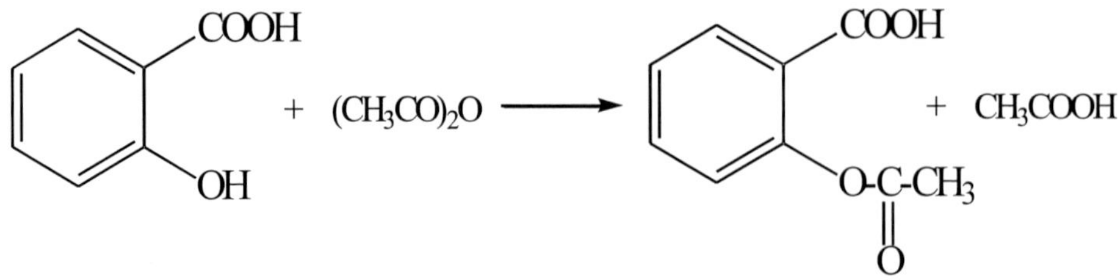

But in 1894, Felix Hoffmann, a chemist working for Bayer & Co., studied this reaction in the hope of synthesizing a substance to alleviate his father's arthritis pain that was more palatable than other medications used at that time. The new drug exceeded expectations, and Bayer received a new product that gained worldwide acceptance. The name "aspirin" was derived as follows: the letter "a" is taken from the word acetyl; "spir" from the name of the *Spiraea ulmaria* (meadowsweet) plant, from which in 1831 Swiss pharmaceutist Johann Pagenstecher extracted salicylic aldehyde; and "in" was a suffix commonly applied to medications. In 1835, German chemist Karl Lowig isolated salicylic acid, from which the name "spirovic" acid is derived. Scientists in different countries continue to advance the synthesis of manifold derivatives on the basis of salicylic acid and are conducting thorough investigations of their pharmacological properties. According to the latest data, derivatives of salicylic acid have been applied to bioregulators, which synthesize in an organism and take part in forming its protective functions.

Sulfanilamide was synthesized in 1908. It is a medical product whose mechanism of action in detail is well known. Its antibacterial properties were discovered in 1936, when sulfanilamide was observed to increase the durability of wool coloring by introducing a sulfamid group to azo dye, which led to the synthesis of the dye, prontozil:

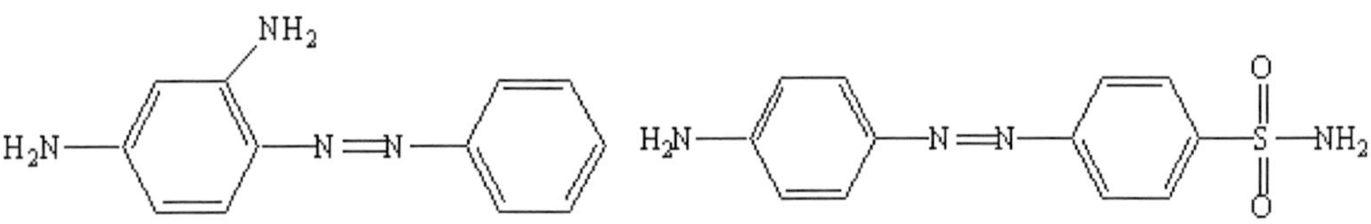

Azo dye Prontozil

Tests of prontozil in vivo demonstrated antibacterial activity, though it was not effective during in vitro testing. The reason for this was unknown at that time, but it was later discovered that the metabolism of prontozil in an animal organism results in the formation sulfanilamide. German chemists, however, did not attach importance to the difference between in vivo and in vitro tests, but French chemists at the Pasteur Institute paid attention to this fact and, in synthesizing various kinds of azo dye, established that only introduction of a sulfamid group into a molecule was accompanied by the appearance of antistreptococcic activity. Moreover, they established that the structure of a second fragment of azo dye did not play an essential role and that sulfanilamide itself possesses the same activity as the source dye.

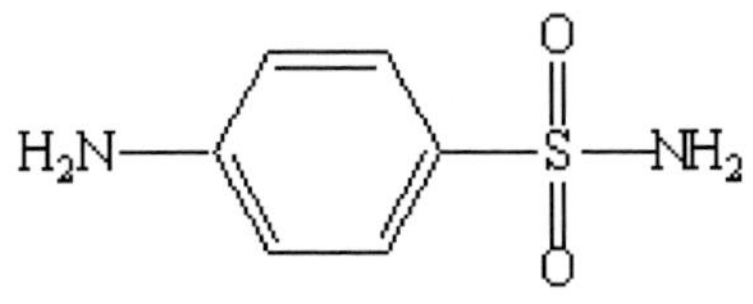

Sulfanilamide

Simultaneously with synthesis, sulpha drugs were analyzed and a connection between their chemical structure and physiological action was established. Principles are summarized as follows:

1. The physiological activity of sulfanilamide stipulates the presence of a sulfanil-radical in the molecule.

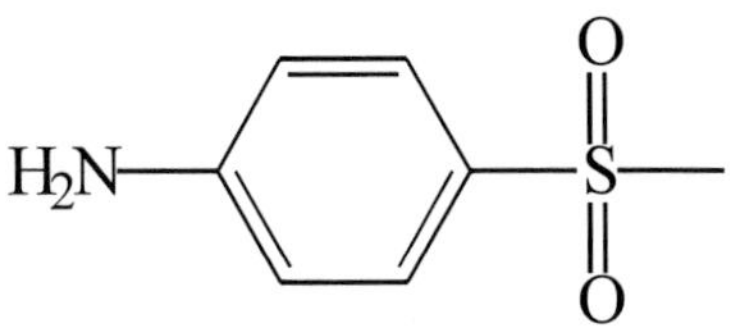

2. Transfer of an amino group from position 4 to other positions of the aromatic nucleus leads to complete loss of physiological activity.
3. Any analogs of sulfanilamide with replacement of an amino group in position 4 may be physiological active only if in an organism a free amino group may be formed.
4. Introduction in an aromatic cycle of supplementary assistants either eliminates or decreases physiological activity.
5. With the introduction of different radicals to a sulfamide group of a molecule, physiological activity may be changed depending on the character of a radical either as an increase or a decrease.
6. Prolongation of action increases with the presence in a molecule of a methoxy group. It is supposed that a methoxy group ensures the bonding of sulfanilamide with plasma proteins, which stipulates preparation for prolongation of action.

Sulfanilamide is an antibacterial that contributes to the synthesis of folic acid, which is extraordinarily important for the ability of bacteria to survive. Animal cells do not synthesize folic acid, but it is a necessary component for their functions. This is why sulfanilamide is toxic for bacteria but not for humans.

Folic acid consists of three fragments: derivates of pteridine; *p*-aminobenzoin acid; and the very widespread amino acid, glutamine. Sulfanilamide joins in the biosynthesis of folic acid substitute, *p*-amino-benzoin acid, because of their structural likeness, which causes errant fermentation responsible for the connection of all three parts of the molecule. Therefore, this results in "false" folic acid, which is not capable of carrying out vital functions of true folic acid in bacteria. This discovery of the secret antibacterial activity of sulfanilamide led to the first modern antibacterial preparation.

Folic acid

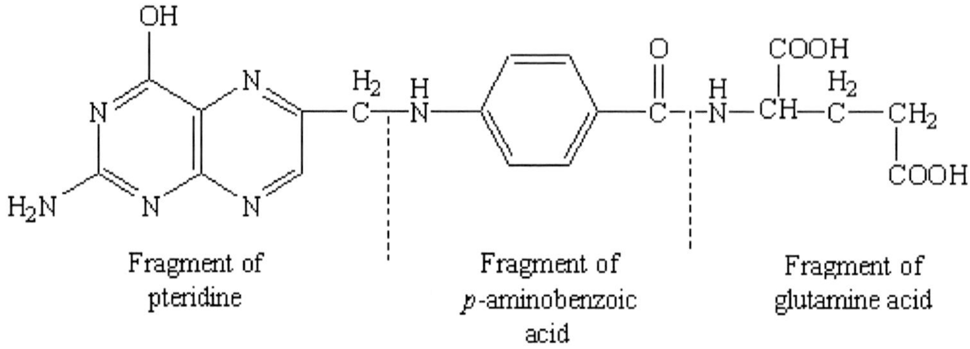

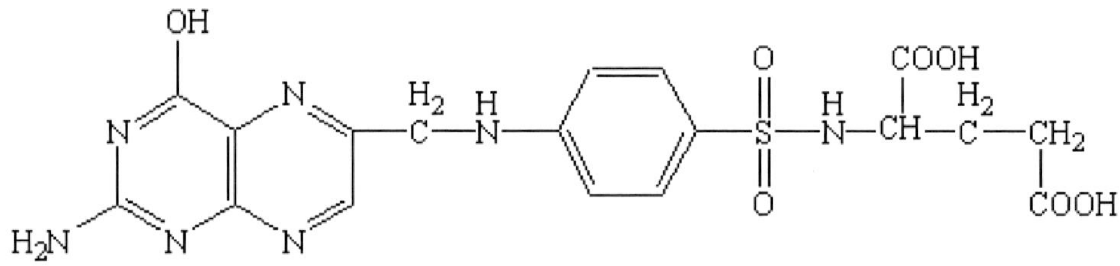

"False" folic acid, containing of sulfanilamide

12.5.2. Antibiotics

The next giant step forward in the discovery of new physiological active substances and their use in medicine was the discovery of antibiotics—in particular, penicillin. Usually, an antibiotic is defined as a substance that synthesizes in microorganisms and is capable of killing them or preventing other microorganisms from developing. A fortunate accident allowed English bacteriologist Alexander Fleming in 1929 for the first time to observe the antimicrobial activity of penicillin and propose its use as an antiseptic. The possibile use of penicillin for medical treatment of infectious diseases was established in 1940 by Howard Walter Florey and Ernst Boris Chain after extracting natrium salt of penicillin (though it contained admixtures), which possessed powerful antistaphylococcic activity. In the beginning of 1941, penicillin was used for the first time on a human (a police constable from Oxford who had fallen ill), which began the triumphant path of this antibiotic. War led to the application of penicillin as a strategic product, which led to intensive research in the definition of the structure and elucidation of the possibility to produce the antibiotic in large quantities. Only in 1945, with the help of X-ray structure analyses, was the structural formula of penicillin finally determined. The exceptional lability and extraordinary sensitivity of the molecule even to slight alteration in experimental conditions that stipulate the presence of a 4-member cyclic amid group not found earlier in natural substances made this work difficult. After establishing the structure, many attempts were made to find other susceptible bacteria. At the present time, many strains are known. The sulphanyl amide mechanism action stipulates a distinction between bacterial and animal cells. The bacterial cell wall carries out base functions that defend against osmotic pressure changes in the environment. Animal cells do not have walls—they have only cell membranes. Penicillin prevents the formation of new cell walls, which are necessary for the growth and reproduction of bacteria. A breach in the cell wall or its absence may result in bacterial cell rupture and leak of its contents into the environment, which immediately initiates the natural protection mechanism of an organism, whereby antibodies penetrate the bacteria and destroy it. Penicillin is effective almost exclusively against gram-positive organisms. The cell walls of gram-negative bacteria do not take on color in the presence of Gram stain, which is evidence of the difference in structure of the cell walls of gram-positive and gram-negative bacteria—specifically, the participation of gram-positive bacteria in reaction with transpeptidase in the cell wall. In parallel with work on penicillin, scientists searched for other natural antibiotics. Once of the sources of new antibiotics proved to be a group of soil microbes—streptomycetes (a genus of the Actinomycetales order). In 1940, Selman Waksman reported the antibacterial properties of actinomycin; in 1942, streptotricin; and in 1943, streptomycin. At first, streptomycin seemed to be a promising antibiotic, since it was effective against both gram-positive and gram-negative bacteria. However, it was soon discovered that in the course of medical treatment the bacteria often became resistant to streptomycin. It is used today as a highly effective treatment for tuberculosis. The discovery of penicillin and streptomycin led to a powerful push for a search for new antibiotics. In the following 65 years, oen thousand new antibiotics were discovered, but only some were found to have important use. The popularity of streptomycin in therapeutics lost ground mostly because of the discovery of a new class of antibiotics—tetracyclines. The first antibiotic in this class, aureomycin (Duomycin), was isolated in 1949 from streptomycetes; however, its structure had nothing common with the structure of streptomycin. The new antibiotic represented a derivative of naphthacene: 7-chlortetracycline, one of several substances with an atom of chlorine found in nature.

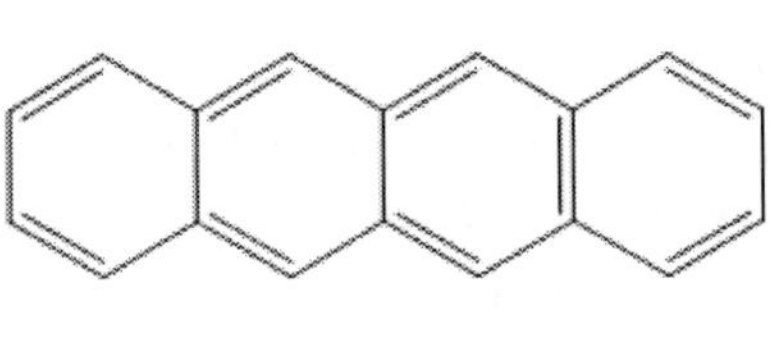
Naphthacene

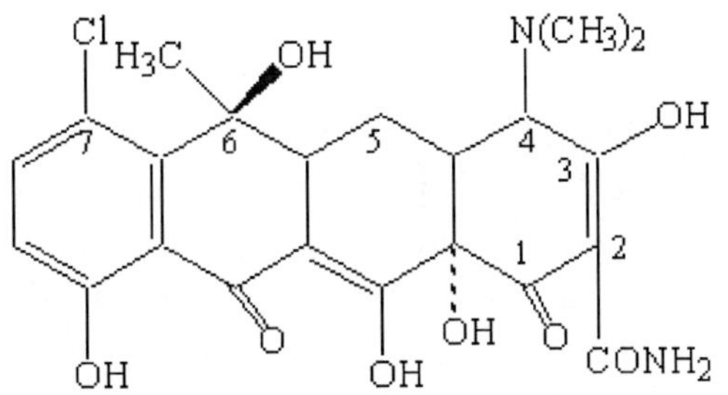

7-chlortetraciclyne (aureomycin, Duomycin)

It was discovered that for antibiotic activity the presence of chlorine in position 7 is not essential for tetracycline as a valuable medicine preparation. Further investigations in the modification of the structure of tetracycline found high activity in more simple structures (for example, 6-demethyl-6-dezoxy-tetracycline). Complete synthesis of this substance was realized by Robert Burns Woodward in 1962 and independently by M.M. Shemiakin et al. in the same year. For clinical use, tetracycline produces economical bacterial fermentation. The spectrum of action of tetracycline is wider than that of other antibiotics and is effective not only against gram-positive and gram-negative bacteria, but also against spirochetes, rickets and even some varieties of viruses. Another antibiotic produced by streptomycetes possessing a wide spectrum of action is chloramphenicol. As in the case of aureomycin, it is a representative of a rare natural substance containing chlorine, and, as in the case of aureomycin, the presence or absence of an atom of chlorine in the molecule is not indicative of antibacterial activity.

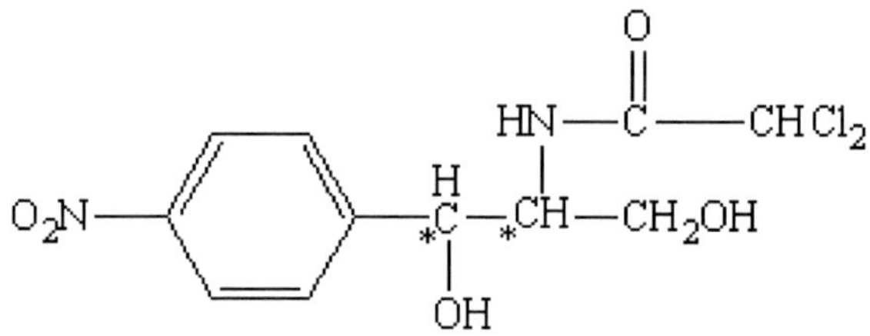

Chloramphenicol

A molecule of chloramphenicol contains two asymmetrical atoms of carbon (distinguished by asterisks in the diagram above) and, since each such asymmetrical center may be in two configurations, perhaps four stereoisomers have been identified and named because of their likeness to the sugars triose and eritrose: D-treo, L-treo, D-eritro and L-eritro forms (see Chapter 6). After the synthesis process, among all possible stereoisomers of chloramphenicol it was discovered that only one of the stereoisomers—namely, L-treoform, possessed antibacterial activity. It was noticed that only D-penicillamine was used as a medicinal remedy, since the L-isomer is not activated and is highly toxic for an organism. Those and still many other similar facts once more confirmed the long-well-known truth held by all toxicologists, synthetists and pharmacologists: the most powerful PhAS will be found only by absolute compliance with molecular structure in drugs or poisons designed for a specific target (receptor, biochemical reaction, or other mechanism) in an organism. This compliance probably demands the presence in a molecule of a PhAS of not only a physical formula (the presence of all necessary chemical elements in the required correlations), but certainly the definite concrete, spatial stereo formula (configuration). This position applies to optical and to *cis-, trans-, treo-* and *eritro*-isomers. In other words, an indispensable condition of effective interaction between a compound with its biotarget is a stereo-complimentary structure—an accordance between structure and conformation of a molecule of a compound and conformation with a definite part of a reaction. Their joining and consistent interaction requires a character of forces connecting their surfaces—van der Vaals force, electrostatic forces and hydrogen bonds. Van der Vaals force between atoms are weak and are displayed only in direct proximity. Small alterations in the structure of a compound (or cellular metabolite) break the stereo-complimentary intereaction between a compound and the active center of fermentation. Therefore, an analog of a compound or an analog of a cellular metabolite because of structural likeness add to the fermentation, but not complimentarily. In this case, the interaction between fermentation and a compound does not take place, but the active part of fermentation acts as a block (impeding access for a stereo-complimentary compound). If we examine the presence not only of one PhAS but the possible presence of other PhAS in food, beverages, smoke or even special injections (for example, poisons and antidotes), there are important implications not only regarding their competition for a target, but their actions on each other. The action of a PhAS may be either intensifying or weak. We have cited many examples of one biologically-active compound (poison, medicine, enzyme, etc.) slow down the removal of another substance, which in the case of medicine raises the risk of overdose. Many doctors at the present time overprescribe antibiotics, some of which should not be combined, affecting the quality of medical treatment. Antibiotics have an influence on the action of medications from other pharmaceutical groups—for example, hypertonic medical treatments, antihistamines and dysrythmia preparations. During administration of tetracycline, it is necessary to a bstain from milk products and fruits. Orange juice is prohibited with aspirin therapy. It is well known that caffeine enters into the composition of many analgesics (cytromone and sedalgine) because of its tendency to intensify the action of other PhAS. It was recently found that caffeine lowers the toxic action of paracetomol on the liver. Grapefruit juice is at the top of the list of dangerous substances that interact with medications, especially with calcium channel blockers. Such a combination often leads to death. Grapefruit juice can increase blook levels of cyclosporine in organ transplant patients taking this medication, an anti-rejection drug. Alcohol in various forms, from pure alcohol to weak alcoholic beverages such as beer, also influence the action of PhAS. Preparations for medicinal treatment of alcoholism—thiuram (disulphiram) and calcium cyanamide—cause a severe adverse reaction when a person consumes alcohol. The extraordinary properties of calcium cyanamide were discovered when supervisors at a nitrogenous fertilizer production plant noticed that employees were avoiding alcoholic beverages. Those who drank alcohol suffered from abrupt blood flow to the face, abundant perspiration, frequent palpitations, increased respiratory rate and sickness. It is dangerous to combine alcohol with sleep medications and tranquilizers. There is also an unexpected interaction between alcohol and clofeline, an antihypertension medication.

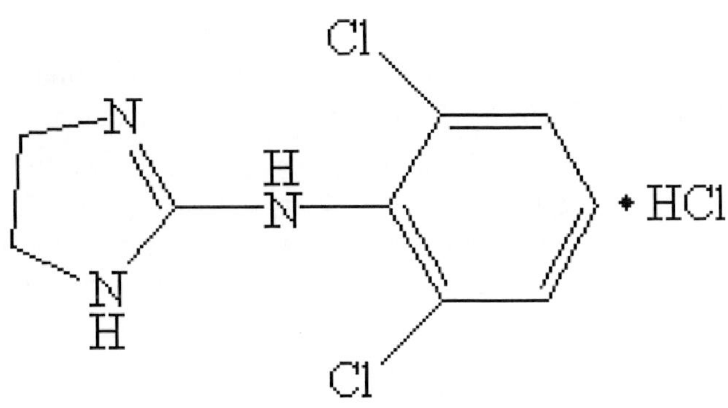

Clofeline

People not only fall into a deep sleep, but have no recollection afterwards of what had taken place. This fact is often used in the plots of detective novels. Clofeline has also been established as a remedy for tobacco dependence.

12.6. Bioregulators and Their Modifications

PhAS cited and briefly examined in this chapter have include products found in nature (plants, mushrooms and soil) and their analogs, which are cleanly synthetic "invented" structures not protein in origin. From examination of warm-blood animal organisms, up to 10,000 enzyme bioregulators with various chemical natures and functional purposes have been identified, produced and used. Bioregulators under consideration for study include those involved in growth and regeneration of tissues, body temperature, blood pressure, thought processes, ability, emotions, etc. And though in normal conditions these substances are present in tissues of organisms in extraordinarily low concentrations, they ensure effective vital action in individual organs (biosystems) and entire organisms. The increased attention devoted to bioregulators in recent years is apparently connected with two factors: a) prospective creation on their basis of a new generation of drugs with increased specificity and effective action without undesirable side effects; and b) prospective creation of biochemical or hormonal weapons, interest in which may be increased because of the Chemical Weapons Convention of 1993, which completely prohibits traditional chemical weapons. Bioregulators occupy an intermediate step between toxins and chemical warfare agents and are not formally prohibited under either chemical or biologic weapons conventions. Investigations and production of bioregulators and their structural modifications for public health may be used to disguise work dedicated to the creation of biochemical weapons, evading the laws of the conventions.

Among all number of molecules that are synthesized in living organisms, we shall briefly discuss the most well-known of two classes of bioregulators: steroids and polypeptides.

12.6.1. Steroids

Steroids, as bioregulators, fulfill different specific biological functions, but have a united principle: a molecule with a carbonic skeleton. Diverse steroids are produced by an organism in different quantities from insignificantly little but with powerful physiological action (for example, sex hormones) to comparatively abundant steroids, e.g., cholesterol, the purpose of whose synthesis is not distinct even today. Steroids possess an interesting property: their structure depends on the type of living organism they are found in. Plant-derived steroids do not join in the metabolism of an animal organism; if a supplementary quantity of steroids is necessary, then it the animal must obtain the needed amount by eating another animal, but not vegetation. This fact abruptly differs from the well-known and long-ago established astounding unity of life that stems from the universal anaerobic metabolism of any organism—for example, in the case of glucose. Exceptionally specialized, some fermentations participate in an organism's metabolism. For example, fermentations are responsible for the synthesis of cholesterol, a steroid that composes most gallstones but is actually present in all tissues of an organism, especially in nerve and brain tissues (approximately one sixth of their total weight), in blood (sometimes spreading in arterial walls, a possible cause of atherosclerosis). There are eight stereogenic centers for cholesterol. Owing to the presence of asymmetrical centers in the structure of cholysterine, the number of possible stereoisomers is 2^8, or 256 stereoisomers. In spite of the discovery of pure cholesterol in 1812, its chemical structure was not completely defined until 1932, but for specification of other details of its structure, another 23 years was required. Also, in the presence of a complicated system of rings and large numbers of asymmetrical centers (that is, stereoisomers), one of the difficulties in determining the structure cholesterol owed to the fact that the base part of the molecule is saturated hydrocarbon. The low ability of compounds in this class to react created complications for chemists in traditional methods of analysis—i.e., by decomposing to fragments that can be identified. Because cholesterol contains four carbonic rings, one can establish its molecular formula as $C_{27}H_{46}O$, since the formation of a ring reflects the formula of the molecule; thus, formation of a double bond decreases the number of hydrogen atoms in the formula to two. For example, the formula of pentane is C_5H_{12}, but the formula of cyclopentane and pentene is C_5H_{10}. The branching of the chain has no influence on the physical formula. A double bond can be distinguished from the cycle by interaction with hydrogen, measuring its quantity used for saturation of a molecule, consequently enabling definition of the number double bonds in a molecule. One mole of cholesterol absorbs only one mole of hydrogen; therefore, it contains only one double bond. The physical formula of unsaturated alcohol (cholesterol containing one hydroxyl group) is written as $C_nH_{2n}O$, but the composition of a molecule cholesterol corresponds to the formula $C_nH_{2n-8}O$; that is, it contains eight fewer hydrogen atoms in comparison with alcohol, with an opening chain having one double bond and, consequently, its composition consists of four rings. Information about the size of the ring is gained by carrying out oxidation with an open ring, the results of which are dicarbo acids. By successively pyrolizing these acids, a five-member ring was formed corresponding to anhydride, a six-member cycle of which is cyclopentanone. These products are easy to identify. This method was used to study the structure of cholesterol, and between the third and fourth cycle the correct answer was found. This fact in 1928 lead to a proposed structure of cholesterol. Although erroneous, this work earned a Nobel Prize for the scientist, Adolf Windaus, who suggested it.

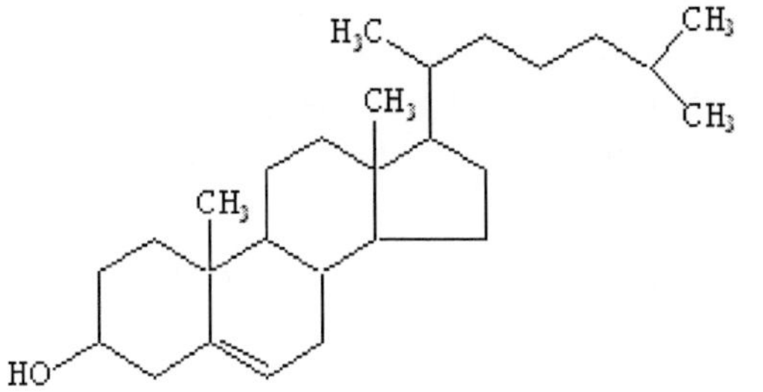

Cholesterol

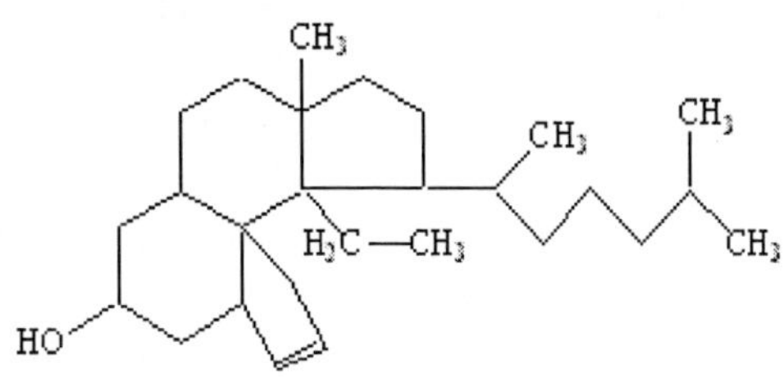

Erroneous structure of cholesterol

Soon after, it was discovered that dehydrogenization of cholesterol by selenium leads to the well-known structures of chrysene and methylcyclopentanphenantrene.

At last, in 1932, the correct structure of cholesterol was determined, which lead to the perfectly logical question: How is such a complicated molecule formed in an organism? This question had become more intriguing after it was discovered that the biological synthesis of cholesterol may be realized when the source of carbon atoms is only one fragment: an acetate ion. What takes place? An exhaustive answer to this difficult question, however, is sufficiently simple, since the synthesis of cholesterol resembles the synthesis of natural rubber with isoprene.

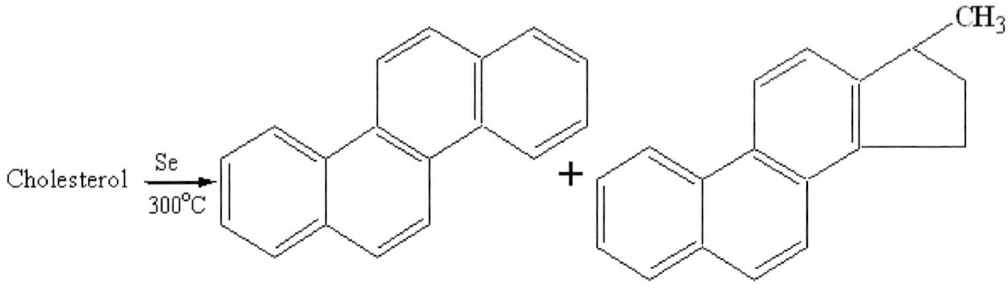

Chrysene Methylcyclopentanphenantrene

At first, three acetate ions join to form a carbon oxide, isoprene. Six links of isoprene add one to another to synthesize another substance (squalene) with a long open chain containing six double bonds. Then, squalene is cyclized with participation of double bonds to form the steroid lanosterol, a predecessor of cholesterol. Undoubtedly, this row of reactions, beginning with acetic acid and resulting in a steroid, strongly distinguishes itself by ordinary chance reactions in collision with molecules that are taken up in nonbiologic systems. As cited above, these reactions possess a high degree of stereo specification for their catalytic enzymes, which strictly and securely direct reactions and result in only definite stereoisomers that are selected from possible thousands. This is the miracle of natural organic synthesis. The proof of reactions in the biosynthesis of cholesterol was obtained mainly in experiments making use of marked atoms with corresponding radioactive isotopes. After fulfillment of this very important work, Konrad Bloch and his collaborator, Feodor Lynen, were awarded the Nobel Prize in 1964.

The biosynthesis of cholesterol in animal tissues is a highly productive process. The general maintenance of cholesterol in humans, for example, is an average of 200 grams. And although its ultimate use is not known, it has been established that during metabolism it disintegrates, making gallic acid and steroidal hormones. However, the requirement of these compounds is small in comparison with the quantity of cholesterol synthesized. Nevertheless, it has been discovered that cholesterol is synthesized and used as a precursor to vitamin D_3. This fact marked the beginning of the use of steroids in medicine. Then, yet another direction was taken in the use of steroids: as sex hormones, at first, in the prevention of pregnancy; sex stimulators; and other treatments. Among numerous bioregulators of an organism, a prominent place is occupied by female (estradiol) and male (testosterone) hormones.

The modification of steroidal structures has produced synthetic products that have advantages over natural substances, since they render much more powerful action by oral administration (per os). Fifty years ago, it was discovered that a state of temporary sterility in women could be supported artificially.

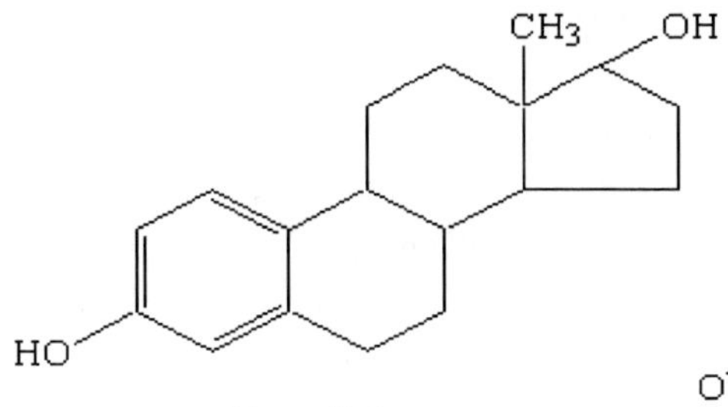

Estradiol

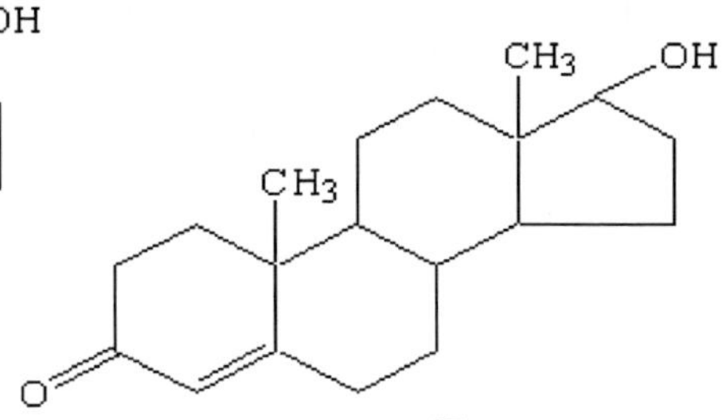

Testosterone

This led to the creation of the now-popular oral birth control method. Introducing sex hormones or their analogs even to castrated or sexually immature animals causes a corresponding effect. Introducing even only 0.1 mkg (a quantity not noticeable with the naked eye) of estrone (a product of the oxidation of estradiol in ketone) into female mice in which the ova have been removed leads to the beginning of sexual maturity, and castrated roosters, after injection of testosterone, grow a comb. Synthetic preparations are called estrogens or progestins depending upon which natural hormone they like. One from the wide-spread synthetic estrogen represents 17-etine (acetylene derivate -C≡CH)-estradiol. A state of temporary sterility of women is reached by suppressing ova production by inhibiting the distribution of follicle stimulating hormone (FSH). Inhibition of FSH may be reached in two ways: introduction of estradiol for suppression of the development of ovarian follicles, or introduction of progesterone (a pregnancy hormone) for suppressing the production of FSH by the anterior pituitary gland. Progesterone is structurally closer to the male hormone (testosterone) than to the female (estradiol). And although progesterone and estradiol act in different ways, they lead to the same result—temporary sterility of women as a consequence of the creation and support of the hormonal state of pseudo pregnancy.

12.6.2. Polypeptides and Lipids

Together with enzymes and hormones with the structure of steroids and other nonproteins, a vast group PhAS among bioregulators are composed of peptides. One molecule discovered long ago and well known for inducing pain is the nanopeptide (that is, a peptide containing nine amino acids), bradykinin. This compound is formed with a blood plasma protein at the sites of wounds and injuries in an organism. A leading role in establishing three measures of space conformation of bradykinin and interrelations with biologic activity belongs to several groups of Soviet biochemists: in Moscow, U. Ovchinnikov and V. Ivanov et al.; in Minsk, S. Galaktionov et al.; and in Riga, G. Chipens, F. Mutulis and others. The history of this and other questions regarding the synthesis of polypeptides and bioregulators (the drug, dizain) in the pursuit of new drugs is brilliantly set forth by Gregory V. Nikiforovich in his popular-science book, *Almost Natural Drugs,* in which bradykinin is prominently featured.

This peptide forms at the shortened tail of a gigantic molecule of protein and enters into the hemoglobin complex, which realizes the transfer of oxygen from the lungs to all tissues of an organism. Intravenous injection of bradykinin into guinea pigs cause bronchospasm, an acute constriction of the muscles of the larynx, resulting in labored respiration and afterwards leads to suffocation. Interest has been generated by the observation that a small dose of aspirin a few minutes before injection of bradykinin fully wards off bronchospasm. Apparently, aspirin blocks the action of bradykinin on the way to bonding with some (but not all) types of receptive centers, causing inflammatory response and pain.

Another example of a highly active peptide bioregulator was discovered in 1988—endothelin, a molecule that contains 29 amino acid residues.

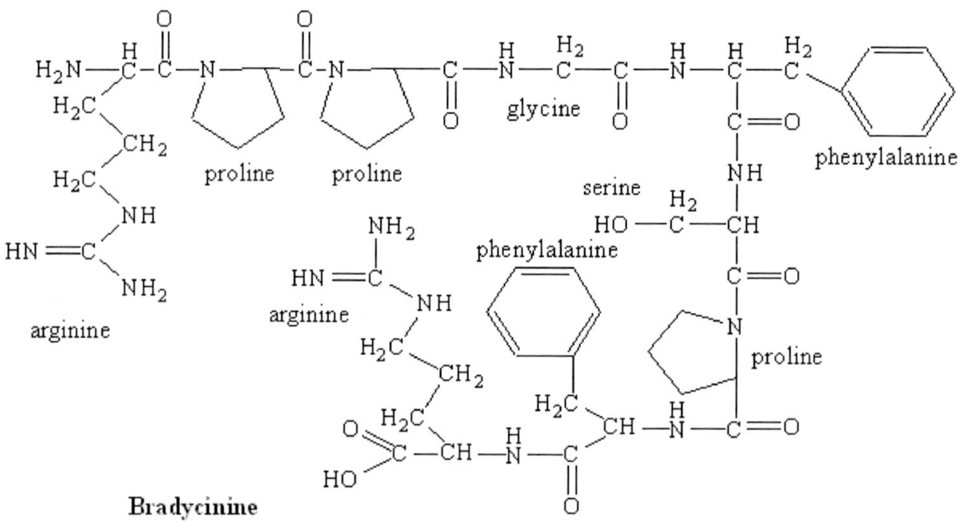

Bradycinine

This is among the strongest compounds that influence the vaso- and bronchoregulating centers. A dose of 0.002 mg/kg (rats, intravenous) of endothelin leads to an increase in arterial pressure and a decrease in the frequency of palpitation during bronchospasm. Two groups of scientists from Japan and the United States each independently found an extraordinary structural and functional likeness with rapid-acting cardiotoxines (sarapho-toxines) taken from the venomous cave snake, *Atractaspis engaddensis*.

Among regulator peptides, substances were discovered with expressly emetic (vomit-inducing) properties. They include a series of neuropeptides: angiotencine-P, nevrotencine, nethionine-ankephaline, leucine-ankephaline, vazopressine, oxitocine, bombenzine, tirotropine-rilizine hormone, gastrine and other vaso-intestinal peptides, which in doses of 0.3–0.35 mg/kg (dogs, intravenous) cause an emetic reaction lasting 0.5–5 min. The higher emetic activity is displayed in the endogenic regulator-peptide RUU, discovered by Canadian scientists, which contains 36 residues of amino acids (molecular mass 4309.8). The threshold dose for dogs of purified RUU is $4.3 \cdot 10^{-4}$ mg/kg, but the effective dose $ED_{50} = 1.4 \cdot 10^{-3}$ mg/kg. The threshold dose is 10 times more effective than the well-known emetic apomorphine. An injection of an effective dose of RUU (ED_{50}), usually causes, within 2–3 min, one emetic episode with a duration of 15 sec, after which the animal returns to normal. By comparison, the well-known emetic of bacteriological origin—staphylococci enterotoxine B (see Chapter 10)—has a latent period lasting 40 min, but emesis lasts a few hours. Until the 1990s, the majority of scientists came to the conclusion that many peptide bioregulators contain small structural fragments that possess the activity of the initial peptide bioregulator, which require the original spatial complementarities to specific receptors. Such fragments are not found in nature and may be used as initial material for constructing and producing analogs, some of which have toxicity close to that of neuro-paralytic warfare agents. The fruitfulness of such an approach may be illustrated with the example of synthesis of analogs of a regular peptide—cholecystokinin (CCK)—with active short chains and stable against metabolism, which in its native form leads to a state of panic. In nature, there are two spreading forms of this peptide—CCK-8 and CCK-33—contain 8 and 33 residues of amino acids, respectively. C. Monmighu from Canada found that shorter fragments of molecules of these peptides—CCK-4 (Trp-Met-Asp-Phe-NH_2)—also show high activity when injected into animals and humans. In doses of 20–100 mg in humans it causes panic in healthy volunteers lasting 1–4 min. It was found that in a molecule of peptide CCK-4, bonding receptors use only triptophane (Trp) and phenylalanine (Phe). Using this information about the relationship between the structure and properties, this series of "peptoidentical" analogs of CCK-4 was created: tret.trichlorbutyloxycarbonyl-D, L-metyltriptophanephenylethylamide:

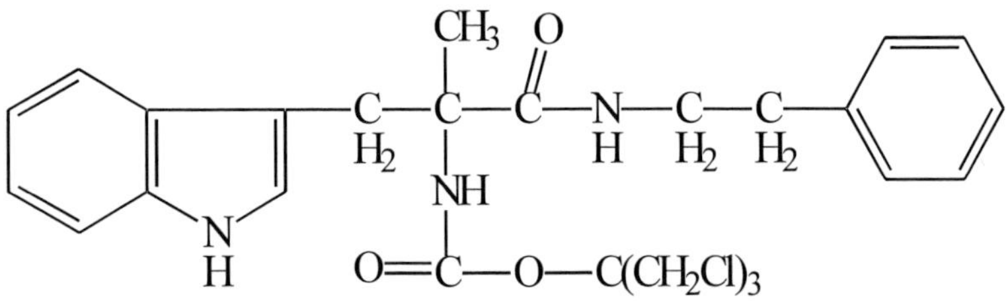

This analog preserves the high biological activity, increased metabolic stability and lipophility, and the ability to overcome the hematoencephalic barrier. It also has greater affinity toward receptors. A characteristic peculiarity of endogenic bioregulators appears to be very low stability. In warm-blooded animals, by process of metabolism, they undergo rapid destruction by catabolizing fermentation. For increasing the life span of bioregulators in an organism, it is necessary at the same time to introduce inhibitors of such fermentations. On the other hand, inhibitors of fermentations alone may cause intense action in PhAS, the presence of which in an organism may bring an imbalance with pathologic consequences simultaneously by accumulation of endogen bioregulators. Together with peptides, large groups of highly activity bioregulators have a mixed structure, the most active among which are lipids and phospholipids. Lipid bioregulators include metabolites of arachidonic acid (prostaglandins, tromboxanes, prostaciklines, lipoxines, leukotrienes) and PAF (platelet-activating factor). These compounds render negative action in cardiovascular and respiratory systems and participate in the formation and preservation of such pathological states as inflammation, allergy, shock, ischemia, poisoning and others. The strongest cardiovascular action, for example, is demonstrated by leukotrienes that possess peptidoleukotrienes C_4 and D_4. The activity of these leukotrienes is demonstrated in submicrogramic injected or inhaled doses. Leukotriene C_4 in a dose of $1 \cdot 10^{-7}$ mg/kg decreases cardiac output by half, but as an aerosol causes brochospasm in humans of average weight in a dose of 0.001–0.01 mg.

PAF (1-hexa (octa)decyl-2-acetyl-glicero-3-phosphorilcholine) applies to endogen phospholipidic bioregulators. PAF causes acute impairment of cardiovascular and respiratory functions. An intravenous lethal dose of PAF is 0.015 mg/kg, and death occurs in 6–7 min because of respiratory arrest. PAF in a dose of 0.0055 mg in pigs causes systemic hypotension, collapse and death. Intratracheal administration of PAF in baboons leads to immediate bronchospasm in doses as small as $6 \cdot 10^{-5}$ mg/kg. Experiments on human volunteers with intratracheal administration of PAF in doses of $4 \cdot 10^{-5}$–$12 \cdot 10^{-3}$ mg/kg causes bronchospasm and other symptoms characteristic of asthma, allowing consideration of PAF as the strongest-acting bronchospasmic compound.

At the present time, investigations into the area of bioregulators have already produced not only scientific but practical interest. Because of the considerable progress in the areas of molecular biology and biotechnology reached in the last 10 years, it has become sufficiently practical to make use of bioregulators as a basis for the development of new drugs. On the other hand, interest in bioregulators as a possible basis for new biochemical weapons necessarily attracts public attention. It is necessary to continue to focus attention and further efforts on prohibition of these compounds for humanitarian purposes, and on the creation of a system of effective control.

About the Authors and Editor

The authors have been friends since their student days. They simultaneously graduated from St. Petersburg State Technological Institute in 1962 and have worked in Volgograd. In 1968, they earned Cand. Chem. Sci. scientific degrees and in the beginning of the 1990s they defended their doctoral theses. Both take a great interest in fishing and hunting.

Zotov Stanislav Borisovich is a doctor of technical sciences and professor at Volgograd State Technical University. In addition to his academic appointment, he has 40 years of experience as specialist in chemistry and technology of bioactive substances at the Scientific Investigative Centre of Volgograd OAO "Khimprom." He is a member of the doctoral faculties of chemistry and technology at VSTU.

Tuzhikov Oleg Ivanovich is a doctor of chemical sciences and professor at Volgograd State Technical University. He is specialist in the areas of chemistry and technology of high molecular compounds and bioactive substances. He is also a member of the doctoral faculties of chemistry and technology at VSTU.

Recent publications of the authors during the past three years include the following:

1) Zotov S.B., Tuzhikov O.I. *Poisons: Physiological active substances*. Ed. by Zotov, S.B. First edition. Volgograd. VolgGTU. RPK Polytechnic, 2005. 204 pp. (Russ.).
2) Tuzhikov O.I., Khokhlova T.V., Bondarenko S.N., Zotov S.B. and others. *Elastomers and plastics of the lowered combustibility*. Ed. by O.I. Tuzhikov. Volgograd. RPK Polytechnic, 2005. 214 pp. (Russ.).
3) *Chemical Physics of Pyrolysis, Combustion and Oxidation*. Editors: A.A. Berlin et al. NY. Nova Science Publishers, 2005. 214 pp.
4) Zotov S.B., Lavrent'ev A.N., Grigor'eva A.V. Engineer-chemical aspects of problem dumped chemical weapon. *Khim. prom. Segodnia*, 2006. No. 9. pp. 24-33. (Russ.).
5) Uskach Y.L. Zotov S.B., Popov U.V., Kolotilina T.V. Termodestruction of nonutilizited liquid organic waste. *Chemical technology: Collection of reports International conference by Chemical technology*. ChT'07. V.3 / Ed. by A.A. Berlin, N.A. Khalturinskiy, A.A. Voshkin. M. Lenand, 2007. pp. 249-252. (Russ.).
6) Zotov S.B., Tuzhikov O.I., Uskach Y.L. Problems of destruction steadfast organic pollutants of environment. *Khim. prom. Segodnia*, 2009. No. 2, pp. 17-24. (Russ.).

General Bibliography

Chapter 1

Graves R. *The Greek Myths*. M., Progress, 1992. (Russ., Engl. version is also available).

Kun N. *Legends and myths ancient Greeks*. M., 1975. (Russ.).

Losev A.F. *Gamer*. M., 1960. (Russ.).

Taho-Godi A.A. *Mythology Greeks*. M., 1989. (Russ.).

Chapter 2

Blyth A.W., Blyth M.W. *Poisons - their effect and detection*. London. Ch. Griffin and Co. 1906.

Figurovskiy N.A. *Essay general history of chemistry. From antiquity to beginning XIX century* M., Nauka, 1972. (Russ.).

Gadaskina I.D., Tolokoncev N.A. *Poisons – yesterday and today: Essays about history's poisons*. L., Nauka, ser. "From molecules to organism," 1988. (Russ.).

General history of chemistry. Beginning and development chemistry from antiquity to XVII century, M., Nauka, 1980. (Russ.).

Golikov S.N. *Poisons and antipoisons*. M., Znanie.1968. (Russ.).

Halstead B.W. *Poisonous and venomous marine animals of the world*. USA. Goverment printing, office, Washington, vol. 1 – 3, 1965 - 1970.

Leykin U.I., Oksengendler G.I., Chkhartishvili V.I. Venomous marine animals. *Marine collection,* 1981. No. 2, 68 (Russ.).

Losev A.F., Taho-Godi A.A. *Aristotle*. M., Detskaiya literatura. 1982. (Russ.).

Narcotics and poisons: Psychodelics and toxic substances, venomous animals and plants. Staff V. I. Petrova, T. I. Revyko. Minsk. Literatura, 1996. p. 592. (Russ.).

Solov'ev U.I. *History of chemistry. Development chemistry from antiquity to XVII century*. M., Prosvestchenie, 1976. (Russ.).

Starkov O. A. *Parasites and venomous animals in "Canon medical science" Abuali ibn-Sino*. Duschanbe, Donisch, 1980. (Russ.).

Sultanov M.N. *Bites of venomous animals*. M., Medicine. 1977. (Russ.).

Talizin F.F. *Venomous animals of land and marine*. M., Znanie. 1970. (Russ.).

Chapters 3 and 4

Agricola G. *About mining affair and metallurgy*. Ed. by S.V. Shukhardin., M., AN SSSR, 1962. (Russ.).

Azimov A. *Brief history chemistry. Development of ideas and representations in chemistry*. Translation with English. M., Mir, 1983. (Russ., Engl. version is also available).

Bikov G.V. *Aleksandr Mikhaiylovich Butlerov. Essay life and activity*. M., AN SSSR, 1961. (Russ.).

Bikov G.V. *August Kekule. Essay life and activity*. M., Nauka, 1964. (Russ.).

Bikov G.V. *History of organic chemistry. Discover more importance organic compounds*. M., Nauka, 1978. (Russ.).

Bikov G.V. *History of stereochemistry organic compounds*. M., Nauka, 1966. (Russ.).

Dobrotin R.B., Solov'ev U.I. *Vant-Goff*. M., Nauka, 1977. (Russ.).

Dorfman Y.G. *Lavuasiet*. M., Nauka, 1962. (Russ.).

Emsley J. *The Elements of Murder: A History of Poisons*. New York, Oxford University Press, 2005.

Figurovskiy N.A. *Dmitriy Ivanovich Mendeleev*. M., AN SSSR, 1961. (Russ.).

Fischer E. *Selected Works*. M., Nauka, 1979. (Russ.).

Musabekov U.S. *Ustus Libih*. M., AN SSSR, 1962. (Russ.).

Pagel W. *Paracelsus. An introduction to Philosophical Medicine in the Era of the Renaissance*. Basel, Karger, 1958.

Shamin A.*N. Chemical synthesis of protein (historical essay)*. M., Nauka, 1969. (Russ.).

Shamin A.N., Jabrailova N.A. *Development chemistry aminoacids*. M., Nauka, 1974. (Russ.).

Shamin A.N. *History chemistry of protein*. M., Nauka, 1977. (Russ.).

Solov'ev U.I., Trifonov D.N., Shamin A.N. *History of chemistry. Development general directions of contemporary chemistry*. M., Prosvestchenie, 1978. (Russ.).

Chapter 5

Barlow R. *Introduction in Chemical Pharmacology*, M., IL, 1959. (Russ.).

Brekhman I.I. Person and biological active substances. M., Nauka, 1980. (Russ.).

Gabuda S.P. Bonding water. Facts and hypotheses. Novosibirsk. Nauka, 1982. (Russ.).

Golikov S.N. Guidance by toxicology chemical warfare agents. M., Medicina, 1972. (Russ.).

Guidance by forensic-medical expertise poisonings. Ed. Berezhnoy et al. M., Medicina, 1980. (Russ.).

Kagan U.S. Toxicology phosphororganic pesticides. M., Medicina, 1977. (Russ.).

Kharkevich D.A. Ganglionaric remedys, M., Medgiz, 1962. (Russ.).

Kutcenco S.A. *Bases of Toxicology*. S-Pb. Foliant. 2004. p. 720. (Russ.).

Oksengendler G.I. Poisons and antipoisons. L., Nauka, 1982. (Russ.).

Petrov R.V. *Conversations about new immunology*, Second Ed. M., "Molodaya gvardiya" 1978. (Russ.).

Stripp R.A. *The Forensic Aspects of Poisons*. NY. Infobase Publishing. 2007.

Zalninsh K.K., Pavlova L.P. Water – source of life. Monografia / IVS RAN, S-Pb. SPGUTD. 2005. p. 293. (Russ.).

Chapter 6

Amici M., Dallanoce C., Angeli P., Marucci G., Cantalamessa F., De Micheli C. Synthesis and pharmacological characterization of new chiral derivatives of muscarine and allo-muscarine. *Il Farmaco*, 2000. Vol. 55, Issue 8, P. 535-543.

Amici M., Micheli C., and other. Synthesis and pharmacological investigation of cholinergic ligands structurally related to muscarone. *European Journal of Medicinal Chemistry*, 1989. Vol. 24, Issue 2, P. 171-177.

Amici M., Micheli C., Molteni G., Pitrd D., Carrea G., Riva S., Spezia S., Zetta L. Chemoenzymatic Synthesis of the Eight Stereoisomeric Muscarines *J. Org. Chem.* 1991. Vol. 56. P. 67-72.

Amouroux R., Gerin B., Chastrette M. Une nouvelle synthese totale de la L(+) et de la D(-)-muscarine. *Tetrahedron*, 1985. Vol. 41, Issue 22, P. 5321-5324.

Amouroux R., Gerin B., Chastrette M. Une synthese simple et tres stereoselective de la d,l-muscarine. *Tetrahedron Letters*, 1982. Vol. 23, Issue 42, P. 4341-4344.

Angeli P., Cantalamessa F., Cavagna R., Conti P., Amici M., Micheli C., Gamba A., Marucci G. Synthesis and Pharmacological Characterization of Enantiomerically Pure Muscarinic Agonists: Difluoromuscarines. *J. Med. Chem.* 1997. Vol. 40, No. 7, P. 1099-1103.

Angle S.R., El-Said N.A. Stereoselective Synthesis of Tetrahydrofurans via Formal [3+2]-Cycloaddition of Aldehydes and Allylsilanes. Formal Total Synthesis of the Muscarine Alkaloids (-)-Allomuscarine and (+)-Epimuscarine. *J. Am. Chem. Soc.* 2002. Vol.124, No. 14. P. 3608-3613.

Baccount. *Ann.Chim. (France).* 1811, 79, 25; 1811, 80, 272; 1813, 87, 237.

Balenovich. *Arhiv. Kem.* 1955, 27, 105.

Boukouvalas J., Radu I. A concise asymmetric synthesis of (+)-muscarine from (S)-γ-hydroxymethyl-γ-butyrolactone. *Tetrahedron Letters*, 2007. Vol. 48, Issue 17, pp. 2971-2973.

Clark Still W., Schneider J.A. Chelation-Controlled Synthesis of (±)-Muscarine. *J. Org. Chem.* 1980. Vol. 45, No. 16, P. 3375-3376.

Corrodi H., Hardegger E., Kögl F. Über Muscarin. 8. Mitteilung. Herstellung von racemischem Allomuscarin. *Helv. Chim. Acta*, 40, 2454 (1957).

Corrodi H., Hardegger E., Kögl F., Zeller P. Synthese von Stereoisomeren des Muscarins. *Experientia*, 13, 138 (1957).

Corrodi H., Steiner K., Halder N., Hardegger E. Über Muscarin. 12. Mitteilung. Synthese des DL-2-Methyl-muscarons, des DL-2-Methyl-muscarins und des DL-2-Methyl-epimus-carins. *Helv. Chim. Acta*, 44, 1157 (1961).

Cox H.C. *Helv. Chim. Acta*, 41, 229 (1958).

Dagaev S.G., Kosmachov A.B., Libman N.M. and others. Method quantitative estimation electoral blockade of muscarinic choline-receptors M_4-subtype in the condition intact organism. *Bull. Experim. Biolog. I Medicine.* 2003. No. 5, P. 524-526. (Russ.)

Eugster C. H. "Chemistry of muscarine." Collection "Uspekhi organicheskoy khimii" v.2. M., *Mir*, 1964. (Russ.)

Eugster C. H., *Helv. Chim. Acta*, 41, 205 (1958).

Eugster C. H., *Helv. Chim. Acta*, 41, 583 (1958).

Eugster C. H., *Helv. Chim. Acta*, 41, 705 (1958).

Eugster C. H., *Helv. Chim. Acta*, 41, 886 (1958).

Eugster C. H. Rev. Chemistry active beginning of mushroom *Amanita muscaria. Fortschr. Chem. organ. Naturstoffe*, 27. Wien, 1969. p.261-321. (Ger.)

Eugster C. H. Synthese des d,l-Muscarins (kurze Mitteilung). 6. Mitteilung über Muscarin. *Helv. Chim. Acta*, 40, 2462 (1957).

Eugster C. H. Zur Konstitution des Muscarins. 3. Mitteilung über Muscarin. *Helv. Chim. Acta*, 39, 1023 (1956).

Eugster C. H., Allner K. Thiomuscarine. Über Wasserstoffbrücken in β-Hydroxyfuranen und β–Hydroxythiophanen. *Helv. Chim. Acta*, 45, 1750 (1962).

Eugster C. H., Waser P. Isolierung von Muscarin aus Inocybe Patouillardi (Bres.) 4. Mitteilung über Muscarin. *Helv. Chim. Acta*, 40, 888 (1957).

Eugster C. H., Waser P.G. Zur Kenntnis des Muscarins. *Experientia,* 1954, 10, 298.

Ewins A. J. The Constitution of Pseudo-Muscarine ("Synthetic Muscarine"). *J. Biochem.*, 1914, 8, 209.

Farina A., Meille S.V., Resnati G. The crystalline conformation and packing of fluoro-muscarine and allo-fluoro-muscarine iodides: The effect of hydroxyl group substitution by fluorine. *Journal of Fluorine Chemistry*, 1996. Vol. 80, Issue 1, P. 47-52.

Fourneau E. *Ann. Pharm. France* 3, 114, 1945.

Fourneau E. *Bull. Soc. Chim. Biol.* Paris, 1944, 26,516.

Fourneau J.P., Rybak B. Mise au point d'une nouvelle technique de titration sur coeur ouvert de mammifere des effets muscariniques a partir d'une nouvelle serie de composes parasympathomimetiques. *Life Sciences*, No. 5, 185-193 (1962).

Givens R.S., Rademacher D.R. Further studies on carbocyclic analogs of muscarine/ Oxidation of desethermuscarine to desethermuscarone. *J. Med. Chem.* 1974. Vol. 17, No. 4, P. 457-459.

Gryszkiewicz-Trochimowski E. *Bull. Soc. Chim. France*, No. 5, 603 (1958).

Gwido Zwicky, Waser P. G., Eugster C. H. Synthese und pharmakologische Eigenschaften des Desmethylmuscarons und der stereoisomeren Desmethylmuscarine Die Basen-stärken der isomeren Normuscarine. 11. Mitteilung über Muscarin. *Helv. Chim. Acta*, 42, 1177 (1959).

Hardegger E. Furter H., Kiss J. Über Muscarin. 10. Mitteilung. Herstellung des unnatürlichen 2R, 3S, 5R-(-)-Muscarins aus 2-Desoxy-D-ribose. *Helv. Chim. Acta*, 41, 2401 (1958).

Hardegger E., Lohse F. Über Muscarin. 7. Mitteilung. Synthese und absolute Konfiguration des Muscarins. *Helv. Chim. Acta*, 40, 2383 (1957).

Harnack E. *Arch. Exp. Path. Pharm.* 1875, 4, 168.

Hartung J., Kneuer R. Synthesis of enantiopure (2R)-configured muscarine alkaloids via selective alkoxyl radical ring-closure reactions. *Tetrahedron: Asymmetry*, 2003. Vol.14, Issue 19, P. 3019-3031.

Hulme E.C., Birdsall N.J.M., Buckley N. J. Muscarinic receptor subtypes. *Ann. Rev. Pharm. Toxicol.* 1990. Vol. 30, P. 633-673.

Jellinek F. The structure of muscarine. *Acta Cryst.* 10, 277, 1957.

Kilimov A.P., Svechnicova M.A., Shevchenko V.I., Kvasnuk-Mudriy F.V., Zotov S.B., Smirnov V.V. Infrared specters ordinary cycle ethers and their derivatives. Comm. 2. Characteristical absorb mono and disubstituente 1,4-dioxane». *ibid.* No. 2, 208 (1969). (Russ.).

Kilimov A.P., Svechnicova M.A., Shevchenko V.I., Kvasnuk-Mudriy F.V., Zotov S.B., Smirnov V.V. Infrared specters ordinary cycle ethers and their derivatives. "Comm.1. Peculiarities skeleton vibrations tetrahydrofuranic cycle," *Khimiya Heterociclicheskikh Soedineniy (KhHS)*, No. 4, 579 (1967). (Russ.).

King H. The isolation of muscarine, the potent principle of Amanita muscaria. *J. Chem. Soc.,* 1922, 121, 1743.

Kiss J., Furter H., Lohse F., Hardegger E. Über Muscarin. 11. Mitteilung. Synthese von bisquaternären, dem Muscarin ähnlichen Verbindungen. *Helv. Chim. Acta,* 44, 141 (1961).

Knight D.W., Staples E.R. Stereocontrol of 5-endo-trig cyclisations by hydroxyl groups: a formal short synthesis of (+)-muscarine. *Tetrahedron Letters*, 2002. Vol. 43, Issue 38, P. 6771-6773.

Kogl F. *Rec. Trav. Chim.*, 76, 109, 1957.

Kogl F., Duisberg H., Erxleben H. Untersuchungen über Pilzgifte. I. Über das Muscarin. *Liebigs Ann.,* 1931, 489, 156.

Kögl F. Cox H.C., Salemink C.A. Über Muscarin. Synthese eines Gemischs von Muscarin und seinen stereoisomeren Formen. *Experientia,* 13, 137, (1957).

Kosmachov A.B., Belyev V.A., Filko O.A. and others. Role blockade separate subtypes of muscarinic receptors in the realization of antidotal effect M-cholinolitics by intoxication of dimethyldichlorvinilphosphate. *Experim. and clinic. Pharmacol.* 1999. No. 4. P. 55-58. (Russ.)

Kuehl F., Lebel N., Richter J.W. Isolation and Characterization Studies on Muscarine. *J. Am. Chem. Soc.*, 1955, 77, 6663.

Kvasnuk-Mudriy F.V., Smirnov V.V., Zotov S.B. Synthesis 5-substituente-2-dimethylamino-methyl-tetrahydrofuranes, *ibid.* Coll. No. 2, 15 (1970). (Russ.).

Kvasnuk-Mudriy F.V., Smirnov V.V., Zotov S.B. Synthesis in series aminomethylderivatives tetrahydrofurane. *ibid.* Coll. No. 2, 19 (1970). (Russ.).

Kyung Ho Kang, Mi Young Cha, Ae Nim Pae, Kyung Il Choi, Yong Seo Cho, Hun Yeong Koh, Bong Young Chung. Synthesis of (+)-muscarine from (S)-(−)-5-hydroxymethyl-2(5H)-furanone. *Tetrahedron Letters,* 2000. Vol. 41, Issue 42, P. 8137-8140.

Maekawa H., Ichihara A., Matsumoto T. The Synthesis of dl-Muscarine and dl-Allomuscarine. *Bull. Chim. Soc. Japan*, 38, 1161 (1965).

Matsumoto T., Maekawa H. Eine neue Synthese des D,L- und D,L-allo-Muscarins. *Angew. Chem.* 70, 507 (1958).

Moskvichev U.A., Feldblum V.Sh. *Chemistry in our life*. Monografia. Yaroslavl. Izd-vo YaGTU, 2007. (Russ.).

Mudriy F.V., Smirnov V.V., Zotov S.B. Investigation in district myscarine. 1. Synthesis mixture racemates of muscarine and it stereoisomers. *ibid.* No. 5, 579 (1970). (Russ.).

Neurotransmitters, drugs and brain function. Ed. R.A. Webster. Chichester, UK. John Wiley and Sons, 2001.

Pirrung M.C., De Amicis C.V. Total synthesis of the muscarines. *Tetrahedron Letters*, 1988. Vol. 29, Issue 2, P.159-162.

Pochet S., Huynh-Dinh T. Stereospecific Synthesis of Muscarines and Allomuscarines in D and L Series. *J. Org. Chem.* 1982. Vol. 47, No. 2, P.193-198.

Popsavin V., Beric O., Popsavin M., Radic L., Csanádi J., Cirin-Novta V. A Divergent Synthesis of (+)-Muscarine and (+)-epi-Muscarine from D-Glucose. *Tetrahedron,* 2000. Vol. 56, Issue 32, P. 5929-5940.

Price Ch., Oae Sh. *Sulfur Bonding*, NY, 1962.

Rogers E. F., Bovet D., Longo V.G., Marini-Bettolo G.B. Alkoxytrimethylammonium salts and muscarine. *Experientia,* 1953, 9, 260.

Schmiedeberg, Koppe. *Das Muscarin*. FCW Vegel Leipzig, 1869.

Shapiro G., Buechler D., Hennet S. Synthesis of enantiomerically pure muscarine analogs. *Tetrahedron Letters,* 1990. Vol. 31, Issue 40, P. 5733-5736.

Smirnov V.V., Antonova N.G., Zotov S.B., Kvasnuk-Mudriy F.V., Sitanova N.A., Cyclic ethers and acetalies. 1. Synthesis aminoderivatives methyl-1,4-dioxane. *Zh. Org. Khimii*, **4**, 1740 (1968). (Russ.).

Smirnov V.V., Antonova N.G., Zotov S.B., Kvasnuk-Mudriy F.V., Sitanova N.A., Cyclic ethers and acetalies. Comm.3. 2,6-derivatives 1,4-dioxane. *Khimiya Heterociclicheskikh Soedineniy (KhHS),* No. 3, 318 (1970). (Russ.).

Smirnov V.V., Zotov S.B., Kvasnuk-Mudriy F.V. Synthesis 2,2,5,5-tetramethyltetrahydro-tiophene., *ibid.* No. 1, 173 (1968). (Russ.).

Sosunov A.A. About some peculiarity's reactionability trialkylsulphonium compounds. *Dissert. of candidate chem. science*, Odessa State University, Odessa, 1972. (Russ.).

Sundelin K. G.R., Wiley R.A., Givens R.S., Rademacher D.R. Synthesis and biological activity of some carbocyclic analogs of muscarine. *J. Med. Chem.* 1973. Vol. 16, No. 3, P.235-239.

Timoney R. F. Structural requirements of muscarine, 1,3-dioxolane and their analogues for agonist activity at cholinergic receptors. *International Journal of Pharmaceutics*, 1983. Vol. 15, Issue 3, P. 223-234.

Waser P.G. Chemistry and pharmacology of muscarine, muscarone, and some related compounds. *Pharmacol. Rev.*, 13, 465, (1961); Toxicological Reviews, No. 2, 465, (1962).

Wess J. Molecular biology of muscarinic acetylcholine receptors. *Crit. Rev. Neurobiol.* 1996. Vol. 10, P. 69-99.

Zotov S.B., Smirnov V.V., Kvasnuk-Mudriy F.V. Cyclic ethers and acetalies. 2. Sulphurcontaining derivatives 1,4- dioxane. *ibid.* **4,** 1776 (1968). (Russ.).

Zotov S.B., Smirnov V.V., Kvasnuk- Mudriy F.V., Schevchenko V.I. Synthesis 2,6-derivatives 1,4-dioxane. Comm.3, *ibid.* Coll. No. 2, 260 (1970). (Russ.).

Zotov S.B., Smirnov V.V., Kvasnuk-Mudriy F.V., Shevchenko V.I. Synthesis 2,6-derivatives 1,4-dioxane. Comm. 2, *ibid.* No. 6, 1124 (1967). (Russ.).

Zotov S.B., Smirnov V.V., Kvasnuk-Mudriy F.V. Synthesis 4-alkyltiomethyl-2-methyl-1,3-dioxolanes., *ibid.*, Coll. No. 2, 257 (1970). (Russ.).

Chapter 7

Andreeva E., Nirthanan S., Cohen J.B., Pedersen S.E. Site Specificity of Agonist-Induced Opening and Desensitization of the Torpedo californica Nicotinic Acetylcholine Receptor. *Biochemistry,* 2006. V. 45. No. 1. P. 195-204.

Boehm R. Ueber Curare und Curarealkaloide. *Arch. Pharm.*, 235, 660, 1897.

Bovie D. *Thankful poison curare.* Article in coll. «Science and humanity», M., 1964. pp. 92-101. (Russ.).

Camps P., El Achab R., Görbig D.M., Morral J., Munoz-Torrero D., Badia A., Banos J.E., Vivas N.M., Barril X., Orozco M., Luque F.J.. Synthesis, in Vitro Pharmacology, and Molecular Modeling of Very Potent Tacrine-Huperzine A Hybrids as Acetylcholinesterase Inhibitors of Potential Interest for the Treatment of Alzheimer's Disease. *J. Med. Chem.* 1999. V. 42. No. 5. P. 3227-3242.

Chemistry biological active nature compounds. Ed. by N.A. Preobrahzenskiy and R.P. Evstigneeva, M., Khimiya, 1970. (Russ.).

Craig L.E. Curariform activity and chemical structure. *Chem. Rev.* 42, 285-410, 1948.

New curarelike and ganglioblocking drugs. Ed. by D.A. Kharkevich. M., Medicina, 1970. (Russ.).

Dutcher J.D. Curare Alkaloids. II. The Purification of d-Tubocurarine Chloride and the Isolation of d-Chondocurarine. *J. Am. Chem. Soc.* 1952. V.74, P. 2221-2225.

Gmiro V.E. Synthesis and investigation of drug substances with disulphide bond. *Avtoreferate diss.* Science leader N.V. Khromov-Borisov. L., L.Ch.Ph.I., 1970. (Russ.).

Hunt R. *Arch. Intern. pharmacodynamia.* 12, 447, 1904.

Hunt R. Renshaw R.R. Ethers of choline and allied compounds. *J. Pharmacol. Exp. Ther.* 58, 140, 1936.

Hunt R. Renshaw R.R. The physiological action of some homologues of betaine and choline esters. *J. Pharmacol. Exp. Ther.* 37, 309, 1929.

Hunt R., Renshaw R.R. On some effects of arsonium, stibonium, phosphonium and sulfonium compounds on the autonomic nervous system. *J. Pharmacol. Exp. Ther.* 25, 315, 1925.

Khromov-Borisov N.V. Structure of d–tubocurarine. *Pharmac. and toxicol.* No. 5, 583, 1972. (Russ.).

King H. Curare alkaloids. Part I. Tubocurarine. *J. Chem. Soc.*, 1935, 1381.

King H. Curare alkaloids. Part II. Tubocurarine and bebeerines. *J. Chem. Soc.*, 1936, 1276.

Nassif-Makki T., Ch. Tränkle, D. Zlotos, G. Bejeuhr, A. Cambareri, C. Pfletschinger, E. Kostenis, K. Mohr, U. Holzgrabe. Bisquaternary Ligands of the Common Allosteric Site of M2 Acetylcholine Receptors: Search for the Minimum Essential Distances between the Pharmacophoric Elements. *J. Med. Chem.* 1999. V. 42. No. 5. pp. 849-858.

Pharmacology miorelacsantes. Ed. by D.A. Kharkevich. M., Medicina, 1989 (Russ.).

Physiological role acetylcholine and searchs new drug substances. Coll. art. by Ed. M.Y. Mikhelson, L., 1957. (Russ.).

Tumiatti V., Rosini M., Bartolini M., Cavalli A., Marucci G., Andrisano V., P. Angeli, Banzi R., Minarini A., Recanatini M., Melchiorre C.. Structure-Activity Relationships of Acetylcholinesterase Noncovalent Inhibitors Based on a Polyamine Backbone. 2. Role of the Substituents on the Phenyl Ring and Nitrogen Atoms of Caproctamine. *J. Med. Chem*. 2003. V.46. No. 6. P. 954-966.

Wieland H., Bahr K., Witkop B. Über die Alkaloide aus Calebassen-Curare. *Justus Liebigs Annalen der Chemie*. 547, 156, 1941.

Wintersteiner O., Dutcher J.D. Curare alkaloids from chondodendron tomentosum. *Science*, 97, 467, 1943.

Chapter 8

Daly J.W. Biological active alkaloids from poison frogs (Dendrobatidae). *J. Toxicol.: Toxin Rev.,* 1982, v. 1, No. 1. P. 33–86.

Daly J.W., Witkop B., Bommer P., Biemann K. Batrachotoxin. The Active Principle of the Colombian Arrow Poison Frog, Phyllobates bicolor. *J. Am. Chem. Soc*., 1965. 87, 124.

Daly J.W., Witkop B. *Venomous animals and Their Venoms*, vol. III, Academic Press, NY, 1971.

Fruentov N.K. *Medicine plants of Far East.* Khabarovsk. Khabarovskoe knizhnoe izdatelstvo. 1987. (Russ.).

Fruentov N.K., Kadaev G.N. *Venomous plants*. Khabarovsk. Khabarovskoe knizhnoe izdatelstvo. 1971. (Russ.).

Genry T.A. *Chemistry plant alkaloids*. Ed. by V.M. Rodionov and N.S. Vulfson. M., Khimizdat, 1956. (Russ. Engl. version is available).

Gorunova S.V., Demina I. S. *Seaweeds – springs toxic substances*. M., Nauka, 1974. (Russ.)

Hashimoto Y. Marine toxins and other bioactive marine metabolites. *Jap. Sci. Soc. Press*, Tokyo, 1979, v. 23. pp. 1–369.

Kao C.Y. Tetrodotoxin, saxitoxin and their significance in the study of excitation phenomena *Pharmacol. Rev.,* 1966. 18, 997.

Karle I.L., Karle J. Structure of batrachotoxin A. *Acta Cryst*. B, 1969. 25, 428.

Karle J., Karle I.L. The symbolic addition procedure for phase determination for entrosymmetric and non-centrosymmetric crystals. *Acta Cryst.* 1966. 21, 849.

Mosher H.S., Fuhrman F.A., Buchwald H.D., Fischer H.G. Tarichatoxin-Tetrodotoxin: powerful neurotoxin. *Science*, 1964. 144, No. 3622, 1100.

Natural toxins. Proc. 6-th Inter. symp. on animal, plant and microbial toxins (Uppsala, 1979). Pergamont Press, Oxford, 1980.

Orlov B.N., Gelashvili D.B., Ibragimov A.K.*Venomous animals and plants of SSSR*. M., Vissh. shkola, 1990. (Russ.).

Plant Toxicology. Ed. by Hock B., Elstner E.F., N.Y., Marcel Dekker. 2005.

Tamura C., Amakasu O., Sasada Y., Tsuda K. The crystal structure of derivatives of tetrodotoxin. I. Tetrodonic acid hydrobomide. The crystal structure of derivaties of tetrodotoxin. II. Diacetylanhydrotetrodotoxin hydroiodide. *Acta Cryst.,* 1966. 21, 219, 226.

Tokuyama T., Daly J.W., Witkop B., Karle J., Karle I.L. Structure of batrachotoxin A, of new steroidal alkaloid. *J. Am. Chem. Soc.*, 1968. 90, 1917.

Tokuyama T., Daly J.W., Witkop B. Structure of batrachotoxin and partial synthesis batrachotoxin, its analogs and homologs. *J. Am. Chem. Soc.*, 1969. 91, 3931.

Toxins of animals and plant origin. Eds. de Vries A., Kochva E., v. 1–3, N.Y., Gordon and Breach, 1971–1973.

Tsuda K. Über Tetrodotoxin, Giftstoff der Bowlfische. *Naturwissenschafte*. 1966. 53, 171.

Unusov S.U. *Alkaloids* (Handbook). Tashkent, FAN, 1981. (Russ.).

Vick J.A., Wiles J.S. Pharmacological and toxicological studies palytoxin. *Army Res. and Development,* 13, No. 5, 70 (1972).

Woodward R.B., Gougoutas J.Z. The Structure of Tetrodotoxin. *J. Am. Chem. Soc.*, 1964. 86, 5030.

Chapter 9

Barkagan Z.S., Perfil'ev P.P. *Venomous snakes and Their Venoms*. Barnaul, Altayskoe knihznoe izd-vo, 1967. (Russ.).

Behringer H. Die Krötengifte: Neuere Ergebnisse der chemischen und pharmakologischen Forschung. *Angew. Chem.*, 1943. 56, 83.

Berger K.J., Guss D.A. Mycotoxins revisited: Part I. *J. Emerg. Med.*, 2005, 28, 53.

Berry C.L. The patology of mycotoxins. *J. Pathol.*, 1988. 154, No. 4, 301-311.

Black R.M., Upshall D.G. Assessing the danger. *Chemistry in Britain*, 1988. 24, No. 7, 656-664.

Brem A.Y. *Life animals*, vol. 5, Earthaquatic and reptile. L., Lening.obl. izd-vo, 1931. (Russ.).

Ciegler A. Micotoxins: a new class of chemical weapons. *Nuclear. Biol. and Chem. Defence and Technol.,* 1986. 1, No. 1, 52-57.

Defense against Bioterror: Detection Technologies, Implementation Strategies and Commercial Opportunities. Proceedings of the NATO Advanced Research Workshop on Defense against Bioterror: Detection Technologies, Implementation Strategies and Commercial Opportunities, held in Madrid, Spain from 8 to 11 April 2004. Series: NATO Science for Peace and Security Series. Subseries: NATO Science for Peace and Security Series B: Physics and Biophysics. Morrison, D.; Milanovich, F.; Ivnitski, D.; Austin, Th.R. (Eds.) Springer. Printed in the Netherlands. 2005. 340 pp.

Gill D. M. Bacterial Toxins: a Table of Lethal Amounts. *Microbiolog. Rev*. 1982. V. 46. No. 1. 86-94.

van Heyningen W.E. *Bacterial Toxins*, Bleckwell, Oxford, 1950.

Maricovskiy P. I. *Tarantula and caracurte*. Frunze. Izd-vo AN Kirgiz. SSR, 1956. (Russ.).

Marki F., Witkop B. The venom of the Colombian arrow poison frog Phyllobates bicolor. *Experientia*, 1963. 19, 239.

Mazokhina-Porshnykova N.N. *Suppression excitants of botulism in food-stuffs*. M., Agro-promizdat, 1989. (Russ.).

Orlov B.N., Gelashvili D.B. *Zootoxinology (Venomous animals and their venoms)*: Uch. posobie. M., Vissh. shkola. 1985. (Russ.).

Orlov B.N., Omarov Sh.M. Gelashvili D.B., and other. Chemistry and pharmacology poison of bee. *Pharmacol. and toxicol.* 1978. No. 3. pp. 358–369. (Russ.).

Orlov B.N., Egorov V.V. Gelashvili D.B. Biological basis's action on organism venom of scorpions. *Biol. nauki*. 1981. No. 2. pp. 45–56. (Russ.).

Pigulevskiy S.V. *Venomous animals. Toxicology spine*. L., Medicina, 1966. (Russ.).

Pigulevskiy S.V. *Venomous animals. Toxicology spineless*. L., Medicina, 1975. (Russ.).

Piller C.H., Yamamoto K.R. *Gene wars: military control over new genetic technologies*. NY, Morrow, 1988.

Seager L.D., Wood Ch. D. *Proc. Soc. exp. Biol. Med.*, 111, 120 (1962); C.A. 15513, 1963.

Tucker J.B. Toxins: "Gray Area" Weapons, *Gene Watch*, 1985. 2, No. 2, 10-12.

Venomous animals and their venoms. Eds. Bucherl W., Buckley E. E. N.Y– London, Acad. Press, v. 1. 1968; v. 2, 3. 1971.

Zakharov V.I. *Poison of toad*. Kishinev. Karty moldavenyske. 1960. (Russ.).

Chapter 10

Akimov P. Truth and lie about binary programme USA. *Zarubezh. voen. obozr.*, 1987, No. 7, P. 11-14. (Russ.).

Alexandrov B.N., Emelyanov B.I. *Chemical Warfare Agents*. Sec. Edition. M., Voenizdat. 1990. (Russ.).

Analgesics from chemistry and pharmacology to clinical application. Ed. by Buschmann H. Wiley-VCH, Veinheim. 2002.

Antonov N.S. *Chemical weapons on the boundary of two century's*. M., Izd. gruppa "Progress," 1994. (Russ.).

Antonov N.S. *Chemical weapons condemn, but process must accelerate*. Mezhdunarodnaya zhizn, 11-12, 1992, P. 47-56. (Russ.).

Antonov N.S. Decline chemical weapons? *Voenniy vestnik*, 1992, No. 11, P. 1-8. (Russ.).

Chemical Stockpile Disposal Program Final Programmatic Environmental Impact Statement. *Report Department of Defense USA*. January 1988.

Chemical warfare agents: chemistry, pharmacology, toxicology, and therapeutics. Editors, J.A. Romano Jr., B.J. Lukey, H. Salem / 2nd ed. CRC Press, Taylor and Francis Group. NY. 2008. -744 p.

Colapzet I.A., Deamantides G., Spenser H.K. Synthesis and pharmacological evaluation of 4,4-disubstituted piperidines. *J. Med. Chem.*, 1989, 32, No. 5, P. 968-974.

Convention about prohibition work out, production, accumulation and application chemical weapons and about it destruction (corr. version 8 aug. 1994). PTS PC OPCW, 1994. 191 p. (Russ.).

Demakhin A.G., Oliskevich V.V., Silnyagin O.A. and others. Technological aspects alteretion reactional masses, production by detoxication lewisite in arseniccontent goods production. *ibid.* 2007, v.51, No. 2. P. 29-31. (Russ.).

Ecstasy: the complete guide. Ed. by J. Holland. Rochester. Park Street Press. 2001.

Ellison D.H. *Handbook of chemical and biological warfare agents.* New York. CRC Press. 2000.

Ember L.R. Pentagon Pressing Hard for Binary Chemical Arms Funds. *Chem. and Eng. News,* 1985, **63**, No. 8, P. 26-29.

Feldman P.L., James M.K. Synthesis and pharmacological evaluation of ultrashort to long-acting opioid analgetics. *J. Med. Chem.* 1991, 34, No. 7, pp. 2202-2208.

Franke S. *Lehrbuch der Militarchemie*. Vol. 1. Berlin, MV, 1976. (Ger, Russ. version is also available).

Franke S. Franc P. Varnke. *Lehrbuch der Militarchemie*. Vol. 2. Berlin, MV, 1976. (Ger, Russ. version is also available).

Gosh R., Newman J.F., *Chem. and Ind.*, 1955, 5, 118.

Gosh R. (I.C.I. Ltd.). New basic esters of thiophosphonic acids and salts thereof. British patent 738839, 1955; 797603, 1955.

Hardman E.F., Domino E.F., Selvers M.H. General pharmacological actions of some synthetic tetrahydrocannabinol derivatives. *Pharmacol. Rev.* 1971, 23, No. 4, pp. 295-313.

Hoenig S.L. *Compendium of chemical warfare agents*. New York. Springer, 2006.

Hydro W.R. Novel process for synthesis of a liquid irritant (1-methoxy-cycloheptatriene). U.S. pat. 4249025, 1981.

Introduction to Military Toxicology: a crush course. Pharmacology Department, University of Bristol. 2001.

Kapashin V.P., Shevchenko A.V., Shvedov A.F. New Russian objects by destruction of chemical weapons. *ibid.* 2007, v.51, No. 2. P. 9-11. (Russ.).

Karakchiev N.I. *Military Toxicology and Protection against Nuclear and Chemical Weapons*. M.; Medicina, 1988. (Russ.).

Kehner G.B. *Date rape drugs*. Philadelphia. Chelsea House Publishers. 2004.

Ketchum J.S. *Chemical warfare secrets almost forgotten*. Santa Ros, California. Chem. Books Inc. 2006.

Kholstov V.I., Fokin E.A., Spirande V.V., Martinov M.V. and others. Chemical disarmament. Practice guarantees fulfillment conventional obligations by prohibition of chemical weapons and it destruction. *Ross. khim. Zh. (Zh. Ross. khim. ob-va im. D.I. Mendeleev)*, 2007, v.51, No. 2. P. 4-8. (Russ.).

Kolodkin V.M., Murin A.V., Petrov A.K., Gorskiy V.G. *Quantity estimation of risk chemical crash*. Ed. by V.M. Kolodkin. Izhevsk. Izdatelskiy dom "Udmurdskiy universitet." 2001. 228p. (Russ.).

Larchenkov D.V., Shvedov A.F. Phenomenological model of estimation and prognosis by technical state longtime storage chemical ammunition. *ibid.* 2007, v.51, No. 2. P. 31-33. (Russ.).

Lavrent'ev A.N. Would be release jinnee in 1995 year? *Newspaper «Vecherniy Peterburg»*, No. 129 (19719). 04.06. 1992. P. 2. (Russ.).

Lavrent'ev A.N. Krutikov V.I. Chemical Warfare Agents, drowning in Baltic Sea. Risks real and imaginary. *Izvestiya Sankt-Peterburgskogo gosudarstvennogo tekhnologicheskogo instituta (tekhnicheskogo universiteta)*. 2007. No. 1 (27). P. 73-77. (Russ.).

Lazur'evskiy G.V., Nikolaeva L.A. *Cannabinoides (narcotic substances of hemp)*. Kishinev. Izd. "Shtinica." 1972. (Russ.).

Mather L.E. Clinical pharmacokinetics of fentanyl and its newer derivatives. *Clin. Pharmacokinetics*, 1983, 8, P. 422-446.

Mechling R. *Marijuana*. Philadelphia. Chelsea House Publish. 2003.

Meselson M. The role of chemical defense in chemical warfare. Chemical Deterrence and Chemical Disarmament. *Chemical weapons convention bulletin*, 1991, No. 11, pp. 17-19.

Miller J.I., Dudley G.E., Blackwell P.A. Preparation of 3-quinyclidinyl benzilate. U.S. pat. 3899497, 1975.

Milshtein, G.I., L.I. Spivak. *Psychotomimetics*. L., Medicina, 1971. (Russ.).

Nagorniy S.V., Miroshnikova O.I., Silant'ev V.F., Tidgen V.P., Cibulskaya E.A. Problems decrease risk intoxications by destruction chemical weapons. *Ross. khim.Zh. (Zh. Ross. khim. ob-va im. D.I. Mendeleev)*, 2004, v. 48, No. 2, P. 61-64. (Russ.).

Nemec V.G., Sochilin E.G. *Chemistry Warfare Agents*. M.-L., Gos. nauch. tekhn. izd-vo khim. literaturi, 1941. (Russ.).

Nikolaev A.I. *Military aspects security Russian Federation*. Mezhdunarodnaya zhizn, 9, 1993, pp. 16-20. (Russ.).

Ocean dumping of chemical monitories: environmental effects in Arctic Seas. MEDEA Office, MS Z059 1820 Dolley Madison Blvd. McLean, Virg. 22012, 1997, 241p.

Onaivi E.S. *Biology of marijuana*. London, NY. Taylor and Francis. 2002.

Pac Z.P. Destruction of chemical weapons stockpiles in Russia: difficulties and perspectives. *The VII International Symposium on Protection against Chemical and Biological Warfare Agents*, Stockholm, Sweden, June 2001. Stockholm, 2001.

Paka V.T. Drowning chemical weapons: state of problem / *Ross. khim.Zh. (Zh. Ross. khim. ob-va im. D.I. Mendeleev),* 2004, v. 48, No. 2, P. 99-109. (Russ.).

Petrov A.N., Sofronov G.A., Nechiporenko S.P., Somin I.N. Antidotes phosphororganic chemical warfare agents. *Ross. khim. Zh. (Zh. Ross. khim. ob-va im. D.I. Mendeleev*), 2004, v. 48, No. 2, P. 110-116. (Russ.).

Petrov S.V. Principal problems of destruction chemical weapons in RF. *Ross. khim. Zh. (Zh. Ross. khim. ob-va im. D.I. Mendeleev),* 1993. v.37, No. 3, P. 5-7. (Russ.).

Petrunin V.A., Demiduk V.V. and others. Creation of system inspection safety object by destruction chemical weapons in settlement Gorniy / Medical and biological problems, binding with destruction chemical weapons: *Thesis's report Intern. Symposium, 26-28.08.2003*. Volgograd, 2003. P. 259-260. (Russ.).

Petrunin V.A., Sheluchenko V.V., Demiduk V.V. Safe, reliable and ecological clean contemporary two-stage Russian technology destruction chemical weapons / *Third public attends about problem by destruction chemical weapons:* Coll. materials, 8-10.07.1997. Kurgan, 1997.P. 58-64.; *Fourth public attends about problem by destruction chemical weapons:* Coll. materials, p. Kizner. 27-28.05.1998. Izhevsk, 1998. P. 55-62. (Russ.).

Ris'ev O.A. *Shungit – national stone of Russia*. St. Peterburg, SP "Minimax," 1997.

Ris'ev O.A. *Shungit – stone of health*. S-Pb. OOO "TESSA." 2001. 126 pp. (Russ.).

Robinson J.P. *Binary nerve gas weapons*, Chapter 2 in Chemical Disarmament. New Weapons for Old Sweden, SIPRI.

Rothschild, J.H. *Tomorrow's Weapons*. M., Voenizdat. 1966. (Russ., Engl. version is also available).

Sabalichka F. *Chemical opening of poison*. Transl. with Ger. Kharkovskoe gos. nauchno-tekhnich. izd-vo Ukraini, 1934. (Russ.).

Saunders B.Ch. *Chemistry and Toxicology organic compounds phosphorus and fluorine*. M., Izd-vo IL, 1961. (Russ., Engl. version is also available).

Shkodich P.E., Klauchek V.V. Basis ecological-hygienical of demands to introduce first in Russia object by destruction of chemical weapons / *Povolzh. ecolog. vestnic*. 2004. Issue 10. P. 310-317. (Russ.).

Shkodich P.E., Klauchek V.V. Hygienical aspects destruction of chemical weapons in RF / *Hygiena i sanitariya*, 2003. No. 4. P. 47-50. (Russ.).

Shkodich P.E., Klauchek V.V., Delaru V.V. *Chemofobia*. M., Izd-vo IGEM RAN, 1997. (Russ.).

Shkodich P.E., Zheltobrukhov V.F., Klauchek V.V. *Ecological-hygienically aspects of problem destruction of chemical weapons*. Monographia. Volgograd. Izd-vo VolGU, 2004. 236 p. (Russ.).

Shulga V.Y., Petrunin V.A., Imasheva M.A., Khudenko A.V. Toxicological aspects safe destruction of stocks Chemical Warfare Agents and liquidation ex-objects their production on territory RF / *Thesis's report 2-th congress of toxicologist Russia*, 10-13.11.2003. M., 2003. P. 297-298. (Russ.).

Sigolaeva L.V., Kurochkin I.N., Eremenko A.V., Sokolovskaya L.G., Makhaeva G.F., Maligin V.V., Richardson R., Makover A., Sheller F., Gachok I.V., Varfolomeev S.D. Biosensors for analysis activity neurotoxic esterase as biomarker toxic action neuropatogenic phosphororganic compounds. *Ross. khim. Zh. (Zh. Ross. khim. ob-va im. D.I. Mendeleev)*, 2004. v. 48, No. 4. pp. 65-72. (Russ.).

Skorobogatov A.G., Ferezanova M.V., Mandich V.G., Scherbakov A.A. Model transfer of toxic compounds in water objects. *ibid*. 2007, v.51, No. 2. P. 74-77. (Russ.).

Smith B.M. Catalytic methods for the destruction of chemical warfare agents under ambient conditions. *Chem. Soc. Rev*. 2008. v. 37. P. 470-478.

Smith J.E., Moss M.O. *Mycotoxins. Formation, analysis and significance*. John Wiley and Sons, 1985.

Spiers E.M. *Chemical weaponary*. A. Continuing Challenge. McMillan, 1989.

Stock T., Lohs K. *Characteristics of Chemical warfare agents and toxic armament wastes / The Challenge of old Chemical Munitions and toxic Armament Wastes*/ Oxford. 1997. P. 15-34.

Suzuki O., Watanabe K. *Drugs and poisons in humans*. Springer-Verlag Berlin, Heidelberg. 2005.

Tammelin L.E. *Arkiv főr Kemi*. 1958, 12, 287.

Tammelin L.E. Dialkoxy-phosphorylthiocholines, alkoxy-methylphosphoryl-thiocholines and analogous choline esters. *Acta Chem. Scand*. 1957, 11, P. 1340-1349; pp. 1738-1742.

Tammelin L.E. Methyl-fluoro-phosphorylcholines. Two Synthetic Cholinergic Drugs and Their Tertiary Homologues. *Acta Chem. Scand.* 1957, 11, P. 859.

Tuteljan V.A., L.V. Kravchenko. *Mycotoxins (Medical and Biological Aspects*). M.; Medicina, 1985. (Russ.).

Umarov A.A., Kutyanin L.I. *New defoliants: search, property, application.* M., Khimia, 2000. (Russ.).

Utkin A.U., Liberman B.M., Kondrat`ev V.B. and others. Mathematical description processes detoxication phosphor organic warfare agents. *ibid.* 2007, v.51, No. 2. P. 12-18. (Russ.).

Utkin A.U., Kholodova V.A., Chebotaev and others. Chemistry and technology destruction "viscous" lewisite. *ibid.* 2007, v.51, No. 2. P. 19-23. (Russ.).

Veselovskaya N.V., Kovalenko A.E. *Narcotics – property, action, pharmacokinetics, metabolism.* M., Triada-X, 2000. (Russ.).

Wannemacher R.W. Jr., Bunner D.L., Dinterman R.E. Transdermal toxicity of several natural toxins from marine and aquatic environmental. *Toxicon.* 1989, 27, No. 1, P. 85.

Zotov S.B., Lavrent'ev A.N., Grigor'eva A.V. Engineering-chemical aspects of problem drowning chemical weapons. *Khimicheskaya promishlennost segodnya.* 2006. No. 9. P. 24-33. (Russ.).

Chapter 11

American Conference of Governmental Industrial Hygienists (ACGIH): *1994–1995. Threshold Limit Values for Chemical Substances and Physical Agents and Biological Exposure Limits.* Cincinnati, OH, ACGIH, 1994.

Bernardiner M.N., Sanfirov E.S. Alteration by high temperatures and harmless toxic wastes, contaning chlororganic compounds / *Khim. prom.*, 1996. No. 6. pp. 60-67. (Russ.).

Bernardiner M.N., Shurgin A.P. *Fire alteration and harmless industrial wastes.* M., Khimia. 1990. 352 pp. (Russ.).

Bondarev L.G. *Microelements – good and harm.* M., Znanie, 1984. 144 pp. (Russ.).

Chang M.B., Huang T.F. The effects of temperature and oxygen content on the PCDD/PCDFs formation in MSW fly ash. *Chemosphere.* 2000. V.40, Iss.2. pp. 159-164.

Filatov B.N., Danilina A.E., Mikhaylova G.M., Kiseleva M.F. *Dioxin. Medical-ecological aspects.* Ed. by P.E. Shkodich. M., 2-th tipographia FU "MB i EP", 1997. 134 pp. (Russ.).

Harmful compounds in environment. Handbook from 11 books. Ed. V.A. Filov, U.I. Musiychuk, B.A. Ivin. S-Pb. Izd. "Professional." 2004. (Russ.).

Harmful compounds in industry. Handbook ed. 7th. In 3 volumes. Vol. 3. Inorganic and element organic substances. Ed. by N.V. Lazarev and I.D. Gadaskina. L., Khimia, 1977. (Russ.).

Hathaway G.J., Nick H. Proctor. *Proctor ahd Hughes' Chemical Hazards of the Workplace,* Fifth Edition, 2004. Hoboken, New Jersey. John Wiley and Sons, Inc., 785 pp.

Hygienical quotes chemical substances in environment. Handbook by ed. V.V. Semenova. S-Pb. Izd. "Proffesional." 2004. 764 pp. (Russ.).

IARC Monographs on the Evaluation of Carcinogenic Risks to Humans. V. 1–83. Lyon, France, International Agency for Research on Cancer, 1972–2002.

Isidorov V.A. *Introduction in chemical ecotoxicology*: Text-book. S-Pb. Khimizdat, 1999. 144 pp. (Russ.).

Izrael Y.A. *Ekology and control state natural environment*. M., Gidrometeoizdat, 1984. 560 pp. (Russ.).

Izrael Y.A. *Problems guarding of natural environment and ways their decision*. L., Gidrometeoizdat, 1984. (Russ.).

Khudoley V.V., Livanov G.A., Kolbasov S.E., Fridman K.B. *Danger of dioxins in city*. S-Pb., NII Khimii S-PbGU. 2000. p. 173. (Russ.).

Klyuev N.A. Control superecotoxicantes in environment and sources their appearance. *J. Anal. Khimii.* 1996. V.51, No. 2. pp. 163-172. (Russ.).

Konorev O.A., Zanaveskin L.N., Suris A.L., Uskach Y.L. Alteration wastes oxidation chlororganic industry by method catalytic oxidation. *Ecology and industry Russia*, 2003. Jan., pp. 8-11, 48. (Russ.).

Latt A., Riko-Latt I., Perez E., Krutikov V.I., Amada B. Application organizing molecular system for chemical decomposes warfare agents. *Ross. khim. Zh. (Zh. Ross. khim. ob-va im. D.I. Mendeleev*), 2007, V.51, No. 6. pp. 36-43. (Russ.).

Lobacheva G.K., Guchanova I.Zh., Guchanova A.I. *Ekology and motor transport*: Text-book. Ed. by G.K. Lobacheva. Volgograd, Izd-vo VolGU, 2004. (Russ.).

Mariani G., Benfenati E., Fanelli R. Concentrations of PSDD in different points of modern refuse incinerator. *Chemosphere*.1990. 21, No. 4-5.507-517.

Melnikov N.N. *Pesticides. Chemistry, technology and application*. M., Khimia. 1987. 712 pp. (Russ.).

Savel'ev A.N. Methods utilization chlororganic wastes and their economical estimation. *Khim. prom.*, 2006. No. 2. pp. 73-82. (Russ.).

Solov'ev N.V., Strelchuk N.A., Ermilov P.V., Kaner B.L. *Basses techniques safety and against fire in chemical industry*. M., Khimiya, 1966. (Russ.).

Toxic substances in environment. Steady organic soils (SOS). http://www.bellona.ru/ Casefiles/stockholm 2001.

Uskach Y.L., Zotov S.B., Popov U.V., Kolotilina T.V. Termoalteration of nonutilization liquid organic wastes. *Chemical technology: Coll. thesis's reports Inter. conference by chem. tech.* KhT'07. v.3. Ed. by A.A. Berlin, N.A. Khalturinskiy, A.A. Voshkin. M., LENAND, 2007. pp. 249-252. (Russ.).

Yak H.K., Lang Q., Wai C.M. Relative Resistance of Positional Isomers of Polychlorinated Biphenyls toward Reductive Dechlorination by Zerovalent Iron in Subcritical Water. *Environ. Sci. Technol*. 2000. V. 34. Iss. 13. pp. 2792-2798.

Yufit S.S. *Dioxins: principal notions and problems*. M., Khimia. 1996. (Russ.).

Zharov O.A., Zharov A.V., Gromak A.I. Energy effective application plasmotron for harmless dangerous wastes. *Thesis's reports Russian scientific practical conference* "Energy resource savings in constriction and housing-commune complex-2004." Yaroslavl, 20-21 October 2004. (Russ.).

Zotov S.B., Tuzhikov O.I., Uskach Y.L. Problems destruction steady organic contaminants of environment. *Khimicheskaya promishlennost segodnya*. 2009. No. 2, p. 17-24. (Russ.).

Zanaveskin L.N., Aver'yanov V.N. Carbon tetrachloride. Methods alteration in ecological safety products and perspectives their development (Rew.). *Khim. prom.*, 2002. No. 9. pp. 4-21. (Russ.).

Zanaveskin L.N., Konorev O.A., Aver'yanov V.A. Methods alteration by oxidation and detoxic chlororganic wastes. Policy to resource savings and ecology safety. *Khim. prom.*, 2002. No. 2. pp. 3-19. (Russ.).

Chapter 12

Akhrem A.A., Titov U.A. *Full synthesis of steroids*. M., Nauka, 1967. (Russ.).

Antonov N.S. In ban chemical weapons. (*Press Conference, March, 1982),* Novosti Press Agency Publishing House, Moscow, 1982.

The art of drug synthesis. Ed. by D.S. Johnson, J.J. Li. Hoboken. John Wiley and Sons, Inc. 2007. 276 pp.

Atkinson E.K., Ballock F.I., Ganchelli F.E. Emetic activity of N-substituted norapomorphines. *J. Med. Chem.* 1975. 18, No.10. pp. 1000-1003.

Bajgar J., Fusek J. et al. Acute toxicites of dialkylaminoalkyl-(dialkylamido)-fluorophosphates. *Physiol. Res.* 1992. 41. P. 399-402.

Basig M. Bicyclische Phosphorsaure ester – potentielle chemische Kampfstoffe. *Militartechnik,* 1985. No. 1. pp. 42-43.

Casida I.E., Lowell J., Lawrence. Structure – Activity correlations for interactions of bicyclophosphorous esthers and some polychlorocycloalkane and perethroid insecticides with the brain-specific t-butylbicyclophosphorothionate receptor. *Environ. Health perspect.*, 1985. 61. pp. 123-132.

Courtwright D. T. *Forces of Habit. Drugs and the Making of the Modern World*. Cambridge, Mass.: Harvard University Press, 2001.

Davenport-Hines R. *The Pursuit of Oblivion. A Global History of Narcotics*. New York: Norton, 2002.

Diaz J.H. *Color atlas of human poisoning and envenoming*. CRC Press, 2006. 560 pp.

Fedorov L.A. *Dioxins – ecological danger: retrospective and perspectives*. M., Nauka, 1993. (Russ.).

Fizer L., Fizer M. *Steroids*. M., Mir, 1964. (Russ.).

Foster O.M. *Designer drugs*. Philadelphia. Chelsy House Publish. 2004.

Golovko A.I., Golovko S.I., Zefirov S.U., Sofronov G.A. *Toxicology GAMK-litics*. S-Pb., Niva, 1996. (Russ.).

Goodman M., Morehouse F. *Organic molecules in action*. Trans. with Eng. M., Izd-vo "Mir," 1977. (Russ., Engl. version is also available).

Janssen P.A.J., Gardocki J.E. Method for producing analgesia. Pat. USA No.3141830, 1964.

Kobylecki R.I., Guest J.C., Lewis J.W. Morphine derivatives. Pat. UK No. 1587831, 1977.

Kolman Ya., Rem K.-G. *Visual biochemistry*. Transl. with Gem. M., Mir, 2000. (Russ.).

Lisina S.V., Brel A.K., Spasov A.A., at al. Synthesis and febrifuge activity new derivatives salicylic acid. *Khim. - pharm. Zh.* 2008.V.42. No. 10. pp. 27-29. (Russ.).

Loginova N.V. *Introduction in Pharmaceutical chemistry*: Text-book. / N.V. Loginova, G.I. Polozov. Minsk, BGU, 2003. 250 pp. (Russ.).

Mashkovskiy M.D. *Drugs*. In 2nd vol. M., Medicina, 1987. (Russ.).

Mechling R. *Hallucinogens*. NY. Chelsy House Publish. 2003.

Middleton W.J. Fluorothiocarbonyl compounds. III. Diels-Alder reactions. *J. Org. Chem.* 1965. 30, No.5. pp. 1390-1394.

Middleton W.J. Bingham E.M. Fluorine-conteining 1,1-dicyanoethylenes: their preparation, Diels-Alder reactions and derived norbornenes and norbornanes. *J. Fluorine Chem.*, 1982. 20, No. 3. pp. 397-418.

Morozov I.S., Petrov V.I., Sergeeva S.A. *Pharmacology of adamantanes*. Volgograd, Volg. med. academia, 2001. (Russ.).

Nikiforovich G.V. *Almost nature drugs*. M., Molodaya gvardiya, 1986. (Russ.).

Paterson J.R., Baxter G., Dreyer J.S. et al. Salicylic Acid sans Aspirin in animals and man: Persistence in fasting and biosynthesis from benzoic acid. *J. Agric. Food Chem.* 2008. V. 56. No. 24. pp. 11648-11652.

Piller C.H. Iamamoto K.R. *Gene wars; Military control over new genetic technologies*, New York, Morrow, 1988.

Schmidhammer H., Schrat A. Synthesis and biological evaluation of 14-alkoxymorphinans. *Helv. Chem. Acta*, 1990. 73, No. 6, pp. 1784-1787.

Sinkkonen S., Paasivirta J. Degradation half-life times of PCDDs, PCDFs and PCBs for environmental fate modeling. *Chemosphere*. 2000. V.40, Iss.9-11. pp. 943-949.

Tucker J.B. "Gene wars," *Foreign Policy*, 1984, No. 57, P.63.

Wingard L.B., Narisimha K. Preparation of a fentanyl ligand for the opiate receptor. *Govt. Repts.*, 1988. 88, No. 14. pp. 170.

Winstein S. Bicycloheptadien dibromides. *J. Am. Chem. Soc.*, 1961. 83, No. 6. pp. 1516-1517.

Index

A

B

C

D

E

G

H

I

J

K

L

N

S